# Field Epidemiology

# Field Epidemiology

## Third Edition

Edited by

## Michael B. Gregg

OXFORD
UNIVERSITY PRESS
2008

OXFORD
UNIVERSITY PRESS

WA
39
F453
2008

Oxford University Press, Inc., publishes works that further
Oxford University's objective of excellence
in research, scholarship, and education.

Oxford New York
Auckland   Cape Town   Dar es Salaam   Hong Kong   Karachi
Kuala Lumpur   Madrid   Melbourne   Mexico City   Nairobi
New Delhi   Shanghai   Taipei   Toronto
With offices in
Argentina   Austria   Brazil   Chile   Czech Republic   France   Greece
Guatemala   Hungary   Italy   Japan Poland   Portugal   Singapore
South Korea   Switzerland   Thailand   Turkey   Ukraine   Vietnam

Published by Oxford University Press, Inc.
198 Madison Avenue, New York, New York 10016
www.oup.com

Library of Congress Cataloging-in-Publication Data

Field epidemiology / edited by Michael B. Gregg. -- 3rd ed.
p.; cm.
Includes bibliographical references and index.
ISBN 978-0-19-531380-2 (cloth )
1. Epidemiology. 2. Epidemics. I. Gregg, Michael B.
[DNLM: 1. Epidemiologic Methods. 2. Epidemiology--organization & administration. WA 950 F453 2008]
RA651.F495 2008
614.4--dc22
2007040284

9 8 7 6 5 4 3 2 1
Printed in the United States of America
on acid-free paper

This book is dedicated to the memory of

Alexander D. Langmuir

Originator, teacher, and practitioner of field epidemiology,
whose wisdom, vision, and inspiration have profoundly
strengthened the practice of public health
throughout the world.

# PREFACE

Over the past several decades, epidemiology has become increasingly complex, theoretical, and specialized. While many epidemiologists are still engaged in the investigation of infectious disease problems, others are addressing newer challenges such as homicides, unwanted pregnancies, environmental exposures, and natural disasters. Computers now make it practical to analyze data in seconds that it might otherwise take weeks or months to calculate. Whole new books have appeared covering such areas as pharmacoepidemiology, perinatal epidemiology, and occupational epidemiology.

Because of the increasing specialization in the real world of contemporary health problems, there is a need for a clearly written, practical, highly usable book devoted to field epidemiology—the timely use of epidemiology to solve public health problems. This process involves the application of basic epidemiologic principles in real time, place and person to solve problems of an urgent or emergency nature.

This book, intended to meet this ever expanding need, is based both on science and experience. It deals with real problems, real places, and real people: nature's experiment, if you will, rather than carefully designed studies in a laboratory or clinical setting. So, in the lexicon of the epidemiologist, the book will be addressing issues relating to observational epidemiology—not experimental epidemiology.

To a great extent, this book is rooted in the experience of the Centers for Disease Control and Prevention (CDC) over more than 50 years of training health professionals in the science—and art—of field epidemiology. In 1951, Alexander D. Langmuir, M.D., CDC's chief epidemiologist, founded the Epidemic Intelligence Service (EIS), and its two-year on-the-job training program in practical, applied epidemiology. On call around the clock, the trainees, called EIS Officers, have been available on request to go into the field to help local and state officials investigate urgent health problems. Before going into the field, however, EIS Officers receive training at CDC in basic epidemiology, biostatistics, and public health practice. The three-week, 8-hour-a-day course is designed to equip them with the essentials of how to mount a field investigation; how to investigate an epidemic; how to start a surveillance system; and how to apply science, technology, and common sense to meet real-life problems at the grass-roots level of experience.

Based on the collective experience of the EIS Officers and their mentors, this book therefore attempts to describe for the field investigator the relevant and appropriate operations necessary to solve urgent health problems at local, state, provincial, federal, and international levels.

Part I contains a definition of field epidemiology; a brief review of epidemiologic principles and methods, under the assumption that the reader has some knowledge of basic epidemiologic methods; and the practice of surveillance. Part II covers the components of field epidemiology: (1) operational aspects of field investigations; (2) conducting a field investigation—a step-by-step description of what to do in the field; (3) survey and sampling methods; (4) using the computer in field investigations; (5) designing studies in the field; (6) describing epidemiologic data; (7) analyzing and interpreting data; (8) developing interventions; and (9) communicating epidemiologic findings. Part III describes special issues such as (1) dealing with the media; (2) legal considerations; (3) immunization practices and the field epidemiologist; (4) investigations in health care facilities and in Out-of Home care settings; (5) investigations of environmental, occupational, and injury problems; (6) field investigations from the local and state perspective; (7) investigations in international settings, terrorism preparedness, and response to natural disasters. Finally, there is an extensive description of the necessary laboratory support for the field epidemiologist and a "walk-through" exercise in the appendix.

Over the past two decades, it has become clear that the teaching and application of field epidemiology have spread widely throughout the world. This book has been translated into Chinese, Korean, and Japanese (not yet in print), and epidemiologists from several other countries have shown similar interest. Such programs as the Global Health Leadership Officer Programme of the World Health Organization; the Public Health Schools Without Walls, supported by the Rockefeller Foundation; and the Field Epidemiology Training Programs (FETP) started by CDC all attest to the importance and application of field epidemiology in the practice of public health.

While *Field Epidemiology* does, indeed, cater the public health epidemiologists practicing in the United States, it is the hope of the editor and the contributors to this book that our collective efforts will contribute significantly to the understanding and practice of field epidemiology worldwide.

M.B.G.
Guilford, Vermont

C.W.T.*
Atlanta, Georgia

*Carl W. Tyler, Jr., former Director of the Epidemiology Program Office, CDC, who wrote the preface to the first edition of this book.

I wish to acknowledge the dedicated and helpful assistance of Marianne G. Lawrence, B.S., and Floyd Grover in the preparation of this book, and the patience and understanding of my wife, Lila W. Gregg.

# CONTENTS

## III.   SPECIAL CONSIDERATIONS

# CONTRIBUTORS

CONSUELO M. BECK-SAGUÉ, M.D.
Pediatric Infectious Disease
 Consultant
Clinton HIV/AIDS Initiative
Dominican Republic

RICHARD E. BESSER, M.D.
Director
Coordinating Office for Terrorism Preparedness
 and Emergency Response
Centers for Disease Control and Prevention
Atlanta, Georgia

GUTHRIE S. BIRKHEAD, M.D., M.P.H.
Deputy Director
Office of Public Health
New York State Department of Health
Associate Professor of Epidemiology
School of Public Health
University at Albany
Albany, New York

JAMES W. BUEHLER, M.D.
Research Professor
Department of Epidemiology
Rollins School of Public Health
Emory University
Atlanta, Georgia

RALPH L. CORDELL, PH.D.
Director, Office of Science Education
Centers for Disease Control and
 Prevention
Atlanta, Georgia

BRUCE B. DAN, M.D.
Adjunct Professor
School of Public Health & Health Sciences
University of Massachusetts Amherst
Amherst, Massachusetts
Adjunct Associate Professor
Department of Preventive Medicine
Vanderbilt University School of Medicine
Nashville, Tennessee

JEFFREY P. DAVIS, M.D.
Chief Medical Officer and State Epidemiologist
 for Communicable Diseases and
 Preparedness
Division of Public Health
Wisconsin Department of Health and Family
 Services
Adjunct Professor
Department of Population Health Sciences
Adjunct Professor of Pediatrics
University of Wisconsin School of Medicine
 and Public Health
Madison, Wisconsin

ANDREW G. DEAN, M.D., M.P.H.
Consultant in Epidemiology and Informatics
Clinton HIV/AIDS Initiative
Dominican Republic

RICHARD C. DICKER, M.D., M.S.
Professor
Department of Public Health and
    Preventive Medicine
St. George's University School of
    Medicine
Grenada, West Indies

RUTH A. ETZEL, M.D., PH.D.
Medical Director—Research
Southcentral Foundation
Anchorage, Alaska

ROBERT E. FONTAINE, M.D., M.S.
Medical Epidemiologist
Division of Epidemiology and Surveillance
Capacity Development
Coordinating Office for Global Health
Centers for Disease Control and
    Prevention
Atlanta, Georgia

STANLEY O. FOSTER, M.D., M.P.H.
Professor of Global Health
Rollins School of Public Health
Emory University
Atlanta, Georgia

RICHARD A. GOODMAN, M.D., J.D., M.P.H.
Public Health Law Program
Office of the Chief of Public Health Practice
Centers for Disease Control and Prevention
Atlanta, Georgia

MICHAEL B. GREGG, M.D.
Private Consultant in Epidemiology
Epidemiologic Training and
    Disease Surveillance
Guilford, Vermont

ELAINE W. GUNTER, B.S., M.T. (ASCP)
Former Deputy Director
Division of Laboratory Sciences,
    NCEH, Centers for Disease Control
    and Prevention
Atlanta, Georgia

JAMES L. HADLER, M.D. M.P.H.
State Epidemiologist and Director
Infectious Diseases Section
Connecticut Department of Public Health
Hartford, Connecticut

WILLIAM HALPERIN, M.D.,
M.P.H., DR.P.H.
Chair and Professor
Department of Preventive Medicine
    and Community Health
New Jersey Medical School
Chair and Professor
Department of Quantitative Medicine
School of Public Health
University of Medicine and Dentistry
    of New Jersey
Newark, New Jersey

JOAN M. HEROLD, PH.D.
Professor Emerita
Rollins School of Public Health
Emory University
Atlanta, Georgia

JAMES G. HODGE, JR., J.D., LL.M.
Associate Professor, Johns
    Hopkins Bloomberg School of
    Public Health
Executive Director, Center for Law
    and the Public's Health
Core Faculty, Johns Hopkins Berman
    Institute of Bioethics
Baltimore, Maryland

HARRY F. HULL, M.D
President
H.F. Hull and Associates
Consultant in Infectious Disease
    Epidemiology
St. Paul, Minnesota

WILLIAM R. JARVIS, M.D.
President
Jason and Jarvis Associates
Hilton Head Island, South Carolina

JOAN S. KNAPP, PH.D.
Laboratory Reference and
    Research Branch
Division of STD Prevention
National Center for HIV/AIDS, Viral Hepatitis,
    STD, and TB Prevention
Coordinating Center for Infectious Diseases
Centers for Disease Control and Prevention
Atlanta, Georgia

JONATHAN B. KOTCH. M.D., M.P.H.
Professor and Associate Chair
Department of Maternal and Child Health
University of North Carolina
Chapel Hill, North Carolina

VERLA S. NESLUND, J.D.
Vice President for Programs
CDC Foundation
Atlanta, Georgia

JANET K.A. NICHOLSON, PH.D.
Senior Advisor for Laboratory Science
Coordinating Center for Infectious Diseases
Centers for Disease Control and Prevention
Atlanta, Georgia

ERIC K. NOJI, M.D., M.P.H.
James A. Baker III Distinguished Fellow in
    Health Policy
Program in Global Health Security
The Center for Health Innovation
Washington, D.C.

DANIEL M. SOSIN, M.D., M.P.H.
Senior Advisor for Science and Public
    Health Practice
Coordinating Office for Terrorism Preparedness
    and Emergency Response
Centers for Disease Control and
    Prevention
Atlanta, Georgia

STEPHEN B. THACKER, M.D., M.SC.
Director
Office of Workforce and Career
    Development
Centers for Disease Control and Prevention
Atlanta, Georgia

DOUGLAS TROUT, M.D.,M.H.S.
Associate Director for Science
Division of Surveillance, Hazard
    Evaluations and Field Studies
National Institute for Occupational
    and Safety and Health
Cincinnati, Ohio

MICHAEL VERNON, DR. P.H.
Director, Communicable Disease Section
Cook County Department of Health
Oak Park, Illinois

DUC J. VUGIA, M.D., M.P.H.
Chief
Infectious Disease Branch
California Department of Health Services
Berkeley, California

RON WALDMAN, M.D., M.P.H.
Professor of Clinical Population and
    Family Health
Mailman School of Public Health
Columbia University
New York, New York

# I

# BACKGROUND

# 1

# FIELD EPIDEMIOLOGY DEFINED

Richard A. Goodman
James W. Buehler

Despite the actual practice of "field epidemiology" in the United States and other countries for well over a century, definitions for field epidemiology have come to the fore only recently. Although epidemiologists work in field settings in a variety of contexts, the term *field epidemiology* as used in this book describes investigations that are initiated in response especially to urgent public health problems. A primary goal of field epidemiology is to inform, as quickly as possible, the processes of selecting and implementing interventions to lessen or prevent illness or death when such problems arise.

The constellation of problems faced by epidemiologists who investigate urgent public health problems gives shape to the definition of field epidemiology. For example, consider the following scenario: At 8:30 A.M. on Monday, August 2, 1976, Dr. Robert B. Craven, an Epidemic Intelligence Service Officer assigned to CDC's Viral Diseases Division, received a telephone call from a nurse at a veterans' hospital in Philadelphia, Pennsylvania. The nurse called to report two cases of severe respiratory illness (including one death) in persons who had attended the recent American Legion Convention in Philadelphia. Subsequent conversations with local and state public health officials revealed that 18 people who had attended the convention from July 21to July 24 had died during the period from July 26 to August 2, primarily from pneumonia. By the evening of August 2, an additional 71 cases had been identified among legionnaires. As a consequence of this information, a massive epidemiologic investigation was immediately initiated that involved public health agencies at the local, state, and federal levels. This problem became known as the outbreak of Legionnaires' disease, and the investigation of the problem led directly to the discovery of the gram-negative pathogen *Legionella pneumophila*[1,2], enabling further studies of the nature and modes of transmission of this organism and the epidemiology and natural history of *Legionella* infections, as well as more-informed recommendations for prevention.

The Legionnaires' disease outbreak and the public health response it triggered illustrate the raison d'être for field epidemiology. Using this epidemic as an example, we can define *field epidemiology* as the application of epidemiology under the following set of general conditions:

- The timing of the problem is unexpected.
- A timely response is demanded.
- Public health epidemiologists must travel to and work in the field to solve the problem.
- The extent of the investigation is likely to be limited because of the imperative for timely intervention and by other situational constraints on study designs or methods.

While field investigations of acute problems share many characteristics with prospectively planned epidemiologic studies, they may differ in at least three important aspects. First, because field investigations often start without clear hypotheses, they may require the use of descriptive studies to generate hypotheses before analytic studies can be designed and conducted to test these hypotheses. Second, as noted previously, when acute problems occur, there is an immediate need to protect the community's health and address its concerns. These responsibilities drive the epidemiologic field investigation beyond the confines of data collection and analysis and into the realm of public health policy and action. Finally, field epidemiology requires one primarily to consider when the data are sufficient to take action, rather than to ask what additional questions might be answered by the data.

Although the timing of acute public health problems that prompt field investigations is typically unexpected, emergencies often unmask latent threats to health that have gone unrecognized or have been "waiting to happen." For example, sporadic or epidemic illness may be inevitable if restaurants fail to adhere to food-management guidelines, if hospitals fail to properly sterilize or disinfect instruments, if employers fail to maintain workplace safety standards, or if members of social networks engage in unsafe sexual behaviors. As a result, field investigations may prompt both immediate interventions and longer-term recommendations, or they may identify problems that require further study.

The concepts and methods used in field investigations derive from clinical medicine, epidemiology, laboratory and behavioral sciences, decision theory, an expanding array of other scientific disciplines, skill in communications, and common sense. In this book, the guidelines and approaches for conducting epidemiologic field investigations reflect the urgency of discovering causative factors, the use of multifaceted methods, and the need to make practical recommendations.

## DETERMINANTS FOR FIELD INVESTIGATIONS

Health departments may become aware of potential disease outbreaks or other acute public health problems in a variety of ways. Often, astute clinicians recognize unusual patterns of disease among their patients and alert health departments. Alternatively, situations may come to attention because surveillance systems for monitoring disease or hazard trends detect increases, because the diagnosis of a single case of a rare disease heralds a broader problem, or because members of the public are concerned and contact authorities. Not all such alerts represent situations that merit a field investigation, and not all situations that merit an initial assessment warrant a full-scale investigation. Thus, the first step in a field investigation is deciding whether to conduct a field investigation; once it is initiated, decisions must be made at successive stages about how far to pursue an investigation. These decisions are necessary to make the most effective use of epidemiologists' time and other public health resources. In addition to the need to develop and implement control measures to end threats to the public's health, such as the Legionnaires' disease outbreak, other determinants for and factors giving shape to field investigations include: (*1*) program considerations, (*2*) public and political concerns, (*3*) research and learning opportunities, (*4*) legal obligations, and (*5*) training needs.

### Program Considerations

Certain disease control programs at national, state, and local levels have specific and extensive requirements for epidemiologic investigation. For example, as part of the measles-elimination effort in the United States, a measles outbreak is considered to exist in a community whenever one case of measles is confirmed.[3] Accordingly, every case of measles may be investigated in order to identify and immunize susceptible persons and to evaluate other control strategies such as the exclusion from school of children who cannot provide proof of immunity. An additional example is the emergence of A(H5N1) influenza beginning in 1997 in Asia among wild and domestic birds, as well as a limited number of humans, which has prompted multiple field investigations because of concerns about the potential for an influenza pandemic.

Because they can be costly in personnel time and resources, field investigations may detract from other activities. Thus, the capacity to do field work may be limited by competing demands of other programs within an agency, whether at national, state, or local levels. Under these circumstances, failure to investigate a specific problem could result in a public health problem of greater magnitude that, if controlled earlier, would have caused less human and economic loss.

The threat of bioterrorism has added urgency to the need for agencies to investigate outbreaks of unusual disease. For example, the 22 cases of terrorism-related anthrax and five deaths in 2001 were exhaustively investigated[4] and led to massive increases in investments in public health emergency preparedness in the United States. Not surprisingly, the anthrax attacks and other bioterrorism-related concerns have actually brought about a lowering of the threshold of suspicion necessary for triggering a full field investigation.[5, 6]

## Public and Political Concerns

Although the public's perceptions of hazards may differ from those of epidemiologists, these perceptions increasingly drive the political process that results in an investigation or public health action. In some instances, a citizen's alert can lead to recognition of a major public health problem, such as with Lyme disease in Lyme, Connecticut, in 1976.[7] In other cases, however, public concerns and attendant political pressures may lead to investigations that otherwise are premature or unlikely to be fruitful from a scientific perspective, but are critical in terms of community relations. Small clusters of disease (e.g., leukemia or adverse fetal outcomes) are an example of problems that frequently generate great public concern. Small clusters of disease often occur by chance alone, and field investigations are often inconclusive and only occasionally yield new information about etiologic links to putative exposures.[8] However, because community members may perceive a health threat and because certain clusters do represent specific preventable risks, some public health agencies have developed standard procedures for investigating such clusters even though the likelihood of identifying a remediable cause is low.[9]

Determining how long an investigation should be continued sometimes is a matter of public controversy. Moreover, in some situations attempts at thorough epidemiologic investigation can be perceived as community experimentation or bureaucratic delay. For example, in a large *E. coli* enteric disease outbreak at Crater Lake National Park in 1975, a one-day delay in implementing control measures to obtain more definitive epidemiologic data resulted in a congressional hearing and charges of a "cover up."[10]

## Research and Learning Opportunities

Because almost all outbreaks are "natural experiments," they also present opportunities to address questions of importance to both the basic scientist and those in the applied science of public health practice. Even when there is a clear policy for control of a specific problem, investigation may still provide opportunities to identify new agents and risk factors for infection or disease, define the clinical spectrum of disease, measure the impact of new control measures or clinical interventions, assess the usefulness of microbiologic or other biological markers, or evaluate the utility of new diagnostic tests.

Recognition of newly emergent or re-emergent diseases often prompts aggressive investigations because of the potential for extensive, life-threatening illness. Some of these diseases initially are recognized only upon the occasion of an epidemic, even though subsequent investigations and studies allow for retrospective diagnosis of earlier occurrences, as well as more complete characterization of the spectrum of clinical manifestations and epidemiology. For example, as referred to earlier in this chapter, after *L. pneumophilia* was discovered and a serologic test developed, subsequent studies showed that, in addition to the severe illness manifested in the 1976 Philadelphia outbreak, *Legionella* infection commonly results in mild disease or asymptomatic infection. The initial recognition of certain other problems—such as toxic shock syndrome, AIDS, hantavirus pulmonary syndrome, West Nile virus disease, and SARS—also was followed by aggressive investigations that enabled analogous understanding of the natural history and disease spectrum of these infections. One caveat, however, is that dramatic outbreaks and investigations such as these that identify previously unrecognized pathogens and that yield a wealth of new scientific insights are unusual; more commonly, field investigations of outbreaks identify familiar pathogens and modes of transmission.

Some outbreaks that initially appear to be "routine" may lead to important epidemiologic discoveries. For example, in 1983, investigators pursued a cluster of diarrhea cases, an extremely common problem, to extraordinary lengths.[11] As a result, the investigators were able to trace the chain of transmission of a unique strain of multiply-antibiotic resistant *Salmonella* back from the affected persons to hamburger they consumed, to the meat supplier, and ultimately to the specific animal source herd. This investigation played a key role in clarifying the linkage between antibiotic use by the cattle industry and subsequent antibiotic-resistant infection in humans.

## Legal Obligations

Field investigations frequently require access to patients' private records, queries about private behaviors, identification of the missteps of private enterprises putatively responsible for illness, review of these companies' proprietary information, or even the reporting of errors of health-care providers. Each task is clearly necessary to complete an objective, defensible field investigation, but each is also fraught with considerable ethical and legal overtones (see Chapter 14).

Some investigations are likely to be used as testimony in civil or criminal trials.[12] In these situations, investigations may be carried further than would otherwise be done. For example, investigations in situations where criminal actions may be suspected to have played a role[13] may carry additional legal requirements for establishing a chain of custody of evidence, which is necessary for criminal prosecutions. The anthrax attacks of the fall of 2001 and related concerns about bioterrorism have stimulated other advanced and carefully designed legal measures to facilitate joint epidemiologic and criminal investigations. An example of such measures is a protocol developed by the New York City Department of Health and Mental Hygiene, the New York City Police Department, and the Federal Bureau of Investigation to guide the interviewing of patients during joint investigations by public health and law-enforcement professionals representing those agencies.[14]

## Training Needs

By analogy to clerkships in medical school and postgraduate residencies, outbreak investigations provide opportunities for training in basic epidemiologic skills. Just as clinical training often is accomplished at the same time as patient care is provided, training in field epidemiology often simultaneously assists in developing skills in and the actual delivery of disease control and prevention. For example, CDC's Epidemic Intelligence Service Program has provided assistance to state and local health departments while simultaneously training health professionals in the practice of applied epidemiology.[15, 16]

## UNIQUE CHALLENGES TO EPIDEMIOLOGISTS IN FIELD INVESTIGATIONS

An epidemiologist investigating problems in the field is faced by unique challenges that sometimes constrain the ideal use of scientific methods. In contrast to prospectively planned studies, which generally are based on carefully developed and refined protocols, field investigations must rely on data sources that are less readily controlled and that may literally change with each successive hour or day. In addition to potential limitations in data sources, other factors that pose challenges for epidemiologists during field investigations include sampling considerations, the availability of specimens, the impact of publicity, the reluctance of subjects to participate, and the conflicting pressures to intervene.

## Data Sources

Field investigations often use information abstracted from a variety of sources, such as hospital, outpatient medical, or school health records. These records vary dramatically in completeness and accuracy among patients, health-care providers, and facilities, since entries are made for purposes other than conducting epidemiologic studies. Thus, the quality of such records as sources of data for epidemiologic investigations may be substantially less than the quality of information obtained when investigators can exert greater control through, for example, the use of standard, pretested questionnaires, physical or laboratory examinations, or other prospectively designed, rather than retrospective, data collection methods.

## Small Numbers

In a planned prospective study, the epidemiologist determines appropriate sample sizes based on statistical requirements for power. In contrast, outbreaks can involve a relatively small number of people, thereby imposing substantial restrictions on study design, statistical power, and other aspects of analysis. These restrictions, in turn, limit the inferences and conclusions that can be drawn from a field investigation.

## Specimen Collection

Because the field investigator usually arrives on the scene "after the fact," collection of necessary environmental or biological specimens is not always possible. For example, suspect food items may have been entirely consumed or discarded, a suspect water system may have been flushed, or ill persons may have recovered, thereby precluding collection of specimens during the acute phase of illness when some tests are most likely to be informative. Under these conditions the epidemiologist depends on the diligence of health-care providers who first see the affected persons, and on the recall of affected persons, their relatives, or other members of the affected community.

## Publicity

Acute disease outbreaks often generate considerable local attention and publicity. Press coverage can assist the investigation by helping to develop information, to identify cases, or to promote and help implement control measures. On the other hand, such publicity may cause affected persons and others in the community to develop preconceptions about the source or cause of an outbreak, which in turn lead to potential biases in comparative studies or a failure to fully explore alternate hypotheses.

As government employees, field epidemiologists have an obligation to communicate to the public what is known, what is not known, and what actions are being taken to assess public health threats. Many reporters, in turn, endeavor to find and bring this information to the public's attention. That said, reporters in pursuit of the most current information on the investigation may demand a considerable amount of the epidemiologists' time, to the detriment of the field investigation itself. Ensuring that a member of the response team has the time and skills to communicate effectively with reporters can be essential to the success of a field investigation and to disease control and prevention efforts, particularly in high-profile situations. Frequently during the course of an event, as information unfolds and as field epidemiologists test, reject or accept, and reshape and re-test hypotheses, recommendations for interventions may evolve or become more focused. Apprising affected parties and the public of the rationale for these changes is important to assure the credibility of the field epidemiologists and of public health recommendations (see Chapter 13).

## Reluctance to Participate

While health departments are empowered to conduct investigations and gain access to records, voluntary and willing participation of involved parties is more conducive to successful investigations than is forced participation. In addition, people whose livelihoods or related interests are at risk may be reluctant to cooperate voluntarily. This reluctance may often be the case for common source outbreaks associated with restaurants and other public establishments, in environmental or occupational hazard investigations, or among health-care providers suspected as being sources for transmission of infectious diseases such as hepatitis B. When involved parties do not willingly cooperate, delays may compromise access to and quality of information (e.g., by introducing bias and by decreasing statistical power).

## Conflicting Pressures to Intervene

Epidemiologists conducting field investigations must weigh the need for further investigation against the need for immediate intervention, often in the face of strong and varying opinions of affected persons and others in the community. In the absence of definitive information about the source, cause, or potential impact of a problem, implementation of a plausible control measure may be viewed differently by various parties affected by the situation. The action may be welcomed by those who favor erring on the side of protecting health and challenged by those who question the rationale for interventions, particularly if their economic or other personal interests are threatened. Delaying interventions may allow time to obtain more definitive information, but such delays may lead to additional morbidity. While this dilemma is not unique to field epidemiology within the realm of public health practice, the heightened urgency of acute situations can elevate the emotional impact on all involved parties.

## STANDARDS FOR EPIDEMIOLOGIC FIELD INVESTIGATIONS

Field investigations are sometimes perceived as "quick and dirty" epidemiology. This perception may reflect the inherent nature of circumstances for which rapid responses are required. However, these requirements for action do not provide a rationalization for epidemiologic shortcuts. Rather, they underscore for the field epidemiologist the importance of combining good science with prudent judgment. A better description of a good epidemiologic field investigation would be "quick and appropriate."

In judging an epidemiologic field investigation, paramount consideration should be given to the quality of the science. This should not be the sole standard, however, for the full range of limitations, pressures, and responsibilities imposed on the investigator also must be taken into account. The goal should be to maximize the scientific quality of the field investigation in the face of these limitations and competing interests. Thus, the standards for an epidemiologic field investigation are that it: (*1*) is timely; (*2*) addresses an important public health problem in the community, as defined by standard public health measures (e.g., attack rates, apparent or potential serious morbidity, or mortality) or community concern; (*3*) examines resource needs early and deploys them appropriately; (*4*) employs appropriate methods of descriptive and/or analytical epidemiology; (*5*) engages expertise, when indicated, from other public health sciences, such as microbiology, toxicology, psychology, anthropology, informatics, or statistics; (*6*) probes causality to the degree sufficient to enable identification of the source and/or etiology of the problem; (*7*) identifies evidence-based options for immediate control and long-term interventions; and (*8*) is conducted in active collaboration with colleagues who have policy, legal, programmatic, communication, or administrative roles to assure that the evidence from the investigation is used optimally.

## CONCLUSION AND TRENDS

This chapter has provided a definition of and framework for the burgeoning discipline of field epidemiology. A host of key developments in public health practice during the past three decades reflects the growing recognition and formalization of field epidemiology, including the establishment of nearly thirty "field epidemiology training programs" and related applied epidemiology training opportunities in affiliation with ministries of health and other national-level public health agencies around the world.[17–21] Other examples of this trend include the development of field epidemiology courses and tracks within curriculum offerings of schools of public health[22]; the emergence of organizations that promote and/or link national-level field epidemiology programs[21]; and the growth of a body of literature related to field epidemiology worldwide[23]—in particular, translation of this book into Chinese, Japanese, and Korean. CDC's own workforce development program in field epidemiology—the Epidemic Intelligence Service (EIS)—has operated continuously since its creation in 1951 and has helped train more than 3,000 professionals in this discipline.[15, 16, 24]

As the discipline of field epidemiology continues to evolve, new developments and trends are shaping its ongoing incorporation within public health practice. Examples of these developments include:

- The potential for parties affected in outbreaks to threaten or actually bring lawsuits, and, if they do, how threatened or actual litigation could affect an ongoing investigation (e.g., complicate or otherwise interfere with data collection, or create or increase response bias).
- The increasing sensitivity to and awareness of privacy protection considerations and duties under both federal (e.g., the Health Insurance Portability and Accountability Act [HIPAA]) and state law. Even if such considerations of law do not directly affect an investigation, then differing interpretations of and misconceptions about those laws by public health agencies (e.g., misconceptions about whether HIPAA interferes with reporting), health-care providers, and privacy advocates, as well as the potential for litigation, may alter the willingness of affected parties to cooperate.
- The implications for field investigations of the possible evolution of regulatory requirements and their interpretation for making the distinction between public health practice and research, and the resulting effects on needs to obtain Institutional Review Board (IRB) approval, subjects' informed consent, and oversight by community advisory boards, as well as resulting effects on whether public health exemptions in privacy laws can be invoked.
- The increasing awareness of and concerns regarding intentionality as a cause of disease outbreaks, including lower thresholds for considering intentional actions as a primary or contributing determinant for an outbreak and, when criminal or terrorist acts are suspected, the resulting need for public health and law-enforcement agencies to coordinate in investigations.
- Uses during field investigations of Internet-based and other advanced information technologies for conducting surveys or collecting electronically

stored health data. Examples of developments are automated methods for accessing data maintained in electronic medical record systems or regional health information exchanges (see: www.phii.org) and the application of automated systems of "syndromic surveillance," including systems developed by state and local health departments and CDC's national BioSense system (see: www.syndromic.org and www.cdc.gov/biosense).

- The use of new laboratory subtyping methods for infectious pathogens as a means to increase opportunities to detect epidemics when laboratories recognize an increase in isolations of an unusual pathogen, making it possible to detect and investigate smaller clusters sooner and to detect the diffuse multi-state outbreaks that previously would have been unrecognized (parenthetically, the application of these methods further emphasizes the need for close communication between epidemiologists and laboratory scientists).

- The public's increasing expectation of government transparency and timely information about unfolding events, combined with the advent of the 24-hour news cycle and the power of the Internet to transmit instant, if not consistently accurate, information—each of which underscores the heightened importance of communication skills.

Field epidemiology draws upon general epidemiologic principles and methods, and field epidemiologists face questions that are familiar to epidemiologists regardless of where they work, such as whether study methods can be shaped by logistical constraints and the amounts of information necessary to recommend or take action. Likewise, field epidemiologists are affected by trends that influence the practice of epidemiology in general, such as public concerns about the privacy of health information, the increasing automation of health information, and the growth in use of the Internet. Field epidemiology is unique, however, in compressing and pressurizing these concerns in the context of acute public health emergencies and in thrusting the epidemiologist irretrievably into the midst of the administrative, legal, and ethical domains of policy making and public health action.

## NOTE

Portions of this chapter as incorporated in the first and second editions of this book were adapted, with permission of the editors, from: R.A. Goodman, J.W. Buehler, and J.P. Koplan (1990), The epidemiologic field investigation: Science and judgment in public health practice. *Am J Epidemiol* 132, 91–6.

ACKNOWLEDGMENT    The authors gratefully acknowledge the review of the chapter and suggestions offered by Robert Tauxe, M.D., M.P.H.

## REFERENCES

1. Fraser, D.W., Tsai, T.R., Orenstein. W., et al. (1997). Legionnaires' disease: description of an epidemic of pneumonia. *N Engl J Med* 297, 1189–97.
2. CDC (1997). Follow-up on respiratory illness—Philadelphia. *Morb Mortal Wkly Rep* 46, 49–56.
3. CDC (1998). Measles, mumps, rubella—vaccine use and strategies for elimination of measles, rubella, and congenital rubella syndrome and control of mumps: recommendations of the Advisory Committee on Immunization Practices (ACIP). *Morb Mortal Wkly Rep* 47 (No.RR-8), 38–9.
4. Jernigan, D.B., Raghunathan, P.L., Bell, B.P., et al. (2002). Investigation of bioterrorism-related anthrax, United States, 2001: epidemiologic findings. *Emerg Inf Dis* 8, 1019–28.
5. Butler, J.C., Cohen, M.L., Friedman, C.R., et al. (2002). Collaboration between public health and law enforcement: new paradigms and partnerships for bioterrorism planning and response. *Emerg Infect Dis* 8, 1152–6.
6. Treadwell, T.A., Koo, D., Kuker, K., et al. (2003). Epidemiologic clues to bioterrorism. *Public Health Reports* 118, 92–118.
7. Steere, A.C., Malawista, S.E., Snydman, D.R., et al. (1977). Lyme arthritis: an epidemic of oligoarticular arthritis in children and adults in three Connecticut communities. *Arthritis Rheum* 20, 7–17.
8. Schulte, P.A., Ehrenberg, R.L.. Singal, M. (1987). Investigation of occupational cancer clusters: theory and practice. *Am J Public Health* 77, 52–6.
9. CDC (1990). Guidelines for investigating clusters of health events. *Morb Mortal Wkly Rep* 39 (RR-11), 1–16.
10. Rosenberg, M.L., Koplan, J.P., Wachsmith, I.K., et al. (1977). Epidemic diarrhea at Crater Lake from enterotoxigenic. *Escherichia coli*: a large waterborne outbreak. *Ann Intern Med* 86, 714–8.
11. Holmberg, S.D., Osterholm, M.T., Senger, K.A., et al. (1984). Drug-resistant *Salmonella* from animals fed antimicrobials. *N Engl J Med* 311, 617–22.
12. Goodman, R.A., Loue, S., Shaw, F.E. (2006). Epidemiology and the law. In R.C. Brownson, D.B. Petitti (eds.), *Applied Epidemiology: Theory to Practice*, 2nd ed., Oxford University Press, New York. pp. 289–326.
13. Goodman, R.A., Munson, J.W., Dammers, K., et al. (2003). Forensic epidemiology: law at the intersection of public health and criminal investigations. *J Law, Med & Ethics* 31, 684–700.
14. CDC (2004). New York City protocol: http://www2a.cdc.gov/phlp/docs/BTProtocol Cover.PDF; http://www2a.cdc.gov/phlp/docs/Investigations.PDF
15. Langmuir, A.D.. (1980). The Epidemic Intelligence Service of the Centers for Disease Control. *Public Health Rep* 104, 170–7.
16. Thacker, S.B., Dannenberg, A.L., Hamilton, D.H.. (2001). Epidemic Intelligence Service of the Centers for Disease Control and Prevention: 50 years of training and service in applied epidemiology. *Am J Epidemiol* 154, 985–92.

17. White, M.E., McDonnell, S.M., Werker, D.H., et al. (2001). Partnerships in international applied epidemiology training and service, 1975–2001. *Am J Epidemiol* 154, 993–9.
18. Thacker, S.B., Buffington, J.. (2001). Applied epidemiology for the 21st century. *Int J Epidemiol* 30, 320–5.
19. CDC Field Epi Training Program relationships: http://www.cdc.gov/descd/fetp.html
20. World Health Organization: http://www.who.int/csr/labepidemiology/projects/fieldepitraining/en/index.html
21. European Programme for Intervention Epidemiology Training: http://www.epiet.org/
22. University of North Carolina CPHP Certificate in Field Epidemiology: http://www.sph.unc.edu/nciph/fieldepi
23. Dabis, F., Drucker, J., Moren, A. (1992). *Epidémiologie d'intervention*, Arnette, Paris.
24. Langmuir, A.D., Andrews, J.M. (1952). Biological warfare defense: The Epidemic Intelligence Service of the Communicable Disease Center. *Am J Public Health* 42, 235–8.

# 2

# A BRIEF REVIEW OF THE BASIC
# PRINCIPLES OF EPIDEMIOLOGY

Richard C. Dicker

Epidemiology is considered the basic science of public health for good reason. First, epidemiology is a quantitative discipline that relies on a working knowledge of probability, statistics, and sound research methods. Second, epidemiology is a method of causal reasoning based on developing and testing biologically plausible hypotheses about health states and events. Third, as a discipline within public health, epidemiology provides a foundation for directing practical and appropriate public health action based on scientific and causal reasoning.[1]

The word *epidemiology* comes from the Greek words *epi*, meaning "on" or "upon," *demos*, meaning "people," and *logos*, meaning "the study of." In other words, the word *epidemiology* has its roots in the study of what befalls the population. Many definitions of epidemiology have been offered, but the following definition captures the underlying principles and the public health spirit of epidemiology: "Epidemiology is the study of the distribution and determinants of health-related states or events in specified populations, and the application of this study to the control of health problems."[2]

Key terms in this definition reflect some of the important principles of the practice of epidemiology.

*Study.* Epidemiology is a scientific discipline with sound methods of scientific inquiry at its foundation. Epidemiology is data-driven and relies on a systematic and unbiased approach to the collection, analysis, and interpretation of data.

16

Field epidemiologic methods tend to rely on careful observation and use of valid comparison groups to assess whether what was observed, such as the number of cases of disease in a geographical area during a particular week or the frequency of an exposure among persons with disease, differs from what might be expected.

*Distribution.* *Distribution* refers to the frequency and pattern of health events in a population. *Frequency* means, not only the number of health events in a population, but the relationship of that number to the size of the population; that is, the number of events divided by the study population. The resulting proportion or rate allows epidemiologists to compare disease occurrence between different populations. *Pattern* refers to the description of health-related events by time, place, and personal characteristics. Time patterns can use categories such as year, season, week, day, hour, weekday versus weekend, or any other breakdown of time that effectively and objectively displays disease or injury occurrence. Place patterns include geographical variations, urban–rural differences, and the location of work sites or schools. Personal characteristics include demographic factors such as age, gender, marital status, and socioeconomic status, as well as behaviors and environmental exposures.

The above characterization of the distribution of health-related states or events comprises one broad aspect of epidemiology called *descriptive epidemiology*. Descriptive epidemiology provides the What, Who, When, and Where of health-related events.

*Determinants.* *Determinants* are the Why and How—the causes and other factors that influence the occurrence of health-related events. Epidemiologists assume that illness does not occur randomly, but happens only when the right combination of risk factors or determinants accumulates. To search for these determinants, epidemiologists use *analytic epidemiology*—the process of assessing whether groups with different rates of disease have differences in demographic characteristics, genetic or immunological makeup, behaviors, environmental exposures, and other potential risk factors. Epidemiologic studies, such as cohort and case-control studies and the analytic methods used by epidemiologists to identify factors associated with the increased risk of disease, are discussed in Chapters 8 and 10.

*Health-related states or events.* Early in its history, epidemiology tended to focus on epidemics of communicable diseases. Later, epidemiologic thinking was extended to endemic communicable diseases and noncommunicable infectious diseases. By the middle of the twentieth century, additional epidemiologic methods had been developed and applied to chronic diseases, injuries, birth defects, maternal–child health, occupational health, and environmental health. Next, epidemiologists looked "upstream" at behaviors related to health and well-being such as exercise, diet, and seat-belt use. More recently, advances in molecular methods have allowed epidemiologists to examine genetic markers of disease risk. Indeed, the phrase "health-related states or events" can be seen as including anything that affects the well-being of a population. Nonetheless, many epidemiologists still use the term "disease" as shorthand for the wide range of health-related states and events that are studied.

*Specified populations.* Although epidemiologists and direct health-care providers are both concerned with the occurrence and control of disease, they differ greatly in how they view "the patient." The clinician has concern for the health of an individual; the epidemiologist has concern for the collective health of the people in a community or population under study. In other words, the clinician's patient is the individual; the epidemiologist's patient is the community. Therefore, the clinician and the epidemiologist have different responsibilities when faced with a person with, say, diarrheal disease. Both are interested in establishing the correct diagnosis. However, while the clinician usually focuses on treating and caring for the individual, the epidemiologist focuses on identifying the exposure or source of the agent that caused the illness, the number of other persons who may have been similarly exposed, the potential for further spread in the community, and interventions to prevent additional cases or recurrences.

*Application.* Although "-ology" is usually translated as "the study of," the definition given above requires that epidemiology be more than just the academic pursuit of knowledge. Field epidemiology, in particular, embodies the application of the knowledge gained to protect and promote the public's health. Thus, field epidemiology, like the practice of medicine, is both science and art. To make the proper diagnosis and prescribe appropriate treatment for a patient, the clinician combines medical knowledge with experience, clinical judgment, and an understanding of the patient. Similarly, the epidemiologist uses the scientific methods of descriptive and analytic epidemiology as well as experience, epidemiologic judgment, and an understanding of local conditions in "diagnosing" the health of a community and proposing appropriate, practical, and acceptable public health interventions to control and prevent disease in the community.

## USES OF EPIDEMIOLOGY

Epidemiology and the information generated by epidemiologic methods have been put to innumerable uses. Some common uses are described below.

### Assessing the Community's Health

Public health officials responsible for policy development, implementation, and evaluation use epidemiologic information as a factual basis for decision making (we hope!). To assess the health of a population or community, you must identify relevant sources of data and analyze the data by time, place, and person (descriptive epidemiology) to address such questions as, What are the actual and potential health problems in the community? Where are they occurring? Who is at risk? Which problems are declining over time? Which ones are increasing or have the potential to increase? How do these patterns relate to the level and distribution of services available? More detailed data may need to be collected and analyzed to determine whether the health services are available, accessible, effective, and efficient. For example, following hurricanes and other natural disasters, you would conduct rapid health assessments to determine the community's health status and health needs.[3, 4]

## Making Individual Decisions

Many individuals may not realize that they regularly use epidemiologic information to make decisions that affect their health. When a person decides to quit smoking, climb the stairs rather than wait for the elevator, eat a salad rather than a cheeseburger with fries for lunch, or use a condom, he or she may be influenced, consciously or unconsciously, by epidemiologists' assessment of risk. Since World War II, epidemiologists have provided information related to all those decisions. In the 1950s epidemiologists reported the increased risk of lung cancer among smokers.[5, 6] In the 1970s, epidemiologists documented the role of exercise and proper diet in reducing the risk of heart disease.[7, 8] In the 1980s, epidemiologists identified the increased risk of acquired immunodeficiency syndrome (AIDS) infection associated with certain sexual and drug-related behaviors, even before the causative virus had been identified.[9] These and hundreds of other epidemiologic findings are directly relevant to the choices that people make every day, choices that affect their health over their lifetime.

## Completing the Clinical Picture

When investigating a disease outbreak, field epidemiologists rely on health-care providers and laboratory workers to help establish the proper diagnosis of individual patients. But epidemiologists, in turn, contribute to health-care providers' understanding of the clinical picture and natural history of disease. For example, in August of 1999, an infectious diseases consultant in Queens, New York, was asked to examine two patients with encephalitis (inflammation of the brain) accompanied by profound weakness, which was not common. The physician could not make a definitive diagnosis, but she did notify public health authorities. Within weeks, field epidemiologists had identified enough other cases to characterize the spectrum and course of the disease, and laboratorians were eventually able to identify the agent as the West Nile virus, which had never before been identified in North America[10] A few years later, epidemiologists described a clinical manifestation that had previously been poorly characterized—West Nile fever without encephalitis.[11] Epidemiologists have also been instrumental in documenting the spectrum of illness of many noninfectious exposures, such as the numerous conditions related to cigarette smoking, from pulmonary and heart disease, to lip, throat, and lung cancer, to reproductive effects.[12]

## Searching for Causes

Much epidemiologic research is devoted to searching for causes or factors that influence one's risk of disease. Sometimes this is an academic pursuit, but in field epidemiology the goal is to identify a cause so that appropriate public health action can be taken as soon as possible. One can argue that epidemiology can never prove a causal relationship between an exposure and a disease, because much of epidemiology is based on ecological reasoning and statistical associations. Nevertheless, epidemiology often provides enough information to support effective action. Examples date from the removal of the handle from the Broad Street pump following John Snow's investigation of cholera in the Golden Square area of London in 1854,[13] to the withdrawal of a vaccine against rotavirus found by epidemiologists to be associated with an increased risk of intussusception, a potentially life-threatening condition.[14] Just as often, epidemiology and laboratory science converge to provide the evidence needed to establish causation. For example, epidemiologists were able to identify a variety of risk factors during an outbreak of a pneumonia among persons attending the American Legion Convention in Philadelphia in 1976, even though the Legionnaires' bacillus was not identified in the laboratory until almost 6 months later.[15]

## CORE EPIDEMIOLOGIC COMPETENCIES

In 2006, the Council of State and Territorial Epidemiologists adopted a set of competencies for epidemiologists working in public health departments.[16] Among these competencies, the ones that form the core of what epidemiologists do as part of Assessment and Analysis are performing public health surveillance and conducting investigations of acute and chronic conditions or other adverse outcomes in the population. These activities are described below.

## Public Health Surveillance

Public health surveillance is the ongoing, systematic collection, analysis, and interpretation of outcome-specific data essential to the planning, implementation, and evaluation of public health practice, closely integrated with the timely dissemination of these data to those who need to know.[17] The purpose of public health surveillance, which is sometimes called "information for action,"[18] is to portray the ongoing patterns of disease occurrence and disease potential so that investigation, control, and prevention measures can be applied efficiently and effectively. This is accomplished through the systematic collection and evaluation of morbidity and mortality reports and other relevant health information, and the dissemination of these data and their interpretation to those involved in disease control and public health decision-making (see Chapter 3). The design, conduct, and evaluation of surveillance systems require that epidemiologists be competent in design of data collection instruments, data management, descriptive methods and graphing, interpretation of data, and scientific writing and presentation.

## Investigation of Acute and Chronic Health Conditions

Surveillance provides information for action, such as an investigation by the public health department following a report of a single case or multiple cases of a specific disease or event. The investigation is sometimes as simple as a health department employee's calling the health-care provider to confirm or clarify the circumstances of the reported case. Other times it may be as extensive as a field investigation involving the coordinated efforts of dozens of people from multiple agencies to determine the extent of an epidemic and to identify its cause.

The objectives of such field investigations also vary. For some diseases, particularly those spread from person to person, the objective may be to identify people with unreported or unrecognized cases who might otherwise spread infection to others. For example, one of the hallmarks of investigations of persons with sexually transmitted disease is the identification of the cases' sexual contacts. When investigated by local health staff, many of these contacts are often found to have asymptomatic infections they were unaware of, requiring treatment for infections they did not know they had.

For some diseases, the primary objective of an investigation may be to identify a source or vehicle of infection that can be controlled or eliminated. For example, the investigation of a case of *E. coli* 0157:H7 usually focuses on trying to identify the vehicle, such as ground beef or fruit juice or municipal water. By identifying the vehicle, investigators can determine how many other persons might have already been exposed and how many continue to be at risk. When the vehicle turns out to be a commercial product, public announcements and recall of the product may prevent many additional cases.

In some instances, the objective of an investigation may be to learn more about the natural history, clinical spectrum, descriptive epidemiology, and risk factors of an unknown or previously unrecognized condition. Early investigations of the epidemic of severe acute respiratory syndrome (SARS) in 2003 focused on the clinical presentation and time, place, and person characteristics. This information was used to establish a case definition and to characterize the persons and populations at risk. As more was learned about the epidemiology and communicability of the disease, appropriate recommendations regarding isolation and quarantine were issued.[19, 20]

Field investigations of the type described above are sometimes referred to as "shoe-leather epidemiology," conjuring up images of dedicated, if slightly haggard, field epidemiologists pounding the pavement in search of additional cases and clues regarding source and mode of transmission. This approach is commemorated in the symbol of the Epidemic Intelligence Service, CDC's training program for field epidemiologists—a shoe with a hole in the sole.

Surveillance and field investigations sometimes are sometimes enough to identify causes, modes of transmission, and appropriate control and prevention measures. At other times, you may have to use analytic studies. Often, the methods are used in combination—with surveillance and field investigation providing clues or hypotheses about causes and modes of transmission, and analytic studies evaluating the credibility of those hypotheses. Clusters or outbreaks of disease frequently are initially investigated using descriptive epidemiology. The descriptive approach involves the study of disease incidence and distribution by time, place, and person. It includes the calculation of rates and identification of parts of the population at higher risk than others. Occasionally, particularly when the association between exposure and disease is obvious, control measures can be implemented immediately without the need for any type of analytic study. In other situations, when the cause or vehicle is not as obvious from the descriptive epidemiology and environmental investigation, an analytic study can help sort out plausible hypotheses.

While some analytic studies are conducted in response to acute health problems such as outbreaks, many others are planned studies. The hallmark of an epidemiologic study is the use of a valid comparison group. The most common types of analytic studies used in field epidemiology are described in greater detail in Chapter 8.

You must be familiar with all aspects of an analytic study, including its design, conduct, analysis, interpretation, and communication of the findings.

- *Design* includes determining the appropriate study design, writing justifications and protocols, calculating sample sizes, deciding on criteria for subject selection (e.g., developing case definitions), choosing an appropriate comparison group, and designing questionnaires.
- *Conduct* involves securing appropriate clearances and approvals, adhering to applicable ethical principles, abstracting records, tracking down and

interviewing subjects, collecting and handling specimens, and managing the data.

- *Analysis* begins with describing the characteristics of the subjects. It progresses to calculation of rates, creation of comparative tables (e.g., two-by-two tables), and computation of measures of association (e.g., risk ratios or odds ratios), tests of significance (e.g., chi-square test), confidence intervals, and the like. Many epidemiologic studies require more advanced analytic techniques such as stratified analysis, regression, and modeling. Data analysis is described more fully in Chapter 10.

- Finally, interpretation involves putting the study findings into perspective, identifying the key take-home messages, and making sound recommendations. Doing so requires that you be knowledgeable about the subject matter and the strengths and weaknesses of the study.

## THE EPIDEMIOLOGIC APPROACH

As with all scientific endeavors, the practice of epidemiology relies on a systematic approach. In very simple terms, epidemiologists:

- **Count** cases or health events, and describes them in terms of time, place, and person;
- **Divide** the number of cases by an appropriate denominator to calculate rates; and
- **Compare** these rates over time or for different groups of people.

Before counting cases, however, the epidemiologist must decide what is a case. This is done by developing a case definition.* Then, using this case definition, the epidemiologist finds and collects information about the case-patients. Using this information, the epidemiologist describes them collectively in terms of time, place, and person. Next, the number of case-patients is put into perspective by dividing by the size of the population; i.e., calculating a disease rate. Finally, to determine whether this rate is greater than what one would normally expect, and, if so, to identify factors contributing to this increase, the epidemiologist compares the rate from this population to the rate in an appropriate comparison group, using analytic epidemiology techniques.

---

* Some people use the term *case* to refer to the illness, not the person experiencing the illness. A person with the illness is then called a *case-patient*, and the case definition often begins with "illness characterized by ..."

## Defining a Case

Before counting cases, the epidemiologist must decide what to count; that is, what to call a case. To do so, the epidemiologist uses a case definition. A *case definition* is a set of standard criteria for classifying whether a person has a particular disease, syndrome, or other health condition. Some case definitions, particularly those used for national surveillance, have been developed and adopted as national standards that ensure comparability. Use of an agreed-upon standard case definition ensures that classification is consistent, regardless of when or where it occurred, or who identified it. Furthermore, the number of cases or rate of disease identified in one time or place can be compared with the number or rate from another time or place. For example, with a standard case definition, health officials could compare the number of cases of listeriosis that occurred in Forsyth County, North Carolina, in 2000 with the number that occurred there in 1999. Or they could compare the rate of listeriosis in Forsyth County in 2000 with the national rate in that same year. When everyone uses the same standard case definition and a difference is observed, the difference is not the result of variation in how cases are classified.

Whereas case definitions for surveillance tend to focus on clinical features, case definitions for outbreaks often use clinical features plus limitations on time, place, and occasionally person. The clinical criteria usually include confirmatory laboratory tests, if available, or combinations of symptoms, signs, and other findings. For example, the standard surveillance case definition for listeriosis is a clinically compatible illness (infection caused by *Listeria monocytogenes*, which may produce any of several clinical syndromes, including stillbirth, listeriosis of the newborn, meningitis, bacteremia, or localized infections) that is laboratory-confirmed (isolation of *L. monocytogenes* from a normally sterile site).[21] The case definition used during an investigation of a listeriosis outbreak in North Carolina in 2000 included the same clinical component but added restrictions on time (onset of illness between October 24, 2000, and January 4, 2001), place, and person (in a resident of Winston-Salem, North Carolina).[22]

## Counting and Characterizing Cases by Time, Place, and Person

Identifying and counting cases is one of the basic tasks in public health. These counts, usually derived from case reports submitted by health-care workers and laboratories to the health department, allow public health officials to determine the extent and patterns of disease occurrence by time, place, and person. They can also indicate clusters or outbreaks of disease in the community.

## Descriptive Epidemiology

Descriptive epidemiology is usually said to include the "when" (time), "where" (place), and "who" (person) of disease incidence or prevalence in a community. Depending on the circumstances, descriptive epidemiology can also include the "what"; that is, a description of the disease itself, particularly the distribution of clinical features in the population.

In terms of disease occurrence in a population, time can be measured in periods as long as decades or as brief as minutes. Long-term trends in disease occurrence are usually presented by year over one or more decades. Number of cases of a disease that tends to occur during the same time each year is usually presented by week or month to highlight the disease's seasonality. The most appropriate time interval for an outbreak is usually based on the causative agent's incubation period, which can be minutes for a toxin, to hours for *Salmonella*, to weeks for hepatitis B, to years for HIV.

Describing the occurrence of disease by place provides insight into the geographical extent and variation of the health problem. Characterization by place refers not only to place of residence, but to any geographical location relevant to disease occurrence. Such locations can include place of diagnosis or report, workplace, school, hospital wing, or recent travel destinations. "Place" can also refer to broad categories such as urban or rural, hospital-acquired or community-acquired, or domestic versus foreign.

Numerous characteristics of a person can affect risk of illness. These include inherent characteristics (e.g., age, gender, race), biological characteristics (e.g., immune status), acquired characteristics (e.g., marital status), activities (e.g., occupation, leisure activities, use of medications, tobacco, or drugs), or the conditions under which persons live (e.g., socioeconomic status, access to medical care). While age and gender are included in almost all data sets and are probably the two most commonly analyzed "person" characteristics, other person variables can be just as important or even more important for identifying groups with elevated risk of disease.

Compiling and analyzing data by time, place, and person is desirable for several reasons. First, by carefully teasing apart the data by time, place, and person, you will become quite familiar with the data. You will see what variables are available, how the data are coded, the range of values, and which variables have an abundance of missing values. Second, you will learn the extent and pattern of the public health problem being investigated, such as which months, which neighborhoods, and which age groups have the most and fewest cases. Third, you will create a detailed description of the health problem that can be easily communicated with tables, graphs, and maps. Fourth, you can identify areas or groups within the population that have high rates of disease. This information, in turn, not only provides important clues to the causes of the disease that need to be investigated further, but also points out where public health interventions need to be targeted.

## Calculating Rates

Counts are essential for health planning. For example, a health official needs to know counts (i.e., numbers) to plan how many doses of vaccine or hospital beds may be needed.

However, simple counts do not provide all the information a health department needs. For some purposes, the counts or numbers must be considered in light of the size of the population in which the cases occurred. A *rate* is a measure that relates the number of cases during a certain period of time to the size of the population. For surveillance purposes, the period of time is usually the calendar year, the numerator is the number of new cases reported that year, and the denominator is the estimated mid-year population. For example, 44,108 new cases of acquired immunodeficiency syndrome (AIDS) were reported in the United States in 2004.[23] This number, divided by the estimated 2004 mid-year population (290,810,000), resulted in a rate of 15.2 cases per 100,000 population for 2004.

Rates are also useful during outbreak investigations, although they are calculated slightly differently. The rate calculated during an outbreak investigation is usually called an "attack rate," which is the proportion of the population that became ill. It is calculated as the number of new cases divided by the size of the population at the start of the outbreak. The time period is usually the duration of the outbreak, which could be a few days or several weeks. For example, as part of an investigation of an outbreak of botulism among church supper attendees in Texas, investigators conducted a retrospective cohort study of the 38 church supper attendees.[24] Fifteen of the 38 met the case definition for botulism, resulting in an overall attack rate of 15/38 or 40%. However, the attack rate was 15 of 24 (63%) among those who had eaten chili; the attack rate was 0 of 14 (0%) among those who had not.

## Comparing Rates

Rates are particularly useful for comparing the frequency of disease in different locations whose populations differ in size. For example, in 2004, Pennsylvania had over twelve times as many births (144,748) as its neighboring state, Delaware (11,369). However, Pennsylvania had nearly ten times the population of Delaware. So a fairer way to compare the birth picture in Pennsylvania and Delaware is to calculate rates. In fact, that year, the birth rate was greater in Delaware (13.7 per 1,000 population) than in Pennsylvania (11.7 per 1,000 population).[25]

Rates are also useful for comparing disease occurrence during different periods of time. For example, 19.5 cases of chickenpox per 100,000 were reported in 2001, compared with 135.8 cases per 100,000 in 1991.[26] In addition, rates of disease among different subgroups can be compared to identify those at elevated risk of disease. These so-called high-risk groups can be further assessed and targeted for special intervention. High-risk groups can also be studied to identify risk factors that put them at increased risk of disease. While some risk factors such as age and family history of breast cancer may not be modifiable, others, such as smoking and unsafe sexual practices, are. Individuals can use knowledge of the modifiable risk factors to guide their decisions about behaviors that influence their health.

Comparing rates is just one example of the fundamental role of comparison in epidemiology. In fact, much of epidemiology is about comparison—comparing one group or time frame that could be labeled *observed* with another group or time frame that provides the *expected*. For example, to determine whether this week's number or rate of a reportable disease exceeds the normal or expected level, you would compare this week's number or rate with the number or rate reported in previous weeks, or the number or rate reported during the same week last year. Similarly, in an analytic study such as a cohort study or case-control study, one group (the exposed group in a cohort study, the case group in a case-control study) can be thought of as providing the observed quantity (incidence of disease in a cohort study, proportion exposed in a case-control study), while the comparison group (unexposed in a cohort study, control group in a case-control study) provides the expected quantity. The comparison of attack rates for botulism among those who were and were not exposed to (i.e., who did or did not eat) the chili dish at the church supper clearly showed an elevated risk among those who had eaten chili. But is a comparison group really necessary when every case shares a particular exposure? Consider a hypothetical outbreak of gastroenteritis caused by *E. coli* 0157:H7. Suppose that every one of the cases drank the tap water. *E. coli* 0157:H7 can be transmitted by water, so water is a plausible vehicle. Does that mean that the water was the source in this outbreak? Not necessarily. After all, all of the cases breathed the air, but that does not mean that *E. coli* was spread by airborne transmission. A comparison needs to be made of water consumption among the cases (observed) and among controls—those who did not get sick (expected). If water consumption was common among the cases but not among the controls, then water is said to be "associated with" illness and needs to be investigated further. On the other hand, if all of the controls drank the water, then the observed water consumption among cases is exactly what is expected based on the controls' water consumption, and the vehicle is likely to be something else. This central role of comparison in epidemiology in both surveillance and investigation cannot be overstated.

## CONCEPTS OF DISEASE OCCURRENCE

A critical premise of epidemiology is that disease and other health events do not occur randomly in a population, but are more likely to occur in some members of the population than others. As noted earlier, one important use of epidemiology is to identify the factors that increase some members' risk of disease above others'.

## Causation

A number of models of disease causation have been proposed. Among the simplest of these is the epidemiologic *triad* or *triangle*, the traditional model for infectious disease. The triad comprises an external *agent*, a susceptible *host*, and an *environment* that brings the host and agent together. In this model, disease results from the interaction between the agent and the susceptible host in an environment that supports transmission of the agent from a source to that host.

Agent, host, and environmental factors interrelate in a variety of complex ways to produce disease in humans. Different diseases require different balances and interactions of these three components.

### Agent Factors

Narrowly, the word *agent* refers to an infectious microorganism—a virus, bacterium, parasite, or other microbe. Generally, the agent must be present for disease to occur. However, presence of the agent alone is not always sufficient to cause disease. A variety of factors influences whether exposure to an organism will result in disease, including the organism's pathogenicity (ability to cause disease) and dose, and the portal of entry (skin, respiratory tract, etc.).

More broadly, the concept of *agent* includes chemical and physical causes of disease or injury. These include chemical contaminants (such as diethylene glycol that contaminated medications in Haiti and Panama and caused several deaths[27, 28]) and physical forces (such as repetitive mechanical forces associated with carpal tunnel syndrome).

### Host Factors

*Host* refers to the human who can get the disease. Host factors are intrinsic factors that influence an individual's exposure, susceptibility, or response to a causative agent. Opportunities for exposure are often influenced by behaviors such as sexual practices, hygiene, and other personal choices, as well as by age and sex. Susceptibility and response to an agent are influenced by such factors as genetic composition, nutritional and immunological status, anatomical structure, presence of disease or medications, and psychological makeup.

### Environmental Factors

Environmental factors are extrinsic factors that affect the agent and host and the opportunity for exposure. Environmental factors include physical factors such as geology and climate; biological factors such as insect vectors that transmit the agent; and socioeconomic factors such as crowding, sanitation, and the availability of health services.

## The Natural History and Spectrum of Disease

The *natural history* of disease refers to the progression of a disease process in an individual over time, in the absence of treatment. For example, untreated infection with HIV causes a spectrum of clinical problems beginning at the time of serocon-version and terminating with AIDS and, usually, death. Many if not most diseases have a characteristic natural history, although the time frame and specific manifes-tations of disease may vary from individual to individual and are influenced by preventive and therapeutic measures.

Natural history begins with an exposure or accumulation of factors sufficient to begin the disease process in a susceptible host. For an infectious disease, the exposure is a microorganism. For cancer, the exposure may be a factor that initi-ates the process, such as asbestos fibers or components in tobacco smoke (for lung cancer), or one that promotes the process, such as estrogen (for endometrial cancer).

After the disease process has been initiated, pathological changes occur that are usually not apparent to the individual. This stage of subclinical disease, extend-ing from the time of exposure to onset of disease symptoms, is usually called the *incubation period* for infectious diseases and the *latency period* for chronic dis-eases. (Note, however, that the term *latency period* is sometimes used for infec-tious diseases to describe the time from exposure to onset of infectivity; i.e., when the host can transmit the infection to others.) The incubation period may be as brief as seconds for hypersensitivity and toxic reactions to as long as decades for some chronic diseases. Even for a single disease, the characteristic incubation period has a range. For example, the typical incubation period for hepatitis A is about four weeks, but it may be as brief as two weeks or as long as seven weeks. The latency period for leukemia to become evident among survivors of the atomic bomb blast in Hiroshima in 1945 ranged from two to twelve years, peaking at six to seven years.[29]

Although disease is inapparent during the incubation period, pathological changes can sometimes be detected with laboratory, radiographic, or other screen-ing methods. Most screening programs attempt to identify the disease process during this phase of its natural history, since intervention at this early stage is likely to be more effective than treatment given after the disease has progressed and become symptomatic.

The onset of symptoms marks the transition from subclinical to clinical dis-ease. Most diagnoses are made during the stage of clinical disease, when a person experiences symptoms. In some people, however, the disease process may never progress to clinically apparent illness. Others experience clinical illness that can be mild or severe or even fatal. This range of clinical manifestations is called the *spectrum of disease*. Ultimately, the disease process ends in either recovery, disability, or death.

For an infectious agent, *infectivity* refers to the proportion of a population who become infected after being exposed. *Pathogenicity* refers to the proportion of the group of infected individuals who develop clinically apparent disease. *Virulence* refers to the proportion of clinically apparent cases that are severe or fatal.

The natural history and spectrum of disease present challenges to the clinician and to the field epidemiologist. Because the clinical spectrum of many diseases ranges from asymptomatic to severe illness, cases of illness diagnosed by clinicians in the community often represent only the tip of the iceberg. Many additional cases may be too early to diagnose or may never progress to the clinical stage. Unfortunately, persons with inapparent or undiagnosed infections may nonetheless be able to transmit infection to others. Such persons who are infectious but have subclinical disease or are still in the incubating stage are called *carriers*. Frequently, carriers are persons incubating disease or with inapparent infection. Persons with measles, hepatitis A, and several other diseases become infectious a few days before the onset of symptoms. However, carriers can also be persons who appear to have recovered from their clinical illness but unknowingly remain infectious, such as chronic carriers of the hepatitis B virus, or persons who never exhibited symptoms at all, such as the infamous Typhoid Mary. The challenge to public health workers is that these carriers, feeling fine and unaware that they are infected and infectious to others, are more likely to unwittingly spread infection than are people who are ill.

## Chain of Infection

The traditional epidemiologic triad model holds that infectious diseases result from the interaction of agent, host, and environment. More specifically, transmission occurs when an infectious agent leaves its reservoir or host through a portal of exit, is conveyed by some mode of transmission, and enters through an appropriate portal of entry to infect a susceptible host. This sequence is sometimes called *the chain of infection*.

### Reservoir

The *reservoir* of an infectious agent is the habitat in which the agent normally lives, grows, and multiplies. Reservoirs vary by agent, and can be humans, animals, and the environment. The reservoir may or may not be the source from which an agent is transferred to a host. For example, the reservoir of *Clostridium botulinum* spores is soil, but the source of most cases of human botulism is improperly canned food containing *C. botulinum* spores and its toxin.

Many of the common infectious diseases have human reservoirs. Diseases that are transmitted from person to person without intermediaries include the sexually transmitted diseases, measles, mumps, streptococcal infections, and many respiratory pathogens. Because humans were the only reservoir for the smallpox virus, smallpox was eradicated after the last human case was identified and isolated.[30]

Humans are also subject to diseases that have animal reservoirs. Many of these diseases are transmitted from animal to animal, with humans as incidental hosts. The term *zoonosis* refers to an infectious disease that is transmissible under natural conditions from vertebrate animals to humans. Long-recognized zoonotic diseases include brucellosis (cows and pigs), anthrax (sheep), plague (rodents), trichinellosis (swine), tularemia (rabbits), and rabies (bats, raccoons, dogs, and other mammals). Zoonoses newly emergent in North America include West Nile encephalitis (birds), and monkey pox (prairie dogs). Many newly recognized infectious diseases in humans, including HIV/AIDS, Ebola infection and SARS, are thought to have emerged from animal hosts, although those hosts have not yet been definitively identified.

Plants, soil, and water in the environment are also reservoirs for some infectious agents. Many fungal agents, such as those causing histoplasmosis, live and multiply in the soil. *Legionella pneumophila*, the bacterium that causes Legionnaires' disease, is often found in the water of cooling towers and evaporative condensers.

## Modes of Transmission

An agent can be transmitted from its natural reservoir to a susceptible host in a variety of ways. These modes of transmission can be classified as:

- Direct
  - Direct contact
  - Droplet spread
- Indirect
  - Airborne
  - Vehicle-borne
    - Food
    - Water
    - Fomites
    - Other
  - Vector-borne
    - Mechanical
    - Biological

In direct transmission, an infectious agent is transferred from a human, animal, or environmental reservoir to a susceptible host by direct contact or droplet spread. Direct contact occurs through kissing, skin-to-skin contact, and sexual intercourse. *Direct contact* also refers to contact with soil or vegetation harboring infectious organisms. Thus, infectious mononucleosis ("kissing disease") and gonorrhea are spread from person to person by direct contact. Hookworm is spread by direct contact with contaminated soil. *Droplet spread* refers to spray with relatively large, short-range aerosols produced by sneezing, coughing, or even talking. Droplet spread is classified as direct because transmission is by direct spray over a few feet, before the droplets fall to the ground. Pertussis and meningococcal infection are examples of diseases transmitted from an infected patient to a susceptible host by droplet spread.

Indirect transmission refers to the transfer of an agent from a reservoir to a host by suspended air particles, inanimate objects (vehicles), or animate intermediaries (vectors).

Airborne transmission occurs when infectious agents are carried by dust or droplet nuclei suspended in air. Airborne dust includes material that has settled on surfaces and becomes resuspended by air currents, as well as infectious particles blown from the soil by the wind. Droplet nuclei are dried residue of less than 5 microns in size. In contrast to droplets that fall to the ground within a few feet, droplet nuclei can remain suspended in the air for long periods of time and are sometimes blown over great distances.

Vehicles—inanimate objects that can indirectly transmit an agent—include food, water, biological products (blood), and fomites (inanimate objects such as handkerchiefs, bedding, or surgical scalpels). Some vehicles passively carry an agent—as food or water can carry hepatitis A virus. Other vehicles provide an environment in which the agent grows, multiplies, or produces toxin—as an improperly prepared can of food supports production of botulinum toxin by *C. botulinum*.

Vectors such as mosquitoes, fleas, and ticks can carry the agent through purely mechanical means or can support growth or changes in the agent. Examples of mechanical transmission are flies carrying shigella on their appendages and fleas carrying *Yersinia pestis*, the causative agent of plague, in their gut. In contrast, biological transmission occurs when the causative agent of malaria or guinea worm disease undergoes maturation in an intermediate host before it can be transmitted to humans.

## Host

The final link in the chain of infection is introduction of the agent into a susceptible host. Susceptibility of a host to infection depends on the portal of entry (e.g., skin, respiratory tract, or gastrointestinal tract) genetic or constitutional factors, specific immunity, and nonspecific factors that affect an individual's ability to resist infection or to limit pathogenicity. An individual's genetic makeup can either increase or decrease susceptibility. For example, people with sickle cell trait seem to be at least partially protected from one type of malaria. *Specific acquired immunity* refers to protective antibodies that are directed against a specific agent. These antibodies develop in response to infection, vaccine, or toxoid (toxin that has been deactivated but retains its capacity to stimulate production of toxin antibodies) or are acquired by transplacental transfer from mother to fetus or by injection of antitoxin or immune globulin. Nonspecific factors that defend against infection include the skin, mucous membranes, gastric acidity, cilia in the respiratory tract, the cough reflex, and nonspecific immune responses. Factors that may increase susceptibility to infection by disrupting host defenses include malnutrition, alcoholism, and disease or therapy that impairs the immune response.

## Implications for Public Health

Knowledge of the chain of infection, including the portals of exit and entry and modes of transmission, provides a basis for determining appropriate control measures. In general, control measures are usually directed against the segment in the infection chain that is most susceptible to intervention, unless practical issues dictate otherwise. For some diseases, the most appropriate intervention is controlling or eliminating the agent at its source. For a disease with a human host, the patient can be treated to eliminate the source. In the community, soil can be decontaminated or covered to prevent the agent's escape.

Some interventions are directed at the mode of transmission. Interruption of direct transmission can be accomplished by isolating someone with infection or counseling someone to avoid the specific type of contact associated with transmission. Vehicle-borne transmission can be interrupted by eliminating or decontaminating the vehicle. For airborne diseases, strategies are sometimes directed at modifying ventilation or air pressure and filtering or treating the air. To interrupt vector-borne transmission, measures are often directed toward controlling the vector population.

Some strategies that protect portals of entry are simple and effective. For example, a dentist's mask and gloves are intended to protect the dentist from a patient's blood, secretions, and droplets, as well to protect the patient from the dentist. To reduce the risk of West Nile virus infection, persons have been advised to wear long pants and sleeves outdoors, and to use insect repellant.

Finally, some interventions aim to increase a host's defenses. Vaccinations promote the development of specific antibodies that protect against infection. Similarly, prophylactic use of antimalarial drugs, recommended for visitors to malaria-endemic areas, does not prevent exposure through mosquito bites, but does prevent infection from taking root.

## Epidemic Disease Occurrence

### Levels of Disease

The amount of a particular disease that is usually present in a community is referred to as the baseline or *endemic* level of the disease. This level is not necessarily the desired level, which is probably zero; rather, it is the usual, observed level. In the absence of intervention, and assuming that the level is not high enough to deplete the pool of susceptible persons, new cases of the disease would probably continue to occur at this level indefinitely. Thus, the baseline level is often regarded as the expected level of the disease. *Sporadic* refers to a disease that occurs occasionally at irregular intervals. *Endemic* refers to the constant presence and/or usual prevalence of a disease or infectious agent in a population within a geographic area. *Hyperendemic* refers to persistent, high levels of disease occurrence.

Occasionally, the amount of disease rises above the expected level. *Epidemic* refers to an increase, often sudden, in the number of cases of the disease above what is normally expected in that population in that area. *Outbreak* carries the same definition as *epidemic* but is often used for a more limited geographic area. *Cluster* refers to an aggregation of cases grouped in place and time that are suspected to be greater than the expected number. Often, however, the expected number is not known. *Pandemic* refers to an epidemic that has spread over several countries or continents, usually affecting a large number of people.

Epidemics occur when an agent and susceptible hosts are present in adequate numbers, and the agent can be effectively conveyed from a source to the susceptible hosts. More specifically, an epidemic tends to result from:

- a recent increase in amount or virulence of the agent,
- the recent introduction of the agent into a setting where it has not been before,
- an enhanced mode of transmission so that more susceptible persons are exposed,
- an environment conducive to interaction between the host and the agent,
- a change in the susceptibility of the host response to the agent, and/or
- factors that increase host exposure or involve introduction through new portals of entry.[31]

### Epidemic Patterns

Epidemics and outbreaks can be classified according to their manner of spread through a population:

- Common source
  - Point

  – Intermittent
  – Continuous
• Propagated
• Mixed
• Other

A *common-source outbreak* is one in which a group of people are all exposed to an infectious agent or toxin from the same source. If the group is exposed over a relatively brief period, so that everyone who becomes ill develops disease at the end of one incubation period, then the common-source outbreak is further classified as a *point-source outbreak*. The epidemic of leukemia cases in Hiroshima following the atomic bomb blast and the epidemic of hepatitis A among diners who ate green onions at a Pennsylvania restaurant are both point-source epidemics.[29, 32] In some common-source outbreaks, exposure can occur over a period of days, weeks, or longer. A *continuous common-source outbreak*, is one in which the exposure and hence the dates of onset occur over a prolonged period of time. An *intermittent common-source outbreak* is one in which exposure, and hence cases of disease, occur intermittently.

A *propagated outbreak* results from transmission from one person to others. Usually, transmission is by direct person-to-person contact, as with syphilis. Transmission can also be vehicle-borne (e.g., transmission of hepatitis B or HIV by sharing needles) or vector-borne (e.g., transmission of yellow fever by mosquitoes). In propagated outbreaks, cases occur over more than one incubation period. The epidemic usually wanes after a few generations, either because the number of susceptible persons falls below some critical level required to sustain transmission or because public health action is taken that interrupts transmission.

Some epidemics have features of both common-source epidemics and propagated epidemics. The pattern of a common-source outbreak followed by secondary person-to-person spread is not uncommon. These are called *mixed epidemics*. For example, a common-source epidemic of shigellosis occurred among a group of 3000 women attending a national music festival. Many developed symptoms after returning home. Over the next few weeks, several state health departments detected subsequent generations of shigella cases spread by person-to-person transmission from festival attendees.[33]

Finally, some epidemics are neither "common source" in its usual sense nor propagated from person to person. Outbreaks of zoonotic or vector-borne disease can result from sufficient prevalence of infection in host species, sufficient presence of vectors, and sufficient human–vector interaction. Examples include the epidemic of Lyme disease that affected several states in the northeastern United States in the late 1980s and the epidemic of West Nile encephalitis in New York City in 1999.[34, 10]

## SUMMARY

As a discipline within public health, epidemiology includes the study of the frequency, patterns, and causes of health-related states or events in populations, and the application of that study to address public health issues. Epidemiologists use a systematic approach to assess the What, Who, Where, When, and the Why and How of these health states or events. Two essential aspects in this systematic approach entail studying populations and making comparisons. Differences in disease occurrence in different populations are assessed by generating and evaluating hypotheses about risk factors and causes. In carrying out these tasks, you are almost always part of a team. Knowledge of basic principles of disease occurrence and spread in a population is essential for selecting and implementing effective measures to protect and promote the public's health.

## REFERENCES

1. Cates, W. (1982). Epidemiology: applying principles to clinical practice. *Contemp Ob/ Gyn* 20, 147–61.
2. Last, J.M. (Ed.) (2001). *Dictionary of Epidemiology*, 4th ed., Oxford University Press, New York. p. 61.
3. World Health Organization (1999). *Rapid health assessment protocols for emergencies*. World Health Organization, Geneva, Switzerland.
4. Centers for Disease Control and Prevention (2005). Epidemiologic assessment of the impact of four hurricanes—Florida, 2004. *Morb Mortal Wkly Rep* 54, 693–7.
5. Wynder, E.L., Graham, E.A. (1950). Tobacco smoke as a possible etiologic factor in bronchiogenic carcinoma. *JAMA* 143, 329–36
6. Doll, R., Hill, A.B. (1954). The mortality of doctors in relation to their smoking habits: a preliminary report. *Brit Med J* 228(i), 1451–5.
7. Kannel, W.B., Gordon, T., Sorlie, P., et al. (1971). Physical activity and coronary vulnerability: the Framingham Study. *Cardiology Digest* 6, 28–40.
8. Kritchevsky, D. (1977). Dietary fiber and other dietary factors in hypercholesterolemia. *Am J Clin Nutr* 30, 979–84.
9. Peterman, T.A., Drotman, D.P., Curran, J.W. (1985). Epidemiology of the acquired immunodeficiency syndrome (AIDS). *Epidemiol Rev* 7, 1–21.
10. Nash, D., Mostashari, F., Fine A., et al. (1999). West Nile Outbreak Response Working Group. (2001). The outbreak of West Nile virus infection in the New York City area in 1999. *N Engl J Med* 344, 1807–14.
11. Watson, J.T., Pertel, P.E., Jones, R.C., et al. (2004). Clinical characteristics and functional outcomes of West Nile fever. *Ann Intern Med* 144, 360–5.
12. U.S. Department of Health and Human Services (2004). *The health consequences of smoking: a report of the Surgeon General*. U.S. Department of Health and Human Services, Centers for Disease Control and Prevention, Office on Smoking and Health, Atlanta, Georgia.
13. Snow, J. (1936). *Snow on Cholera*. Oxford University Press, London.

14. Murphy, T.V., Gargiullo, P.M., Massoudi, M.S., et al. (2001). Intussusception among infants given an oral rotavirus vaccine. *N Engl J Med* 344, 564–72.

15. Fraser, D.W., Tsai, T.R., Orenstein, W., et al. (1977). Legionnaires' disease: description of an epidemic of pneumonia. *N Engl J Med* 297, 1189–97.

16. CDC/CSTE Development of Applied Epidemiology Competencies. Retrieved November 1, 2006, from http://www.cste.org/comptencies.asp.

17. Thacker, S.B., Birkhead, G.S. (2007). Surveillance. In Gregg, M.B. (ed.), *Field Epidemiology*, 3rd ed. New York: Oxford University Press.

18. Orenstein, W.A., Bernier, R.H. (1990). Surveillance: information for action. *Pediatr Clin North Am* 37, 709–34.

19. CDC (2003). Outbreak of Severe Acute Respiratory Syndrome—Worldwide, 2003. *Morb Mortal Wkly Rep* 52, 226–8.

20. CDC (2003). Severe Acute Respiratory Syndrome (SARS) and coronavirus testing— United States, 2003. *Morb Mortal Wkly Rep* 52, 297–302.

21. CDC (2001). Case definitions for infection conditions under public health surveillance. *Morb Mortal Wkly Rep* 46 (RR-10).

22. MacDonald, P., Whitwam, R.E., Boggs, J., et al. (2005). Outbreak of listeriosis among Mexican immigrants as a result of consumption of illicitly produced Mexican-style cheese. *Clin Infect Dis* 40, 677–682.

23. CDC (2004). Summary of notifiable diseases—United States, 2004. *Morb Mortal Wkly Rep* 53, 18–20.

24. Kalluri, P., Crowe, C., Reller, M., et al. (2003). An outbreak of foodborne botulism associated with food sold at a salvage store in Texas. *Clin Infect Dis* 37, 1490–5.

25. CDC (2001). Summary of notifiable diseases—United States, 2001. *Morb Mortal Wkly Rep* 50, 91.

26. Martin, J.A., Hamilton, B.E., Sutton, P.D., et al. (2006). Births: Final Data for 2004. National Vital Statistics Reports 55, 52.

27. O'Brien, K.L., Selanikio, J.D., Hecdivert, C., et al, for the Acute Renal Failure Investigation Team (1998). Epidemic of pediatric deaths from acute renal failure caused by diethylene glycol poisoning. *JAMA* 279, 1175–80.

28. Barr, D.B., Barr, J.R., Weerasekera, G., et al. (2008). Identification and quantification of diethylene glycol in pharmaceuticals implicated in poisoning epidemics: an historical laboratory perspective. *J Anal Toxicol* 32, 106–115.

29. Cobb, S., Miller, M., Wald N. (1959). On the estimation of the incubation period in malignant disease. *J Chronic Dis* 9, 385–93.

30. Fenner, F., Henderson, D.A., Arita, I., et al. (1988). Smallpox and its eradication. Geneva: World Health Organization.

31. Kelsey, J.L., Thompson, W.D., Evans, A.S. (1986). *Methods in Observational Epidemiology*. Oxford University Press, New York. p. 216.

32. CDC (2003). Hepatitis A outbreak associated with green onions at a restaurant— Monaca, Pennsylvania, 2003. *Morb Mortal Wkly Rep* 52, 1155–7.

33. Lee, L.A., Ostroff, S.M., McGee, H.B., et al. (1991). An outbreak of shigellosis at an outdoor music festival. *Am J Epidemiol* 133, 608–15.

34. White, D.J., Chang, H-G., Benach, J.L., et al. (1991). Geographic spread and temporal increase of the Lyme disease epidemic. *JAMA* 266, 1230–6.

# 3

## SURVEILLANCE

Stephen B. Thacker
Guthrie S. Birkhead

The two previous chapters reviewed the basic principles and practices of epidemiology and their use in a newly defined application of epidemiologic study; namely, field epidemiology. With or without the urgency to investigate, make recommendations, or take specific action, all epidemiologic studies obtain data on a study population and capture facts to analyze. But for the public health epidemiologist and, in particular, the field investigator, getting timely health-related data, either in a hurry (e.g., in response to an obvious or suspected acute public health problem) or on an ongoing basis (e.g., to assess or monitor trends in major public health problems affecting a population), carries a distinct implication—the idea of information for action. So, in this context, the acquisition of information for use in the public health arena has been called *surveillance*.

### DEFINITION

No standard, universally accepted definition of surveillance exists in public health practice. The Centers for Disease Control and Prevention (CDC), however, has promoted the following generally agreed-upon definition:

> Public health surveillance (sometimes called epidemiologic surveillance) is the
> ongoing systematic collection, analysis, and interpretation of outcome-specific data

essential to the planning, implementation, and evaluation of public health practice, closely integrated with the timely dissemination of these data to those who need to know. Outcomes may include disease, injury, and disability, as well as risk factors, vector exposures, environmental hazards, or other exposures. The final link of the surveillance chain is the application of these data to prevent and control human disease and injury.

Some have compared the surveillance system with a nerve cell that has an afferent arm that receives information, a cell body that analyzes the data, and an efferent arm that takes appropriate action. This analogy is particularly appropriate in the context of field investigations of acute public health problems, where, very often, surveillance must be started quickly to get necessary data so that the right action can be taken.[1, 2] Using surveillance to guide immediate public health prevention and control measures is often a major goal of the field epidemiologist.

## BACKGROUND

Following the discoveries of infectious disease agents in the late 1800s, the first use of scientifically based surveillance concepts in public health practice was monitoring contacts of persons with serious communicable diseases such as plague, smallpox, typhus, and yellow fever. A common feature of these diseases is the potential for explosive outbreaks with high case-fatality rates. One purpose of surveillance is to detect the first signs and symptoms of disease and to begin prompt isolation to prevent further spread. For many decades in the United States, early detection and isolation were functions of municipal and state health departments and of foreign quarantine stations—not only of the United States Public Health Service, but of quarantine agencies throughout the world.

In the late 1940s, Alexander D. Langmuir, M.D., then the chief epidemiologist of the Communicable Disease Center (now the Centers for Disease Control and Prevention), began to broaden the concept of surveillance. Although surveillance of persons at risk for specific disease continued at quarantine stations, Langmuir and his colleagues changed the focus of attention to diseases, such as malaria and smallpox, rather than individuals. They emphasized rapid collection and analysis of data on a particular disease with quick dissemination of the findings to those who needed to know.[3]

Now this credo of rapid reporting, analysis, and action applies to nearly 100 infectious diseases and health events of noninfectious etiology at the local, state, and national levels in the United States. Many ongoing systems of reporting have resulted from local or national emergencies, such as poliomyelitis resulting from contaminated lots of vaccine (the so-called Cutter incident of 1955), the Asian influenza epidemic of 1957, shellfish-associated hepatitis A in 1961, toxic shock syndrome in 1980, Hantavirus pulmonary syndrome in 1994 in the Four Corners area (the juncture of New Mexico, Arizona, Colorado, and Utah), widespread outbreaks of *E. coli* 0157:H7 from 1994 to 1999, West Nile encephalitis in the Northeast in 1999 (subsequently spreading across the United States), and SARS and monkey pox in 2003. After the events of September 11, 2001, surveillance systems have been devised to detect hopefully rare, but potentially catastrophic outbreaks of diseases, such as smallpox or anthrax, spread by terrorist groups. And concerns that a human pandemic might arise from the H5N1 avian strain of influenza in 2005 and 2006 led to rapid preparations in many sectors of public health, including the development of specific surveillance systems. These recent catastophes have stimulated significant investment in syndromic surveillance, which applies basic surveillance principles to indicators of disease and injury (e.g., prescription data, emergency-department-visit chief complaint, or 911 calls) in an effort to identify outbreaks at the earliest stages (see Chapter 22). Within days after the investigation of L-tryptophan-associated eosinophilia–myalgia syndrome (EMS) in 1990, a national reporting system was established for a previously rare and nonreportable condition.

## TYPES OF SURVEILLANCE

Surveillance has been classified historically as either active or passive. Passive surveillance (i.e., initiated by the source of the data, often a health-care provider or clinical laboratory rather than the health department) refers to data supplied to a health department based on a known set of rules or regulations that require such reporting. For example, in the United States, certain diseases (mostly communicable diseases but also cancers and certain injuries in some geographic areas) are required by state law or regulation to be reported by practicing physicians to a local health department. In turn, these reports might be sent to state health departments and forwarded to the federal government's CDC. Most surveillance systems throughout the world are passive, because they are cheaper and easier for health departments to operate. However, in general, they also substantially undercount the occurrence of most reportable diseases.

On the other hand, in active surveillance (i.e., surveillance initiated by a health department), which is also based on certain regulations, the health agency regularly or routinely solicits reports from various providers. Active surveillance is most commonly implemented during an epidemic such as the 1976 epidemic of Legionnaires' disease in Philadelphia or the 1990 epidemic of EMS in the United States. A modification of passive and active surveillance is an enhanced passive surveillance system where active follow-up of each case is used to pursue other possible cases (e.g., contact tracing of sexually transmitted disease performed by investigators in local health departments). Thus, the system of surveillance will vary by disease, source of report, need for complete case counting, and sense of urgency, because public health measures often need to be taken in response to each case (e.g., prophylaxis of contacts of cases of meningitis).

The principles and practices relating to surveillance that are discussed in this chapter apply broadly to all surveillance efforts, but because of the time frame involved, some practices are more appropriate when acute disease problems occur in the field: the primary focus of our attention. Other systems are more adaptable to what we refer to as "ongoing" or long-term surveillance practices, where the goal is to monitor trends over time, and often no real sense of urgency exists or no immediate public health response is needed (e.g., cancer surveillance). Obviously, there is a gray area, but the basic differences between acute and long-term surveillance will remain clear and logical.

## PURPOSES OF SURVEILLANCE

Whether investigating an epidemic in the field or implementing a statewide program of prevention, surveillance is a basic tool for the field epidemiologist; it is the cornerstone and the management tool for public health practice. Just as businesses manage their day-to-day affairs by well-recognized precepts and actions, so must those of us in the practice of public health. Good surveillance, like good business practice, provides the data needed to give

- an accurate *assessment* of the status of health in a given population,
- an early warning of disease problems to guide immediate *control measures*,
- a quantitative base to define *objectives* for action,
- measures to define specific *priorities*,
- information to *design and plan* public health programs,
- measures to *evaluate* interventions and programs, and
- information to plan and conduct *research*.

In short, surveillance data provide a scientific and factual basis for appropriate policy and disease-control decisions in public health practice, as well as an evaluation of public health efforts and allocation of resources.

## DATA SOURCES

Before discussing how to start a surveillance system, let us look at some of the kinds of data that are often readily available in the field and where they can be found.

Depending on the problem, the epidemiologist will have to choose which data are most appropriate to collect and understand the strengths and weaknesses of different data sources. If certain information is unavailable, you might have to get it by conducting surveys or administering questionnaires (see Chapter 6).

In any event, every effort should be made to follow a simple, standardized method at the beginning, knowing that, as the health problem becomes more clearly understood or circumstances change during the investigation, you might have to modify the surveillance system accordingly. The growth and acceptance of personal computers and the Internet have made a variety of morbidity and mortality data widely available and readily accessible to the field epidemiologist.[4]

## Mortality Data

Mortality data are regularly available at the local and state level, and because of burial laws, mortality statistics can be used at the local level within a matter of days. Mortality data for selected causes of death are available on a weekly basis from 122 large U.S. cities as part of a national influenza surveillance system. Maintained and published weekly during the influenza season by CDC, in collaboration with local health jurisdictions, these mortality statistics come from cities that represent more than 25% of the nation's population and give a useful, timely index of the extent and impact of influenza at local, state, and national levels.

Medical examiners and coroners are excellent sources for data concerning sudden or unexpected deaths. Data are available at the state or county level and include detailed information regarding the cause and the nature of death that is unavailable on the death certificate. For investigations of acute disease outbreaks, recent mortality data often have to be accessed by hand-tally of death certificates, although electronically filed death certificates are becoming more widely available. These data are especially valuable for surveillance of intentional and unintentional injuries, as well as sudden deaths of unknown cause. However, death certificate data have certain limitations: the lack of standardization in determining and listing the cause of death by physicians, and the limited information on the circumstances of death (i.e., external causes). Nonetheless, for field investigations, death certificates can be used to contact the attending physician and to locate the patient medical record to obtain further information.

Another source is the National Mortality Followback Survey, which is conducted periodically by CDC on a sample of knowledgeable informants to ascertain social and health information on decedents. (*Note:* For this and many of the surveillance systems discussed in this chapter, more information and surveillance data are available on the Internet [see Appendix 3–1]). This data source might be useful to establish baseline expected rates of death for conditions of interest.

Multiple cause-of-death data are generally available with a several-year lag and might also serve as a useful source of expected rates of death against which to judge mortality data used for the surveillance of acute disease problems.

The quality of death certificate data might vary from location to location, state to state, and particularly from country to country. Physicians' assessments of cause(s) of death are divergent at times, and even definitions of death, time of death, and words such as "infant" are subject to variation. Therefore, comparisons of mortality statistics between time frames and across geopolitical boundaries should be made with caution and only after obtaining in-depth knowledge regarding important considerations such as local customs, changes in coding of death certificates, and advances in medical knowledge. In some areas, computerized mortality data on underlying cause of death might not be available for many months after the period of interest; the availability of multiple cause of death listings often takes longer.

## Morbidity Data

Most countries require the reporting of certain diseases (usually infectious) that are considered important to health authorities. In the United States, laws and regulations of each state's health department list from 50 to 130 notifiable diseases (or conditions) that are reportable health events.[5] A complete listing of physician and laboratory disease reporting requirements by state is available at the Council of State and Territorial Epidemiologists homepage: http//:www.cste.org. These data are used routinely and published for surveillance purposes at local, state, and national levels. Virtually all surveillance systems rely on physicians or other health-care providers for these reports. Unfortunately, most infectious diseases are underreported by practicing physicians. Increasing reliance on reporting from clinical laboratories and use of computerized medical record, billing, or managed-care data could improve the completeness of reporting diagnosed cases. Of course, unrecognized or undiagnosed illnesses never enter the reporting loop. However, the severer and rarer the disease, the more sensitive and specific the reports of both infectious and noninfectious conditions tend to be.. In these cases, physicians might be likelier to report because they see the direct benefit of reporting, not only for the sake of public health but also for the benefit of obtaining the assistance and expertise of the health department in confirming the diagnosis and gaining access to appropriate treatment. A good example is surveillance of botulism, where the public health department laboratory may be the only source of specific diagnostic testing to confirm the diagnosis and where the epidemiologist can assist in obtaining botulism antitoxin from the U.S. Public Health Service, the only available source. In this circumstance, emergency department physicians encountering suspected botulism cases will want to call the health department to access these diagnostic and treatment services. Reporting diseases under intensive surveillance (e.g., measles, meningococcal disease, and AIDS in the United States) can reach a sensitivity of more than 90% of diagnosed cases. However, such levels of reporting are uncommon and depend heavily on resource-intensive active surveillance (e.g., in the case of AIDS).

The transition to integrated electronic systems from paper-based systems for disease surveillance has made substantial strides in recent years.[6] As of April 2005, a total of 27 states were using secure, Internet-based systems for entry of notifiable disease reports, and 26 received laboratory test results through automated electronic laboratory results (ELR). When clinicians, laboratories, or local health department investigators enter data securely over the Internet, that information can be available to state or local health departments immediately, avoiding delays caused by mailing forms or backlogs in data-entry processing at health departments. Some states have designed systems that automatically send e-mail and telephone messages to public health officials in the event of an urgent laboratory report such as a case of meningococcal disease.

Using standards and systems to enhance the exchange of information between the clinical sector and public health sector is a principal goal of the National Electronic Disease Surveillance System (NEDSS) and the Public Health Information Network (PHIN). The ELR enhancements have required detailed specifications for the format, data elements, and standard codes. In addition, PHIN specifies the standards for secure transmission of these messages over the Internet; to meet these standards, CDC has provided the PHIN Messaging System for use by public and private partners. Successful ELR reporting provides experience with secure, standards-based, interoperable data exchange, relevant for public health agencies and also for their partners in clinical medicine. Use of secure, Internet-based systems enables public health response 24 hours a day, seven days a week. State health departments have used these systems to manage workloads and increase capacity during outbreaks and to help improve the nation's ability to detect and respond to disease threats.

Other sources of morbidity data can prove useful both in ongoing systems of surveillance and in field situations. Private physicians are contacted by several survey groups. The National Ambulatory Medical Care Survey (NAMCS) is a national probability sample of visits to office-based physicians, which began in 1974. Three thousand physicians have participated in the survey, which has been conducted annually since 1989 by CDC's National Center for Health Statistics (NCHS); data are collected on diagnosis, symptoms, drugs, and referrals. The National Drug and Therapeutic Index, a similar sample, is conducted by a private company, IMS Health. Diagnostic, specialty, therapeutic, and disposition data are available from both of these samples. The Ambulatory Sentinel Practice Network, initiated in 1978 by the North American Primary Care Research Group, is an example of a voluntary office-based system that examines particular health problems selected on a periodic basis. These surveys provide a useful source of baseline data on several conditions but lack the timeliness and full geographic coverage needed to be useful in most local field investigations. Recently, networks of sentinel emergency rooms and travel physicians have collected data on emerging infectious disease threats. These systems provide more rapid data, although they do not cover all geographic areas; they have the advantage of the flexibility to look for new diseases of interest on short notice. One example is the 1999 outbreak of West Nile encephalitis in the northeastern United States, where these networks were mobilized to look for cases of unexplained encephalitis nationwide to gauge the extent of the outbreak.

Health maintenance organizations and other forms of managed care have become a substantial component of health services in the United States. Both managed care organizations and public health practitioners need population-based data on disease, injury, and risk for assessment and planning. This common interest has stimulated collaboration between managed care and public health officials at both the local and national levels for research purposes as well as health promotion and disease prevention. In many areas, this is still an underdeveloped source of surveillance data; however, at the local level, such alliances should prove especially useful to the field epidemiologist.

Hospital data are another useful source of surveillance information. The National Hospital Discharge Survey and the National Hospital Ambulatory Medical Care Survey, conducted by NCHS, provide data abstracted from hospital records. State-specific hospital discharge data are available in many areas. Information typically includes diagnosis, length of stay, operative procedures, laboratory findings, and costs. However, hospital discharge data might be of limited use in detecting or evaluating acute disease outbreaks, because of the lack of timeliness of data collection and the lack of accuracy of diagnostic coding because these data are often collected for billing or administrative purposes.

The National Birth Defects Prevention Network was established in the 1990s to form a national surveillance system based on reports from hospitals and physicians to state health department congenital-malformation registries. These data have been used recently by some states to look for potential birth defects among infants of HIV-infected mothers who took antiretroviral therapy during pregnancy. Natality (birth certificate data) is used to monitor prenatal care practices and adverse birth outcomes. Electronically recorded birth certificates make such information available within a few days of birth, allowing immediate public health questions to be addressed. The National Nosocomial Infection Surveillance System consists of a group of hospitals that voluntarily reports hospital-acquired infections to CDC. These data provide useful baseline rates of infection and an early warning system of regional trends (e.g., hospital-acquired infections that are resistant to antibiotics).

## Laboratory Data

Whether serving the interests of a single hospital, local or state health department, or national or international health agency, the clinical diagnostic laboratory has given the field epidemiologist invaluable information, particularly during infectious disease outbreaks. Now, at the beginning of the twenty-first century, the consolidation of many laboratories into regional ones and the near-universal computerization of laboratory data have substantially increased the usefulness of the laboratory in surveillance efforts. Clinical laboratories are relatively few in number and thus are fairly easy to monitor to ensure mandated reporting is occurring. Establishment of regular, even daily, reporting from large clinical laboratories to state and local health departments, essentially a form of active surveillance, holds promise to provide complete reporting of laboratory-diagnosed cases. In addition to generating disease cases for public health follow-up, recognition of rare or unusual sero- or biotypes, or even simply an increase in demands for laboratory facilities provide essential data for the detection and investigation of epidemics caused by agents such as salmonella, shigella, *Escherichia coli*, and staphylococcus. New molecular fingerprinting techniques, such as pulsed-field gel electrophoresis, can identify clusters of related cases, which may be geographically dispersed and thus not recognized as being related, and can link human isolates to isolates from food, water, or other sources.[7] Ongoing laboratory surveillance of influenza and poliomyelitis isolates as well as laboratory studies of lead and other environmental hazards continue to provide pivotal information for prevention and control. During an influenza pandemic, the laboratory may be critical, at least initially, in documenting the presence of the pandemic strain in a geographic area. With the rapidly increasing sophistication of laboratory methods in environmental health, the laboratory is playing an increasingly important role in field investigations of toxins, such as lead, mercury, pesticides, and volatile organic compounds.

## Individual Case Reports

Because some infectious diseases have high ratios of inapparent-to-apparent disease, a single case should be considered a sentinel health event and should be investigated immediately. A single case of paralytic poliomyelitis or aseptic meningitis commonly represents 100 to 200 other cases of mild-to-subclinical disease elsewhere in the community. One full-blown case of arthropod-borne encephalitis or dengue reflects tens, if not hundreds, of other cases yet unrecognized or unreported. Also, recall the variability of individual response to toxic exposures. A single clinical case of intoxication should alert you to the possibility of unrecognized exposures in the family or in the neighborhood. Similarly, a single case of some chemical or heavy-metal poisoning, such as mercury-induced acrodynia, could be an indication of a potentially widespread risk.

## Epidemic Reporting

Sometimes it is easier, more practical, and more useful to count epidemics rather than single cases of disease. This is particularly true for common diseases that have epidemic potential and for which there is limited public health action that can be taken in response to individual cases; diseases that are poorly reported; and, in some instances, diseases with a wide clinical spectrum. Probably the best example is influenza. One of the time-honored methods of tracking influenza by CDC includes several degrees of involvement, assessed by each state, that describe influenza levels as isolated cases, sporadic outbreaks, outbreaks affecting fewer than one-half of the counties in the state, and outbreaks affecting over one-half of the state's counties. This method is not rigorous science but is extremely useful, nonetheless. Rubella, rubeola, varicella, and dengue can be grossly assessed in this fashion—primarily to inform the public, but also to determine where control or prevention efforts should be directed. In fact, during the successful smallpox eradication program of West Africa in the early 1970s, the field teams stopped counting cases and counted only epidemics, which were defined as one or more cases. Focusing most of the effort on control, much time and effort were saved. The need for epidemic reporting is particularly clear when considering an influenza pandemic on the magnitude of the one that occurred in 1918–1919. Even during the annual influenza season it is not necessary to count every case to determine the status of disease in the population. In a pandemic, surveillance systems will be strained even further by the sheer number of cases as well as the fact that surveillance personnel may themselves be ill or may be reassigned to public health response functions. Under such circumstances, the surveillance parameters will need to be chosen carefully to provide information on aggregate cases, hospitalized patients or those in need of hospitalization, mortality, and so forth. Surveillance data collected will have to be limited to critical elements to avoid overburdening reporters in the medical care system. The surveillance needs and the best surveillance measures in an influenza pandemic are currently the subject of active planning efforts.

## Sentinel Systems

Existing systems of morbidity reporting should be sensitive and specific enough to detect early the appearance of an outbreak. For many reasons, however, not all such systems are that effective. Also, some diseases of public health importance are not reportable conditions. Regardless of the reason for inadequate reporting, there might be times to consider starting a sentinel system—a simple, relatively sensitive way of early detection and monitoring (see Chapter 22).

Again, probably the best example of this kind of surveillance has been that of influenza. Many states do not require that physicians report influenza, so when epidemics are impending and it is considered important to know when they arrive, the state will ask or even pay selected physicians to report influenza cases on a daily basis. In seasonal influenza or in an influenza pandemic, cooperating medical practices can report simply the number of patients with influenza-like-illness (ILI) on a weekly basis. Compared with the baseline number of ILI cases in the particular practice, county or region, and state can provide information on when the epidemic "threshold" has been exceeded. Usually, these kinds of voluntary systems are not statistically valid. Selection is usually based on the willingness of the physician to cooperate and the geographic location, both very practical and compelling criteria. In some countries, because diagnostic capabilities in remote areas barely exist, the sentinel system will merely require reports of "unusual events"; nonetheless, such systems still can be useful. Such systems have the advantages of being low-cost and minimally intrusive on the reporters, while still giving a sense of the impact of disease among the selected populations, which are assumed to be generally representative of the population as a whole.

## Knowledge of Vertebrate and Arthropod Vector Species

In any assessment of zoonotic disease (diseases of animals that also affect humans), you should be aware that an important adjunct to or surrogate for human-disease surveillance is the monitoring of nonhuman vertebrate hosts and species. For example, in many arboviral infections, generally with high inapparent-to-apparent disease ratios among people, humans are incidental or dead-end hosts. Human disease contributes insignificantly to further disease transmission among animals, and human surveillance of these diseases is usually poor or nonexistent, in part because of the high rate of inapparent infections and the specialized laboratory testing needed to diagnose a human case if illness occurs. Eastern equine encephalitis (EEE) is a mosquito-borne viral disease that has a reservoir in birds and infects horses and other vertebrates, including humans, as a dead-end host. A comprehensive surveillance system for EEE involves integrating data from viral culture of captured mosquitoes, regular serologic testing of sentinel flocks of chickens or pheasants kept outdoors, surveillance by veterinarians for EEE-like illness among horses, as well as surveillance of encephalitis cases and deaths among humans. In the 1999 outbreak of West Nile encephalitis, another mosquito-borne viral infection, in New York City, all these surveillance methods were used after the outbreak was recognized. In addition, because this infection resulted in increased mortality of crows and other birds, surveillance of dead birds was very helpful in measuring the geographic extent of the outbreak and in reassuring people in the areas that were not affected.

Similarly, illness among vertebrate or nonvertebrate animals might reflect exposure to environmental toxins or disease-causing agents (e.g., anthrax) before clinical disease appears among human populations. In circumstances where toxic exposures are thought to be increased, regular communication should be established among health officers, the veterinary community, and agencies responsible for monitoring wild and commercial animals as well as insect populations.

## Surveys of Health in General Populations and Special Databases

Although databases containing health or survey information are not frequently used in field investigation settings, several provide baseline or background incidence and prevalence information that might help assess the magnitude of a problem under study. The Behavioral Risk Factor Surveillance System (BRFSS) is a representative telephone survey of health promotion and risk behaviors in the population, which is conducted annually by all states. These data are used to gauge the magnitude and trends of behaviors of public health interest (e.g., smoking) and to measure the impact of public health programs (e.g., programs to reduce sexual activity that places persons at risk for HIV and other sexually transmitted diseases). The survey can be expanded to ask questions of local interest (e.g., insurance coverage for childhood immunizations in New York). BRFSS is used so extensively that some states are now funding county-level versions of BRFSS to provide surveillance data for targeting and evaluating local public health programs.

You can access several other useful databases for surveillance purposes; three are available from CDC. The National Health and Nutrition Examination Survey (NHANES) is a periodic survey that includes clinical examinations and collection of laboratory specimens as well as demographic data and medical histories. NHANES has been conducted three times since 1971 and became an ongoing activity in 1999. The National Health Interview Survey is a continuing survey of about 45,000 civilian households that collects information on illness, disability, health service utilization, and activity restriction.

Before you create a new surveillance system or perform a field study, you should know about several other national surveillance systems with distinctive features that might be useful. The National Cancer Institute funds the Surveillance Epidemiology and End Results (SEER) system, a group of cancer registries in 11 geographic areas of the United States (states and large metropolitan areas) that collects information on cancer, histologic type, site, residence, and relevant demographic information. This information is particularly useful in investigating clusters of cancer in the field. Although the investigation of cancer clusters is often not scientifically fruitful, often it is necessary to address community concerns. The National Electronic Injury Surveillance System (NEISS), sponsored by the Consumer Product Safety Commission (CPSC), is a stratified, random sample of hospital emergency rooms. NEISS collects continuous reports on product-related injuries and has conducted special studies on problems such as fire-related injuries and injuries caused by motor vehicle crashes. In 2000, CPSC and CDC initiated a collaborative effort to include all injuries in the NEISS system. The Fatality Analysis Reporting System (FARS), initiated by the National Highway Traffic Safety Administration (NHTSA), collects information on fatal crashes occurring on public roadways. The National Automotive Sampling System (NASS) is another NHTSA program that includes a random sample of traffic crashes reported by the police in the United States. The Environmental Protection Agency compiles air monitoring data from 51 U.S. areas regarding seven selected air pollutants to monitor compliance with the Clean Air Act. Finally, the National Fire Administration compiles the National Fire Incident Reporting System from local fire departments that report both fire incidents and casualties. These various data sources have been used to combine health event and risk-factor data for surveillance purposes.

Medical school researchers, university hospitals, and voluntary organizations such as the Cystic Fibrosis Foundation collect and maintain incidence and prevalence data on several health conditions that can be sources of valuable information during an investigation in the field.

## Demographic and Environmental Factors

As in all epidemiologic investigations, basic demographic characteristics of the population at risk (i.e., number, age, and sex distribution) are among the many important variables that should be available. Without these data, no rates can be determined. In other words, a denominator must be included to calculate rates of illness or exposure. The U.S. Bureau of the Census is an important source of data from which denominators can be calculated for any analysis of surveillance data (http:\\www.census.gov). These data are collected once every decade, but intercensile estimates are available. In some instances, particularly in developing countries, these data are not readily available, and you must get them yourself during the field investigation. However time-consuming and expensive to acquire, demographic data are indispensable; without them valid comparisons of populations and exposures are impossible.

You might also need to document such characteristics as heat, cold, airflow, humidity, rainfall, and other environmental determinants that predispose to disease or injury during the investigations. Weather data and data concerning air pollutants are available from the U.S. Weather Service for many areas of the country.

## LEGAL CONCERNS

Before establishing any surveillance system—whether it is an emergency system during a field investigation or a process of continued monitoring for months or years to come—you should first be very clear about the legal aspects of such a plan (see Chapter 14). In most instances, surveillance is conducted under the aegis of state health laws passed by state legislatures or regulations developed by health departments or boards of health through an administrative process. So be careful to avoid any activities that violate such requirements.[8] State health commissioners and local health officers are often empowered by these laws and regulations to determine which conditions should be under surveillance and what data may be collected. They are also often empowered to respond to emergency situations with broad powers to collect data and authorize preventive actions. Nongovernmental entities may conduct surveillance, but they should determine the legal basis for such activity and discuss the plan with the appropriate health department before proceeding. In epidemic investigations, the field team is usually given oral approval for setting up emergency surveillance systems, but when long-term programs of surveillance are being considered, it might be necessary to obtain written clearance from the appropriate authorities.

Concerns such as confidentiality and the public's right to know can be in conflict with each other, and you must consider these problems carefully at all steps in the surveillance process. In many cases, health-care providers can be required, by law or regulation, to provide data to a new surveillance system. However, data collection from individual residents is done on a voluntary basis and cannot be compelled. Consent should be obtained at least orally (even in an outbreak setting) to collect data directly from individuals. Any authorization to conduct surveillance should contain strong confidentiality protections, so that data cannot be released in a form that could identify an individual and the data cannot be used for purposes other than the original intent. Similarly, you must recognize who will be affected at each level of surveillance, including individuals in the community such as patients (both in and outside of institutions); physicians, nurses, and others involved in the health-care delivery system; members of the local health department; and, of course, members of your immediate staff. Failure to recognize potential conflicts of interest or lack of acceptability to any of these persons can derail the surveillance process. Policies concerning the release of personal data should be in place for all surveillance data. These policies should specify that individuals cannot be identified without their consent.

## How to Establish a Surveillance System

### Goals

At the beginning, you need to state clearly the purpose of establishing or maintaining a surveillance program. You should know which surveillance data are necessary and how and when they are to be used. A particular surveillance system may have more than one goal, including monitoring the occurrence of fatal and nonfatal disease, evaluating the effect of a public health program, or detecting epidemics for control and prevention activities. These needs might require multiple surveillance systems to monitor a single condition such as data to track morbidity, mortality, laboratory tests, exposures, and risk factors. Regardless of the goal, you must ask (*1*) "What action will be taken?" and (*2*) "What will you or others do with the data and the analyses?" A specific action-oriented commitment is needed.

*Case Study: The West Nile Encephalitis Outbreak.* On August 23, 1999, the communicable disease epidemiologist at the New York City Department of Health (NYCDOH) was contacted by a hospital-based infectious disease physician who had two patients with undiagnosed encephalitis of apparently infectious etiology. In addition to the usual symptoms of encephalitis, one patient had profound muscle weakness, possibly Guillain-Barré syndrome, or less likely, botulism. Viral encephalitis and botulism are reportable conditions in New York State, including New York City, and the legal basis for reporting human cases was the New York State Sanitary Code and New York City Health Code. However, the main reason the physician called was to request assistance in diagnosing botulism and to obtain botulinum antitoxin, if indicated. Because of the unusual nature of the reported illnesses, telephone calls were made by the local health department to several other hospitals in the area, a form of active surveillance (case finding). These calls identified a total of eight patients ill with similar symptoms. Most of the initial patients lived in a two-square-mile area in northeastern New York City.

The initial surveillance goals were to confirm a diagnosis in the initially reported cases and to determine if other cases were occurring. Laboratory specimens were sent via NYCDOH to the New York State public health laboratory and CDC. On September 2, testing revealed evidence of viral encephalitis, first thought to be St. Louis encephalitis, but later determined to be West Nile encephalitis (WNE). WNE is a mosquito-borne viral infection that can be fatal and that had not been seen previously in the Western Hemisphere.

With this initial information, the surveillance goals were expanded to define the geographic extent and time course of the outbreak, to ascertain the populations and areas (including neighboring counties and states) at risk, and to determine the source of the outbreak. This information ultimately led to targeting mosquito-control activities and notifying the public in these areas to avoid mosquito exposure.

Mammal and bird surveillance was initiated in response to reports of a die-off of crows, other birds, and possible disease among horses.

## Personnel

You must know not only who is responsible for overseeing the surveillance activities but also who will be providing the data, collecting and tabulating the data, analyzing and preparing the data for display, and finally, who will be interpreting these data and disseminating them to those who need to know. In the field, you will probably personally know who these persons are; in longer-range systems implemented or orchestrated from some distance, these key persons will probably be names only.

The entire surveillance system in a small area might have only one person doing essentially all these tasks. At the state and national levels, several persons are likely to be involved in the surveillance of specific health events. In an acute outbreak setting, a large number of persons at various professional levels might be involved in starting and conducting the necessary active surveillance. As time progresses and the epidemic becomes better understood, the participants will probably assume a more well-defined role.

*Case Study.* Because of the potential magnitude of the WNE outbreak, a number of public health agencies and public health specialities were involved. The NYC-DOH and the New York State Department of Health worked jointly on surveillance activities, with the state health department coordinating surveillance efforts with neighboring counties and states. The state agriculture department became involved in surveillance for illness among domestic animals. CDC also provided technical assistance on zoonotic and vector surveillance, vector control, and laboratory support. Those with "a need to know" who would use information derived from surveillance included state and city environmental and emergency management agencies as well as political leaders.

## Case Definition

A case definition should be as clear and as simple as possible. Ideally, it should be practical and include quantifiable and, when possible, explicit criteria. Minimal criteria for definition of a case must be made clear and exact, including the essential clinical and laboratory information. During an epidemic investigation, when laboratory data are often unavailable, the case definition is usually broad, sometimes depending only on clinical and epidemiologic criteria. As understanding of the disease process increases, a more refined definition may be used. In this context, you should consider classifying cases by levels of probability (e.g., confirmed case, probable case, or possible case). This method gives you more informative case categories to analyze.

*Case Study.* Early in the expanded surveillance for WNE, clinical and laboratory case definitions for probable and confirmed cases were developed and transmitted by fax to health-care providers in all acute health-care settings. Probable cases had symptoms clinically compatible with encephalitis; confirmed cases required laboratory confirmation. Because public interest was high, many physicians and individuals reported mild, nonspecific illness. To increase the specificity of surveillance, the investigators focused on collection of epidemiologic and laboratory data from patients with the most pronounced symptoms. Clinicians were encouraged to call the health department if they had a suspected case of WNE. In this way, the health department was able to coordinate collection and submission of appropriate clinical specimens for laboratory testing. Positive laboratory tests for WNE were necessary to confirm a case. In addition, laboratory criteria were established for the confirmation of West Nile virus among mammal, bird, and arthropod specimens. After the primary geographic area of the outbreak was defined, surveillance methods were used to determine the impact of control measures in these areas. In addition, suspect cases reported from outside the primary geographic area were prioritized for follow-up to determine if the outbreak was spreading to new areas. After the outbreak was under control, retrospective surveillance of hospital records was conducted in an attempt to determine if a missed "source" case existed (e.g., someone who might have acquired disease through foreign travel).

## The "Human Element" in Surveillance

After you have designed and developed the surveillance system and are prepared to start, consider the human element involved. The system should be acceptable to everyone who plays a part in collection, analysis, dissemination, and use of the data. Be sure to make some personal contact—not only with those who supply the data, but also with those who collect and analyze the data. Successful systems almost always have included personal contact as an essential ingredient. An occasional visit, particularly to persons who provide the data, enhances interest and a sense of purpose; gives faces and names to remember; "humanizes" an otherwise often impersonal activity; gives the participants visibility and recognizes their importance; and makes people glad they belong. In short, all of these ingredients build and support a team, which is absolutely essential in any field investigation. At the beginning, if possible, you should also make contact with potential users of surveillance data to incorporate their needs into the collection, analysis, and dissemination process. From a strict management viewpoint, this means planning for travel costs in the budget.

*Case Study.* During the outbreak of WNE, which had such potential importance and magnitude, the human element in surveillance was critical. From the end of August through September 1999, the NYCDOH assigned staff to maintain regular contact by fax with all hospitals in the city to inform physicians of the current situation, the criteria for diagnosis, the process of specimen submission, and advice on supportive therapy for patients. This communication helped ensure the appropriate diagnosis and reporting of true WNE cases and minimize overdiagnosis. Furthermore, the ability to communicate regularly with other members of the team created a comprehensive and coordinated approach for assessment and control efforts.

Teams for human, mammal, bird, and mosquito surveillance were formed with members from the local, state, and federal levels. Communication within and among these groups was key to successful coordination of surveillance efforts and integration of surveillance data. This communication was achieved by daily, or more frequent, conference calls and e-mail and fax communication. Dissemination of surveillance data was carried out by daily briefings for policy makers and daily press releases for the general public. Three articles in CDC's *Morbidity and Mortality Weekly Report* (*MMWR*) provided authoritative information and interpretation to health-care and public health officials in the region and around the country.

Early in an epidemic investigation, an important part of the human element is to keep an open mind; do not narrow the range of surveillance approaches prematurely. Make certain that you have a solid understanding of the epidemic processes before curtailing particular elements of the surveillance activities.

### Get the System Started

A final element in establishing a surveillance system is the need to get the system going. During an epidemic, this need is obvious. When reports of toxic shock syndrome began to appear in unprecedented numbers in early 1980, it became clear that a surveillance system was essential to assess the magnitude of the epidemic as well as the nature and distribution of cases. The same was true, of course, with AIDS the following year and the eosinophilia–myalgia syndrome ten years later. In any setting, however, try to engender a sense of the health event's importance to stimulate and maintain the team's interest in studying it.

In establishing a long-term or ongoing system, a natural tendency at the start will be to make the system as specific and sensitive as humanly possible. Logical and defensible though this may be, do not let it stand in the way of getting the system off the ground. Many systems have languished for months, even years, because of needless worry over missing or misclassifying a case or two; thus, interest, cooperation, and potential impact were diminished. Get the system moving; get the team energized and committed. You can always refine the system as it progresses. Remember, surveillance is a fluid process: as populations or health problems change, the surveillance system must adapt. If you know this, you will overcome the tendency to wait or postpone starting the system until everything is academically perfect. Finally, because surveillance needs always change, you should also establish some type of ongoing mechanism to monitor and evaluate the surveillance process, including sensitivity and specificity.

*Case Study.* During the WNE outbreak, the need to get the surveillance system up and running efficiently and effectively was obvious to everyone involved. Use of modern electronic and computer technologies such as telephone, fax, and electronic mail enabled surveillance activities to be initiated quickly and to involve almost the entire medical community. A combination of sensitive and specific case definitions was established quickly and modified as needed to ensure comprehensive, yet manageable surveillance. The main participants in the public health system (the NYCDOH, the New York State Department of Health, and CDC) had a long history of collaboration and understood the roles of the various players. However, the ground rules and agreement on the responsibilities for each component of the system still needed ongoing reinforcement. The surveillance systems relied upon during the outbreak were a combination of current, revived, and new systems. Human surveillance for encephalitis in New York City and New York State had been in place for many years, but detection of an event such as WNE highlighted the importance of direct personal connections between state and city health department epidemiologists and practicing physicians. The detection of WNE was an opportunity to reemphasize to the clinical community the importance of reporting clinical syndromes such as encephalitis. This outbreak would not have been recognized by laboratory reporting alone because testing for WNE was not available in New York. However, the role of the New York State and CDC public health laboratories became essential for recognizing and tracking a pathogen not previously known in the western hemisphere.

A combination of local, state, and federal public health laboratory resources is critical for successful surveillance for new and emerging diseases as well as diseases of traditional public health importance. The 1999 WNE outbreak in New York also underscored the importance of mosquito, mammal, and bird surveillance. Surveillance of these species had been done in New York City previously but had been stopped for many years because of an apparent lack of any detected disease.

In the years following the initial outbreak of WNE in the New York City area in 1999, WNE has spread progressively across the country, finally reaching the west coast of the United States in 2005. The lessons learned in setting up the initial surveillance systems in New York were very useful to other states that drew on this experience to establish surveillance systems, in many cases before the advancing disease front arrived. As a result, additional local, state, and federal resources are now being directed to maintain these surveillance activities.[9]

## ANALYSIS AND DISSEMINATION OF SURVEILLANCE DATA

If you are responsible for a surveillance system, be sure to analyze the data appropriately and disseminate them in a timely manner. Programmed data analysis packages are a first step to data analysis, but you should review the results of these analyses and further "customize" the analysis as needed. As with all descriptive epidemiologic data, surveillance information must be analyzed in terms of time, place, and person. Apply simple tabular and graphic techniques for display and analysis (see Chapter 9). More sophisticated methods such as cluster and time-series analyses and computer mapping techniques might be appropriate at some point, but concentrate initially on simple analyses and presentations.

Critical to the usefulness of surveillance systems is the timely dissemination of surveillance data to those who need to know. Publish the data and the analyses together with your interpretation on a regular basis. Whatever format is chosen, be sure to define your audience clearly. The composition of your readers might dictate data collection, interpretation, and the dissemination processes. Distribute the data in a regular and timely manner so that control and prevention measures can be implemented. Because some of those who need to know include policy makers and administrators, people with little epidemiologic knowledge or background, make the reports simple and easy to understand. Finally, in print, recognize those who have contributed to the surveillance effort. People like to see their names in print and people like to belong; it helps justify their role in the prevention process. Recognizing people by name not only gives them credit, but it gives them a degree of responsibility as well.

## Dissemination of Findings During a Field Investigation

In the field setting, particularly in epidemics with large numbers of cases or cases covering large geographic areas, it is often extremely useful to make a surveillance report available daily or semiweekly. The benefits include informing all interested parties; avoiding misinformation and misunderstanding; identifying the players; giving credit to persons who deserve it; identifying who is responsible for what; and creating an extremely useful diary of what was done, why, and what was found. Finally, making a surveillance report available daily or semiweekly is useful for distribution to the media (thus minimizing interviews) and allows them to better inform the public and the medical community. In short, a regular surveillance report serves as an extremely important management and public information tool. Again, however, keep it simple, emphasizing tables, charts, and figures with minimal text. To some degree, let the facts speak for themselves.

## Dissemination of Findings from Ongoing
## Surveillance Systems

Virtually all states and many local health departments publish their own reports at least once per year and disseminate them to health-care providers and other interested parties in their respective locales. CDC also gives information to persons who need to know through the *Morbidity and Mortality Weekly Report* and through the *CDC Surveillance Summaries, MMWR Recommendations and Reports*, the *Summary of Notifiable Diseases*, and special condition-specific reports. All of these publications are available on the Internet at http://www.cdc.gov/mmwr. When personal identifiers are protected appropriately, customized data analyses requested by investigators or the public can be conducted over the Internet. Also, surveillance data are analyzed and published in the medical literature, although the timeliness of these papers might often leave a good deal to be desired.

## ADDITIONAL USES OF SURVEILLANCE DATA

Although we have previously discussed, in general, the purposes of surveillance activities, perhaps it would be useful to outline some additional uses of such systems, particularly those that are long-range.

### Portrayal of Natural History of Disease

Surveillance data are often used to identify or verify perceived trends in health problems. For example, the reported occurrence of malaria in the United States during the previous 50 years has documented the impact of improved diagnosis, importation of cases from foreign wars, and the impact of both increased international travel by U. S. citizens and foreign immigrants (Fig. 3–1).[10] At the local

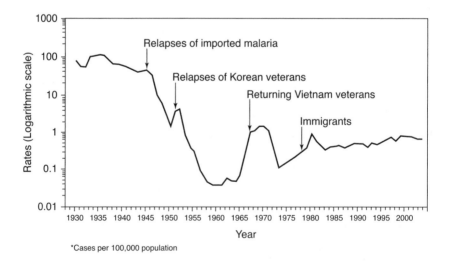

**Figure 3–1.** Rate (cases per 100,000 population) of malaria, by year—United States, 1930–2004. [*Source:* CDC, 2006.]

level (and to a lesser degree the national level), surveillance data are used to detect epidemics that lead to control and prevention activities.

## Test Hypotheses

In the day-to-day monitoring of health problems in a community, you often cannot wait to do special studies. The data that are available must be analyzed. Although the information might not be ideal for analysis, it can often be used to test certain hypotheses. For example, the impact of laws specifying when children enter school in the United States was expected to change the patterns of reported cases of certain diseases by age. Indeed, the peak incidence of measles changed. Before the widespread adoption of these laws in 1980, the peak incidence occurred among children 10 to 14 years of age. Within two years, the peak incidence occurred among children less than five years of age (Fig. 3–2).[11]

## Identify and Evaluate Control Measures

Surveillance data are used to quantify the impact of intervention programs. For example, decreases in poliomyelitis rates occurred following the introduction of both the inactivated and oral polio vaccines (Fig. 3–3).[12] In other examples,

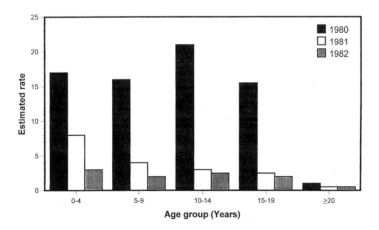

Note: Rates were estimated by extrapolating age from the records of case-patients with known age.

**Figure 3–2.**  Estimated rate (cases per 100,000 population) of measles, by age group—United States, 1980–1982. Rates were estimated by extrapolating age from the records of case-patients. [*Source:* CDC, 1983.]

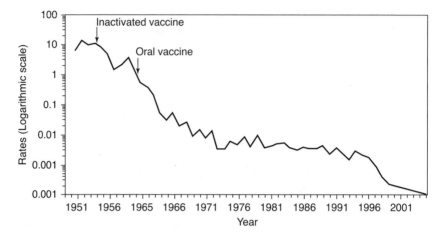

**Figure 3–3.** Rate (reported cases per 100,000 population) of paralytic poliomyelitis—United States, 1951–2004. [*Source:* CDC, 2006.]

broad-based community interventions such as increased legal age of driving and safety-belt laws have had demonstrable effects on mortality.

## Monitor Changes in Infectious Agents

In hospital and health department laboratories, various infectious agents are monitored for changes in bacterial resistance to antibiotics or antigenic composition. The detection of penicillinase-producing *Neisseria gonorrhoeae* in the United States has provided critical information for the proper treatment of gonorrhea (Fig. 3–4).[13] The National Nosocomial Infection Surveillance System monitors the occurrence of hospital-acquired infections, including changes in antibiotic resistance. Another example has been the detection of the continual change in the influenza virus structure, information vital to vaccine formulation.

## Monitor Isolation Activities

The traditional use of surveillance was to quarantine persons infected with or exposed to a particular disease and to monitor their health status. Although this measure is used rarely today, isolation and surveillance are performed on patients with multidrug-resistant tuberculosis and those suspected of having serious, imported diseases such as the hemorrhagic fevers.

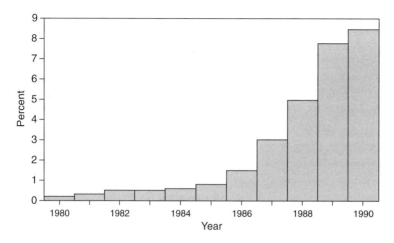

**Figure 3-4.** Percentage of reported cases of gonorrhea caused by antibiotic-resistant strains of *Neisseria gonorrhoeae*—United States, 1980–1990. [*Source:* CDC, 1990.]

## Detect Changes in Health Practices

Surveillance has been used to monitor health practices such as vaccinations, hysterectomy, caesarean delivery, mammography, and tubal sterilization. The surveillance of such practices and health-care technologies has been increasing in public health practice in recent years.[14]

## EVALUATION OF A SURVEILLANCE SYSTEM

This chapter describes the essentials of a surveillance system and how to start and maintain one. It is important to understand the basic levels of evaluation of such systems. They should be evaluated at three levels: (*1*) the public health importance of the health event; (*2*) the usefulness and cost of the surveillance system (e.g., whether it is meeting its goals and at what cost); and (*3*) the explicit attributes of the quality of the surveillance system, including sensitivity, specificity, representativeness, timeliness, simplicity, flexibility, and acceptability.[15, 16]

The decision to establish, maintain, or deemphasize a surveillance system should be guided by assessments based on these criteria. Ultimately, the decision rests on whether a health event under surveillance is a public health priority and whether the surveillance system is useful and cost-effective.

## SUMMARY

Public health surveillance is a basic tool of the field epidemiologist, providing the scientific and factual database essential to informed decision-making and to the conduct of public health prevention and control programs. Surveillance is based on morbidity, mortality, and risk factor data, often from multiple sources. Some data, such as vital statistics, are collected primarily for other uses; other data, such as behavioral risk factors, are collected specifically for the surveillance system.

Surveillance systems are established by the field epidemiologist for specific outcomes, such as a disease or injury, and must have clearly expressed goals. Explicit case definitions are at the core of a surveillance system. The initiation and maintenance of any successful surveillance system will reflect recognition of the human element in surveillance practice: data collection, analysis, and data dissemination. Insensitivity to the persons involved in such a system dooms it to failure.

Surveillance data have many uses but, in general, are needed to assess the health status of a population, to set public health priorities, and to determine appropriate actions. Effective systems of public health surveillance are evaluated regularly on the basis of their usefulness in public health practice.

## REFERENCES

1. Thacker, S.B., Berkelman, R.L. (1988). Public health surveillance in the United States. *Epidemiol Rev* 10, 164–90.
2. Thacker, S.B., Stroup, D.F. (1992). Future directions for comprehensive public health surveillance and health information systems in the United States. *Am J Epidemiol* 140, 383–97.
3. Langmuir, A.D. (1963). The surveillance of communicable diseases of national importance. *N Engl J Med* 268, 182–92.
4. Koo, D., Parrish, R.G., II. (2000). The changing health-care information infrastructure in the United States: opportunities for a new approach to public health surveillance. In S.M. Teutsch, R.E. Churchill (eds.), *Principles and Practice of Public Health Surveillance*, vol. 1, pp. 76–94. Oxford University Press, New York.
5. Centers for Disease Control and Prevention (1997). Case definitions for public health surveillance. *Morb Mortal Wkly Rep* 46, (RR-10) 1–55.
6. Centers for Disease Control and Prevention (2005). Progress in improving state and local disease surveillance—United States, 2000–2005. *Morb Mortal Wkly Rep* 54, 822–5.
7. Bender, J.B., Hedberg, C.W., Besser, J.M., et al. (1997). Surveillance for *Escherichia coli* 0157:H7 infections in Minnesota by molecular subtyping. *N Engl J Med* 337(6), 338–94.
8. Roush, S., Birkhead, G., Koo, D., et al. (1999). Mandatory reporting of diseases and conditions by healthcare professionals and laboratories. *JAMA*, 282, 164–70.

9. Centers for Disease Control and Prevention (2006).Assessing capacity for surveillance, prevention, and control of West Nile virus infection—United States, 1999 and 2004. *Morb Mortal Wkly Rep* 55, 150–3.

10. Centers for Disease Control and Prevention (1999). Summary of notifiable diseases, United States, 1998. *Morb Mortal Wkly Rep* 47, 47.

11. Centers for Disease Control and Prevention (1983). Annual Summary 1983: Reported morbidity and mortality in the United States. *Morb Mortal Wkly Rep* 32, 33.

12. Centers for Disease Control and Prevention (1999). Summary of notifiable diseases, United States, 1998. *Morb Mortal Wkly Rep* 47, 54.

13. Centers for Disease Control and Prevention (1990). Sexually Transmitted Disease Surveillance Morbidity Report.

14. Thacker, S.B., Berkelman, R.L. (1986). Surveillance of medical technologies. *J Public Health Policy* 7, 353–77.

15. Romaguera, R.A., German, R.R., Klaucke, D.N. (2000). Evaluating public health surveillance. In S.M. Teutsch, RE. Churchill (eds.), *Principles and Practice of Public Health Surveillance*, 2nd ed., pp. 176–93. Oxford University Press, New York.

16. Centers for Disease Control and Prevention (2001). Updated guidelines for evaluating public health surveillance systems: recommendations from the guidelines working group. *Morb Mortal Wkly Rep* 50(No. RR-13).

## APPENDIX 3–1 INTERNET SITES FOR THE FIELD EPIDEMIOLOGIST

### DATA SETS

- Behavioral Risk Factor Surveillance System (BRFSS) Available: http://www2.cdc.gov/nccdphp/brfss2/publications/index.asp#search
- National Mortality Follow-back Survey
- Available: http://www.cdc.gov/nchs/about/major/nmfs/nmfs.htm
- National Ambulatory Medical Care Survey (NAMCS)
- Available: http://www.cdc.gov/nchs/about/major/ahcd/ahcd1.htm
- National Hospital Ambulatory Medical Care Survey: 1997 Outpatient Department Summary
- Available: http://www.cdc.gov/nchs/about/major/ahcd/ahcd1.htm
- National Health and Nutrition Examination Survey (NHANES/NCHS)
- Available: http:www.cdc.gov/nchs/nhanes.htm
- National Health Interview Survey (NHIS/NCHS)
- Available: http://www.cdc.gov/nchs/nhis.htm
- National Hospital Discharge Survey
- Available: http://www.cdc.gov/nchs/about/major/hdasd/nhds.htm
- National Nosocomial Infections Surveillance (NNIS)System
- Available: http://www.cdc.gov/ncidod/dhap/nnis/.html

- National Disease and Therapeutic Index (IMS Health) Not Available on the Internet. This item is available for purchase through IMS Health North America
- (http://us.imshealth.com/intersite/default.asp) No price listed.
- National Birth Defects Prevention Network
- Available: http://www.nbdpn.org/
- Surveillance Epidemiology and End Results (SEER) System- National Cancer Institute
- Available: http://seer.cancer.gov/Publications/CSR7393/index.html
- National Electronic Injury Surveillance System (NEISS)—CPSC
- Available: http://www.cpsc.gov/library/neiss.html
- Fatality Analysis Reporting System (FARS)—NHTSA
- Available: http://www.nhtsa.dot.gov/people/ncsa/fars.html
- National Automotive Sampling System—NHTSA
- Available: http://www.nhtsa.dot.gov/people/ncsa/nass_ges.html
- National Fire Incident Reporting System USFA/FEMA
- Available: http://www.nfirs.fema.gov/
- National Weather Service
- Available: http://www.nws.noaa.gov/
- Web-based Injury Statistics Query and Reporting System (WISQARS)
- Available: http://www.cdc.gov/ncipc/osp/data.htm

## INSTITUTIONS AND OTHER ORGANIZATIONS

- Centers for Disease Control and Prevention
- Available: http://www.cdc.gov
- *Morbidity and Mortality Weekly Report (MMWR)*
- Available: http://www.cdc.gov/mmwr/
- Council of State and Territorial Epidemiologists
- Available: http:/www.cste.org
- Bureau of the Census
- Available: http://www.census.gov

# II

# THE FIELD INVESTIGATION

# 4

# OPERATIONAL ASPECTS OF EPIDEMIOLOGIC FIELD INVESTIGATIONS

Richard A. Goodman
James L. Hadler
Duc J. Vugia

An epidemiologic field investigation entails considerably more effort than simply following the recommended, scientifically oriented steps as enumerated and described in Chapter 5. Besides the necessary collection, tabulation, and analyses of the data, there are numerous operational issues that must be addressed. This chapter describes certain critical operational and management principles that apply before, during, and after the field work. These principles encompass the basic steps of: determining whether additional persons from outside the jurisdiction should be invited in; initiating an invitation; evaluating and responding to an invitation; preparing for the investigation through collaboration and consultation; developing and issuing basic administrative instructions prior to departure to the field; and initiating, implementing, and addressing the aftermath of the field investigation. Finally, the chapter concludes with a brief discussion of selected emerging developments in the operational approach to field investigations. The operational considerations addressed in this chapter extend far beyond the scientific work of the investigators. However, if these considerations are not addressed, the field investigation may encounter great difficulty, or may even fail.

This chapter largely addresses work that the *invited* field investigator may have to perform. However, most of the same operational concerns apply to field investigators within a jurisdiction. In addition, it is critical that local and state jurisdiction personnel in positions to call for assistance are able to understand the perspective of those they invite in to assist.

## DETERMINATION OF THE NEED FOR ASSISTANCE

In the United States, the responsibility for public health rests primarily with the state and local agencies. While many investigations may be carried out with local resources, sometimes they require additional assistance. Additional staff and/or expertise may be necessary to fully investigate and respond to complex, large or multijurisdictional problems. When additional help is needed, a process and discussion follow to extend an invitation and define the relative roles of all involved.

## THE INVITATION

An essential consideration is the need to have a formal request for assistance from an official who is authorized to request help. In the United States, usually the state epidemiologist has the authority and responsibility for major epidemiologic field investigations of acute public health problems and for making decisions about whether to investigate independently or to seek help elsewhere. Other persons or organizations may be involved in generating a request, including persons in institutional settings (e.g., nursing homes, hospitals, and businesses), as well as organizational entities with special jurisdiction or authority (e.g., prisons, military facilities, cruise ships, and reservations for Native Americans). For international problems, determining who possesses authority to extend a request may be considerably more complicated and may involve, for example, ministries of health or multinational organizations such as the World Health Organization (see Chapter 21).

The relations between larger and smaller health jurisdictions vary from state to state (or province to province) within countries, as well as from country to country. In general, the larger health jurisdictions help serve the smaller in time of need. Yet the sensitivities between these jurisdictional levels are often delicate, particularly as they relate to perceived competence, local scope of responsibility, and ultimate authority. The health officials of the jurisdiction providing assistance must decide—on the basis of prevailing local–state agreements, as well as their best judgment—what is the most appropriate response.

At the time of the initial request for assistance, the invited field epidemiologists should attempt to determine the answers to three questions.

- First, what is the purpose of the investigation?
  - Is the health department simply requesting more help to perform or complete the investigation?
  - Has the health department been unable to determine the nature or source of the disease or the mode of spread?
  - Does the health department want to share the responsibility of the investigation with others in order to be relieved of political or scientific pressure?
  - When an epidemic is declared or announced by health officials or citizens, is assistance being requested to publicize perceived adverse health conditions, to awaken state or national health leaders, or even to secure funds?
- Second, and clearly related to the first, what specifically is the investigation expected to accomplish? The team may be asked to confirm the findings already collected; collect new or different data for local analysis; or perform an entirely new investigation, including analysis and recommendations.
- Third, can you confirm that the requestor is authorized to invite assistance? Occasionally field studies have been aborted simply because those requesting assistance had no authority to do so, or national teams were investigating without state (or local) permission.

## PRELIMINARY DETERMINATION OF RESPONSIBILITIES

As noted in Chapter 1, there are several reasons why field investigations should be done, if not encouraged. These include, but are not limited to, the need to:

- Control and prevent the occurrence of further disease;
- Provide agreed-upon or statutorily mandated services.
- Increase understanding of the natural history, clinical presentation, and/or epidemiology of the problem under investigation;
- Strengthen surveillance through assessment of its quality; and
- Provide training opportunities in field epidemiology.

During preliminary discussions with the public health official(s) who are requesting assistance with an investigation, the assignment of the following roles and responsibilities should be addressed:

- What resources (including personnel) will be available locally within the jurisdiction requesting assistance?
- What resources will be provided by the visiting team responding to the request?

- Who will direct the day-to-day investigation?
- Who will be the media point person for the investigation team?
- Who will provide overall supervision and ultimately be responsible for the investigation?
- How will the data be shared and who will be responsible for their analysis?
- Will a report of the findings be written? Who will write it, and to whom will it be submitted or circulated?
- If the results of the field investigation warrant publication in a peer-review journal or presentation in another scientific venue, who will be the senior author of the scientific paper?

These are extremely critical issues, some of which cannot be totally resolved before the investigative team arrives on the scene. However, they must be addressed, discussed openly, and agreed upon as soon as possible.

## PREPARATION

### Collaboration and Consultation

Many field investigations require support by a competent laboratory. Even if local laboratories are capable of processing and identifying the nature of specimens, you should immediately, upon being informed of the proposed investigation, contact your counterparts within your support laboratories. The laboratory scientists should be requested to provide any needed guidance and laboratory assistance. Now is the time to obtain assurance of cooperation and commitment rather than during the field investigation or near the end after specimens have already been collected. Not only must the laboratory staff schedule the processing of specimens, they should also be asked to recommend what kinds of specimens should be collected and how they should be collected and processed (see Chapter 24). There also may be substantive basic or applied research questions that could be appropriately addressed and answered during the field investigation. Discuss these issues in detail with these professionals, and make every effort to enlist their interest and support.

Advice on statistical methods also may be sought at this time. The same consideration applies to contacting other health professionals—such as veterinarians, mammalogists, entomologists and vector-control specialists, environmental health specialists, and infection-control practitioners—whose expertise can be crucial to a successful field investigation. Moreover, give consideration to including such professionals on the investigative team. Determine whether they should be part of the initial team so that appropriate data and, particularly, specimens can be collected at the same time as other relevant epidemiologic information. Information specialists can also be extremely important in the overall management of a field investigation (see Chapter 13): because large outbreaks are likely to attract moderate local or regional attention in the media, the presence of an experienced and knowledgeable public information officer (PIO) who can respond to public inquiries and meet the media on a regular basis can be invaluable. In the United States, the inviting local or state health department often has its own PIO who can serve as the media point person for the investigation. Finally, consider including secretarial and/or administrative personnel on the investigating team, both to use their services and to expose them to a real-life situation that will, in turn, enhance their abilities to support future field investigations.

## Basic Administrative Instructions and Notification

Once the field team has been chosen, certain key measures should be taken.

- Identify the team leader and the senior staff to whom s/he should report regularly at the "home base."
- Hold a meeting of all proposed field team members with home-based staff to review known details of the public health problem, the nature of the request for assistance, current knowledge of any suspected pathogen or disease, goals and objectives for the field investigation, and preliminarily agreed-upon roles and responsibilities.
- Try to arrange in advance an initial meeting with the requestor (e.g., the state epidemiologist) or persons either designated or identified by the requestor (e.g., local disease-control director or other official). This will ensure that local authorities are not surprised by an unexpected arrival. In addition, this step underscores for all parties the need for advance planning and orderliness in the investigation—in essence, it sets a tone for the conduct of the investigation.
- Before leaving for the field, a senior member of the team should write a memorandum to the record and/or to relevant key officials. It should summarize how and when the request was made, what information was provided by the requesting health agency, what is the agreed-upon purpose of the investigation, what are the commitments of both the visiting team and the requesting health officials, who is on the field team, and when the latter is expected to arrive in the field. This memorandum should be distributed to key personnel in the offices of the visiting team and the requesting, host agency, and to others who need to know. This kind of communication will serve not only as notification to all concerned, but as a method of preventing redundant responses (i.e., to avoid "crossing wires"). It will also

identify expertise and resources from other programs that may contribute to the investigation. Basic programmatic jurisdictions and interests must also be respected, and some programs and staff simply want to or need to know as a courtesy. Even when a problem does not directly involve a state (for example, as in the case of prison or military facility), a wide array of state and local officials are generally notified because of possible ramifications of the problem for populations in surrounding communities.

- Lastly, before departing for the field, each member of the investigative team should review a basic checklist to ensure they have materials and aids essential for field operations, and have covered fundamental travel and logistical considerations. Such items include, for example, background journal articles, statistical references, laptop computers (already loaded with essential software, such as Epi Info), digital cameras, portable voice recorders, credit cards, and travel and lodging reservations. Finally, each member also should review the need for any necessary personal protective measures, including vaccinations, anti-malarial prophylaxis, antimicrobials or antivirals for post-exposure prophylaxis, and personal protective equipment such as face masks, gloves, and gowns.

## INITIATION OF THE INVESTIGATION

A key concept and philosophy for the field investigation team to keep in mind is the importance of the role of "consultant/collaborator," and what that implies. In general, the guiding principle should be that the team is there to provide help, not simply to "take charge." Equally important is the need to balance the focus of the investigation with the competing priorities in the locality of the requesting jurisdiction. While the immediate problem is the team's sole concern, local health officials must continue to address myriad other priorities and ongoing problems. This dichotomy can be appreciated if the team tries to take the local point of view early in the investigation.

Once on site, the team should meet promptly with the official who requested assistance—usually the state, provincial, or local epidemiologist or a program director. At this meeting, essential steps include the needs to:

- Review and update the status of the problem;
- Identify and review who are the primary contacts;
- Identify a principal collaborator who also can serve as a "guardian angel" during the investigation;
- Identify local resources (e.g., office space, clerical support, assistance for surveys, and laboratory support);

- Create a method and schedule for providing updates to local officials and headquarters;
- Review sensitivities, including potential problems with institutions and individuals (e.g., hospitals, administrators, practitioners, and local public health staff) likely to be encountered during the investigation. Ideally, the team initially should take the time to meet the requesting official—so that key "doors" will be opened—rather than spend valuable time later in the investigation mending bridges.

During the initial meeting between local staff and the visiting team, an appropriate local person should be identified to speak for the entire investigative team. In general, the visiting team should try to avoid direct contact with the news media and should always defer to local health officials (see Chapter 13). The field team is essentially working at the request and under the aegis of the local health officials. Therefore, it is the local officials who not only know and appreciate the local situation but also are the appropriate persons to comment on the investigation. In the most practical sense, the less the media make contact with the visiting team, the more the team can do at its own pace and discretion.

The work required to organize an investigation through this stage (starting travel and convening the initial meeting) is relatively straightforward and uncomplicated. In contrast, however, at least three factors will probably complicate the start of the scientific investigation: (*1*) the effects of a new setting (i.e., visiting team members are outsiders and unfamiliar with the environment); (*2*) the often intense pressure to solve the problem immediately and end the outbreak; and (*3*) the media's queries and other demands for the team's time. Thus, in short order, circumstances may change from tranquility and orderliness to a situation of pressure and confusion. To overcome the myriad potential distractions, team members must maintain the proper perspective by adhering to the basics: focusing the mission to collect data systematically; verifying the diagnosis; and then proceeding through case identification, orientation of data, and development and testing of hypotheses (see chapters 8 and 10). Therefore, at the conclusion of the initial meeting, some team members should try to visit patients to verify the diagnosis through interviews, review of laboratory data, and, if necessary, conducting a physical examination.

## MANAGEMENT

Because of the potential complexity of field investigations, as well as the distracting circumstances under which they are typically conducted, the field team may want to take the following approaches to ensure the systematic and orderly progression of the investigation. First, maintain lists of necessary tasks, check off the actions that have been completed, and update the list at least twice daily. Second, communicate frequently with coworkers, the requesting official, and the person designated to be the media contact; hold a team meeting each day at a regularly scheduled time. The team leader also should communicate with the home base senior staff as frequently as needed. Third, never hesitate to request additional help if required by the circumstances. Fourth, to ensure the investigation will be completed, avoid setting a departure date in advance or succumbing to the pressure of family members to return earlier.

Investigations of large and complex problems may be particularly challenging for field teams and require even more rigorous organization of field operations. The following practical pointers are offered to assist in managing key aspects of the investigation:

- Record the team's decisions as the team makes them—this will help ensure consistency and make the study reproducible, a consideration particularly important in regard to case definitions and why certain criteria were used.
- Remember the need for quality-control measures such as training and monitoring of data collectors and abstractors, conducting error checks and validating data independently, and evaluating non-respondents and missing records.
- Resist collecting more data than are needed (e.g., excessive clinical details).
- Write down the reason the team went to investigate and what was there when the team arrived (i.e., a background section).
- Write while the investigation is ongoing—months later, team members will have forgotten what they did.
- Write the methods while they are being defined and developed by team members—a decision log helps.
- Maintain and retain an inventory of data files.
- Protect the information privacy interests of subjects.
- Because field investigations are difficult, associated with long hours and great stress, field team managers must make a special effort to maintain morale and should find ways to provide encouragement, positive reinforcement, and appreciation to those who participate.

Occasionally, after some time in the field, an investigation does not yield definite results or it identifies additional questions that require one or more investigations to address. At that point, the team leader, in consultation with the home base senior staff, should assess the team's morale and capacity to persevere to determine whether the team should continue its efforts or a fresh team should prepare to come in to extend the investigation.

## DEPARTURE

Upon concluding the on-site field investigation, a departure meeting should be organized to include the requestor, other key officials, and members of the investigation team. In addition to helping to formally conclude the on-site work, the departure meeting enables the team to debrief the requesting official on findings of the investigation, review preliminary recommendations, provide acknowledgments, and express appreciation to local hosts and collaborators. The team should obtain any additional names, titles, and street and e-mail addresses for follow-up communications. If at all possible, the team should leave on site a preliminary report, and at the same time make a commitment to provide a complete written report within an agreed-upon, specified time period.

The departure meeting also may be the most appropriate occasion for planning follow-up activities with the requesting official and organization. Such activities could include additional studies, evaluation of control measures, analysis and maintenance of data collected during the investigation, plans for final reports and manuscripts (including discussion of authorship), and determining who is responsible for each of these different follow-up activities.

## REPORTS

Written summaries of the investigation include both preliminary and final reports. The preliminary report fulfills the immediate obligation to the requesting official and agency. It should include a summary of methods used to conduct the investigation, preliminary epidemiologic and laboratory findings, recommendations, a clear delineation of tasks and activities that must be completed, and appropriate "thank you's." In addition to the preliminary report, which optimally should be delivered to the requestor on departure or from the field within one to two weeks of completion of the investigation, the team should prepare follow-up letters to other principals (e.g., local health officials, co-investigators) to inform them and to reinforce long-term relations.

The final reports should be written as quickly as possible—before team members are called out to another epidemiologic field investigation! The final report should include complete and final data. In addition to a written final report, field investigation team members should consider other methods or forums for communicating the investigation's findings. Options include formal seminars—in person, by teleconference, or by videoconference—where an oral presentation will promote critical feedback; reports for public health bulletins intended for public health practitioners (e.g., CDC's *Morbidity and Mortality Weekly Report*);

comprehensive articles for peer-reviewed journals; and presentations of findings at professional meetings.

## EMERGING DEVELOPMENTS

This chapter has outlined and described operational principles for epidemiologic field investigations. These principles represent a combination of standard management and administrative concepts adapted to the settings and needs of field epidemiology. However, in the closing decades of the 20th century and the beginning of the 21st century, major epidemiologic developments and other events, as well as shifts in societal norms and governmental policies, have had an impact on the operational aspects of field investigations. These emerging developments encompass, but are not limited to, health information privacy, field investigations spanning multiple jurisdictions, investigations of suspected bioterrorism, and use of incident-command system. This chapter concludes by briefly discussing these selected emerging developments.

### Privacy Concerns

Privacy requirements and confidentiality concerns must be adhered to throughout all phases of the field investigation. In addition to federal requirements regarding information privacy (see Chapter 14), each state has its own laws that cover privacy and confidentiality of information obtained during epidemiologic investigations[1]. The stringency of these laws varies by state. The need to adhere to these laws and to respect personal privacy and confidentiality interests also applies when members of the field team write reports and make presentations to groups of people who are not members of the investigation team. Trip reports should be written in a manner that prevents identification of individuals and places that were the subject of or implicated during the field investigation. Once the investigation is complete, all records containing identifying information should be given to the state or local jurisdiction that extended the invitation for management according to the jurisdiction's laws. In addition to protecting the privacy interests of persons who were subjects of the investigation, this approach also minimizes the likelihood that members of the invited field team would possess information that could be subject to subpoena or freedom of information requests that normally would be denied by the state or local jurisdiction.

### Multi-jurisdiction Investigations

As global transport of foods, goods, and humans became rapid and routine, multi-jurisdictional disease outbreaks also have become more frequent.

Contaminated produce from a farm or deli meat from a processing plant can cause a multi-county, multistate, or international food-borne disease outbreak. In the United States, improved surveillance and detection of multi-jurisdictional outbreaks have been facilitated by new tools, such as PulseNet, a national molecular subtyping network,[2] and investigations of multistate food-borne disease outbreaks have become better coordinated across local, state, and federal agencies. The key features of a well-coordinated investigation of a multistate food-borne disease outbreak include rapid communication between local, state, and federal public health officials as soon as possible after recognition of the outbreak, led by a single central group, such as the Foodborne and Diarrheal Diseases Branch at the CDC; participation on regular, weekly teleconference calls to share proposed case definition(s), evolving case counts, laboratory findings, hypotheses, and study instruments; coordination of epidemiologic and laboratory investigations and support, whether provided in the field by some states or centrally by CDC; involvement of food safety regulatory agencies in tracebacks or traceforwards of implicated food(s); and frequent and consistent risk communication to the public and media.[3]

For an acute public health problem involving many jurisdictions, rapid, centralized communication and coordination of field investigations involving key public health officials from all levels is necessary to efficiently define and control the source of the problem. For example, in the multistate outbreak of *E. coli* 0157: H7 infections associated with consumption of fresh spinach in the United States in 2006, CDC held a multistate teleconference within a few days after being alerted by at least two states of small clusters of *E. coli* 0157:H7 infections and CDC PulseNet confirmation of a rare matching PFGE pattern in patients from some of these states.[4] Based on preliminary information shared on this call, the U.S. Food and Drug Administration (FDA) immediately advised consumers to not eat bagged fresh spinach, effectively intervening on the ongoing nationwide outbreak. Days later, parallel laboratory investigations in several states detected the outbreak strain of *E. coli* 0157:H7 in some bagged spinach, and weeks later, two epidemiologic investigations, one led by a state enrolling its own infected residents and the other led centrally by CDC enrolling patients from other states, implicated the same food vehicle.

## Suspected Bioterrorism

Instances of suspected bioterrorism raise a spectrum of general operational and other practical considerations regarding the coordination of concurrent and overlapping investigations involving officials from both public health and law enforcement agencies.[5] A paramount operational consideration involves determining what sector and persons may be in charge of a given site: this is a function of several factors, including the extent to which information and evidence suggest that the site is a "crime scene," as well as the extent to which findings indicate that the site has public health intervention implications in terms of preventing further exposures and identifying and managing persons who may have been exposed prior to the initiation of the investigation.

In addition to the issue of determining who is "in charge" of the site, examples of related and key operational considerations are the approaches to collecting samples from the site of the concurrent investigation and to interviewing persons who may be affected—either with active cases of disease or who may have been exposed—and/or who may be targeted by the criminal investigation as potential suspects. From a public health perspective, the routine epidemiologic investigation may necessitate the collection of biologic specimens from persons (e.g., blood and sputum samples) and environmental samples (e.g., swabs). However, during a concurrent investigation of suspected bioterrorism, when such specimens and samples are being obtained in the setting of a possible crime scene, epidemiology field team members must recognize that physical information-gathering steps taken by law enforcement officials as part of an ongoing criminal investigation must adhere strictly to the process of establishing a "chain of custody of evidence." A key purpose for this process is to ensure that specimens and samples presented as evidence during a criminal prosecution and trial in court can withstand challenge by the defense. The standards required for establishing a chain of custody of evidence for any given sample are rigorous in relation to documenting its precise source, who obtained it, who handled and maintained it, and other factors.

Conducting interviews jointly by public health and law enforcement officials is another example of emerging operational developments that pose new challenges for the epidemiology field team. Under the circumstances of an investigation of suspected bioterrorism or some other problem in which criminal activity may have contributed to the public health problem, epidemiologists and criminal investigators must adhere to procedures that both serve the interests of public health and safety, and respect laws that safeguard the rights of individuals, including persons who are or may become suspects in a criminal investigation. These requirements have prompted some jurisdictions to develop agreements between public health and law enforcement agencies that provide a basis for crafting protocols for joint interviews conducted by representatives of both sectors.[6]

## Incident Command Systems

Finally, whether an acute public health problem is the result of a natural or unintentional occurrence or of suspected bioterrorism, it may be serious enough to involve multiple jurisdictions (i.e., local, state, and federal) and multiple governmental agencies (e.g., emergency medical services [EMS], law enforcement, public health), and may require a standardized, coordinated response encompassing jurisdictions beyond public health. In the United States, the Incident Command System (ICS) is a standardized, on-scene command structure set up to manage incidents across jurisdictional boundaries. ICS allows personnel from various agencies and disciplines to work together in a common management structure with a clear chain of command or unified commands, and provides logistical and administrative support to operational staff. Originally developed in the 1970s to improve management of destructive fires, ICS has been embraced by fire, police, EMS, and military agencies. In recent years, as part of bioterrorism preparedness, public health personnel at local, state, and federal levels have been engaged in emergency preparedness and many are trained in ICS. In addition, ICS increasingly is used at all levels of public health to coordinate responses to large outbreaks or other acute situations with substantial political and public interest.

In the 2001 anthrax attacks in the United States, local, state, and federal public health field investigators worked with investigators from other agencies under ICS set up at state and federal levels "to address the constant emergence of new information, pursue many public health activities simultaneously across multiple investigations, and communicate effectively" while the emergency operations center (EOC) was activated at CDC.[7] On a smaller scale, a local health department in Virginia used ICS to implement a mass tuberculosis-screening program working with community partners and participating agencies to find and test over 2,500 potential contacts of a nurse who died of untreated active tuberculosis.[8] Field investigators should be familiar with both ICS and the EOC, as well as their relationships to the ICS should it be used and to an EOC activated before or during an investigation. In general, use of ICS should simplify the defining of roles for all involved and optimize use of all available resources and expertise across jurisdictions when managing emergency incidents.

ACKNOWLEDGMENTS The authors gratefully acknowledge Michael B. Gregg, Robert A. Gunn, and Jeffrey J. Sacks, whose work on the this chapter in previous editions of this book contributed in part to this chapter.

## REFERENCES

1. Hodge, J.G., Hoffman, R.E., Tress, D.W., et al(2007). Identifiable health information and the public's health: practice, research, and policy. In: R.A. Goodman, R.E. Hoffman, et al. (eds.), *Law in Public Health Practice*, 2nd ed., Oxford University Press, New York. pp. 238–61.
2. Swaminathan, B., Barrett, T.J., Hunter, S.B., et al. (2001). CDC PulseNet Task Force. PulseNet: the molecular subtyping network for foodborne bacterial disease surveillance, United States. *Emerg Infect Dis* 7(3), 382–9.

3. Sobel, J., Griffin, P.M., Slutsker, L., et al. (2002). Investigation of multistate foodborne disease outbreaks. *Public Health Rep* 117, 8–19.
4. CDC (2006). Ongoing multistate outbreak of *Escherichia coli* serotype 0157:H7 infections associated with consumption of fresh spinach—United States, September. *Morb Mortal Wkly Rep* 55, 1045–6.
5. Goodman, R.A., Munson, J.W., Dammers, K., et al. (2003). Forensic epidemiology: law at the intersection of public health and criminal investigations. *J Law Med Ethics* 31, 684–700.
6. CDC (2004). NYC protocol: http://www2a.cdc.gov/phlp/docs/BTProtocolCover.PDF; http://www2a.cdc.gov/phlp/docs/Investigations.PDF.
7. Perkins, B.A., Popovic, T., Yeskey, K. (2002). Public health in the time of bioterrorism. *Emerg Infect Dis* 8, 1015–8.
8. Rendin, R.W., Welch, N.M., Kaplowitz, L.G. (2005). Leveraging bioterrorism preparedness for non-bioterrorism events: a public health example. *Biosecur Bioterror* 3, 309–15.

# 5

# CONDUCTING A FIELD INVESTIGATION

## Michael B. Gregg

This chapter explains how to perform an epidemiologic field investigation. It focuses on a presumed point source (common source) epidemic, recognized and reported by local health authorities to a state (provincial) health department. This is a typical setting that highlights the tasks that you need to perform. Although the context is one of an acute infectious disease epidemic in a community, the epidemiologic and public health principles apply equally well to noninfectious disease investigations.

## BACKGROUND CONSIDERATIONS

### Overall Purposes and Methods

Some purposes of epidemiology include determining the cause(s) of a disease, its source, its mode of transmission, who is at risk of developing the disease, and what exposure(s) predispose to the disease. Fortunately, in many outbreak investigations the clinical syndromes are easily identifiable; the agents can be readily isolated and characterized; and the source, mode of transmission, and risk factors of the disease are usually well known and understood. Therefore, you are often well prepared for the field investigation. However, when the clinical diagnosis and/or laboratory findings are unclear, the task becomes much more difficult. It requires more careful consideration of the clinical presentation of disease in an effort to determine the source, mode of spread, and population(s) at risk. For example, bacterial contamination of food or water is usually manifested by signs and symptoms referable to the gastrointestinal tract. Pathogenic agents transmitted in air often affect the respiratory tract and sometimes the skin, eyes, or mucous membranes. Skin abrasions or lesions may suggest animal or insect transmission. So the clinical manifestations of disease may serve as critical leads.

Regardless of how secure the clinical diagnosis may be, your thought process must include clinical, laboratory, and epidemiologic evidence. Together these provide leads and pathways to take or reject to discover the natural history of the epidemic.

Although you will perform several separate operations, in broad strokes you will really do two things. First, you will collect information that describes the setting of the outbreak; namely, when people became sick, where they acquired disease, and what the characteristics of the ill people were. These are the descriptive aspects of the investigation. Often, simply by knowing these facts (and the diagnosis), you can determine the source and mode of spread of the agent and can identify those primarily at risk of developing disease. Common sense will often give you these answers, and relatively little, if any, further analysis is required.

On occasion, however, it will not be readily apparent where the agent resided, how it was transmitted, who was at risk of disease, and what the exposure was. Under these circumstances, you will have to use a second operation, analytic epidemiology, to provide the answers. And the critical operations here include determining rates and comparing these rates. Virtually all epidemiologic analyses require comparisons, usually groups of persons—ill and well or exposed and not exposed (see Chapter 8). In epidemic situations you will usually compare ill and well people—both believed at risk of disease—to determine what exposures ill people had that well people did not have. These comparisons are made by using appropriate statistical techniques (see Chapters 8 and 10). If the differences between ill and well persons are greater than one would expect by chance, you can draw certain inferences about why the epidemic occurred. In some situations, comparisons can be made between exposed persons and those not exposed to see if there are significant differences in rates of illness between the two groups.

## The Pace and Commitment of a Field Investigation

An underlying theme throughout this chapter is the need to act quickly, establish clear operational priorities, and perform the investigation responsibly. This should not imply haphazard collection and inappropriate analysis of data, but rather the use of simple and workable case definitions, case-finding methods, and analyses (see Chapters 4 and 11).

Data collection, analyses, and recommendations should be performed in the field. There is a strong tendency to collect what you think is the essential information in the field and then retreat to "home base" for analysis—particularly now with the availability of personal computers. Avoid this reflex at all costs. Such action will probably be viewed as lack of interest or concern or even possessiveness by the local constituency. A premature departure also makes any further collection of data or direct contact with study populations and local health officials difficult, if not impossible. Once home, you lose the urgency and momentum to perform, the sense of relevancy of the epidemic, and, most of all, the totally committed time for the investigation. Every field investigation should be completed, not only to the field team's satisfaction, but particularly to that of the local health department as well.

## THE INVESTIGATION

### Introduction

Ten basic tasks will be described in a logical order (Table 5–1). However, you may perform several of these functions simultaneously or in different order during the investigation. Control and prevention measures may even be recommended soon after beginning the investigation simply on the basis of intuitive reasoning or

**Table 5-1.**   The Ten Steps of a Field Investigation

1.  Determine the existence of the epidemic

2.  Confirm the diagnosis

3.  Define a case and count cases

4.  Orient the data in terms of time, place, and person

5.  Determine who is at risk of becoming ill

6.  Develop a hypothesis that explains the specific exposure that caused disease and test this hypothesis by appropriate statistical methods

7.  Compare the hypothesis with the established facts

8.  Plan a more systematic study

9.  Prepare a written report

10. Execute control and prevention measures

common sense. Sometimes the local officials know why the epidemic occurred, and you are there simply to supply a scientific basis for their conclusion.

No two epidemiologists will take the exact same pathway of investigation. Yet, in general, the data they collect, the analyses they apply, and the control and prevention measures they recommend are likely to be similar.

Since, by definition, our example epidemic has resulted from a point source and may be nearly over before the field team arrives, the investigation will in all likelihood be retrospective in nature. This should alert you to some fundamental aspects of any investigation that occurs "after the fact." First of all, because many illnesses and critical events have already occurred, virtually all information acquired and related to the epidemic will be based upon memory. Health officers, physicians, and patients will probably have different recollections, views, or perceptions of what transpired. Information may conflict, may not be accurate, and certainly cannot be expected to reflect the precise occurrence of past events. Like the clinician, you may have to ask patients what they think made them sick, what they think caused the epidemic. Most critically, in parallel with medical practice, action may have to be taken without the benefit of all the desired data (see Chapter 11).

For the young, inexperienced medical epidemiologist steeped in the tradition of molecule and millimole determinations, the "more-or-less" measurements of the field epidemiologist can initially be major hurdles to a successful field investigation. However lacking in accuracy these data may be, they are often the only data you have; and they must be collected, analyzed, and interpreted with care, imagination, and caution. Furthermore, you have not seen the epidemiologic method work in real life. Unlike clinical medicine when in a matter of minutes to a few hours the physical examination usually reinforces the history, and the laboratory results usually reinforce both, there often is no immediate reinforcement of the thought processes and activities in the field. It usually takes several days or a week before data start coming in that begin to reassure you that you are on the right track.

## Determine the Existence of an Epidemic

Local health officials usually will know if more disease is occurring than would normally be expected. Since most local health departments have ongoing records of communicable diseases and certain noninfectious conditions, by comparing weekly, monthly, or yearly data, you can easily determine if the observed numbers exceed the expected level. Although there may not be laboratory confirmation at this time, an increase in reported cases by local physicians is enough evidence to investigate. However, at this time avoid the use of the terms "epidemic" or "outbreak." These words are quite subjective. Local health officials take different views of the normal rise and fall in cases, and whether changes in the pattern merit investigation.

You must be aware of artifactual causes of increases or decreases in reported cases such as changes in local reporting practices, increased interest in certain diseases because of local or national awareness, a new physician or clinic in town, or changes in diagnostic methods. An excellent example of artifactual reporting occurred in southwest Florida in 1977 when a new physician in the community reported many cases of encephalitis in his practice. After extensive field work by local, state, and federal epidemiologists, it was clear there was no epidemic, but simply misdiagnoses by the physician.[1]

Sometimes, however, it may be difficult to document the existence of an epidemic rapidly. You may need to acquire absentee records from schools or factories, records of outpatient clinic visits or hospitalizations, laboratory records, or death certificates. A simple telephone survey of practicing physicians will strongly support the existence of an epidemic, as would a similar rapid survey of households in the community. In such quick assessments, you could ask about signs and symptoms rather than about specific diagnoses. Ask physicians or clinics if they are treating more people than usual with sore throats, gastroenteritis, or fever with rash, as examples, in order to obtain an index of disease incidence. Although not specific for any given disease, such surveys can often establish the existence of an epidemic. Sometimes it is extremely difficult to determine if there is an epidemic. Yet because of local pressures, the team may have to continue the investigation even if they believe no significant health problem exists.

## Confirm the Diagnosis

Confirm the clinical diagnosis by standard laboratory techniques such as serology and/or isolation and characterization of the agent. Do not try to use newly introduced, experimental, or otherwise not broadly recognized confirmatory tests—at least not at this stage in the investigation. If at all possible, visit the laboratory and verify the laboratory findings in person. For example, talk to the technician, check the record books, and look at the gram stain yourself.

Not every reported case has to be confirmed in the laboratory. If most patients have signs and symptoms compatible with the working diagnosis, and, perhaps, 15% to 20% are laboratory-confirmed, you do not need more confirmation at this time. This usually is ample confirmatory evidence. See and examine several representative cases of the disease as well, if at all possible. Clinical assumptions should not be made; the diagnosis should be verified by you or a qualified physician with you. Nothing convinces supervisors and health officers more than an eyewitness confirmation of clinical disease by you and the investigating team.

## Define a Case and Count Cases

Now try to create a workable case definition, decide how to find cases, and count them. The simplest and most objective criteria for a case definition are usually the best (e.g., fever, X-ray evidence of pneumonia, white blood cells in the spinal fluid, number of bowel movements per day, blood in the stool, or skin rash). However, be guided by the accepted, usual presentation of the disease with or without standard laboratory confirmation in the case definition. Where time may be a critical factor in a rapidly unfolding field investigation, use a simple, easily applicable definition—recognizing that some cases will be missed and some non-cases included. For example, in an epidemic of hepatitis A, a history of jaundice, fever, and an abnormal liver enzyme test should be quite adequate to start with. Later you can refine the definition.

Some factors that can help determine the levels of sensitivity and specificity of the case definition are the following:

- What is the usual apparent-to-inapparent clinical case ratio?
- What are the important and obvious pathognomonic or strongly clinically suggestive signs and symptoms of the disease?
- What microbiologic or chemical isolations, identification, and serologic techniques are easy, practical, and reliable?
- How accessible are the patients or those at risk; can they be contacted again after the initial investigation for follow-up questions, examination, or serology?
- In the event that the investigation requires long-term follow-up, can the case definitions be applied easily and consistently by others not on the current investigating team?
- Is it absolutely necessary that all patients be identified during the initial investigation or would only those seen by physicians or hospitalized suffice?

No matter what criteria are used, you must apply the case definition equally and without bias to all persons under investigation.

Methods for case finding will vary considerably according to the disease in question and the community setting. Most outbreaks involve certain clearly identifiable groups at risk; therefore, finding cases will be relatively self-evident and easy. Active, direct contact with selected physicians, hospitals, laboratories, schools, or industries or by using some form of public announcement will find most of the remaining, unreported cases. However, sometimes more intensive efforts—such as physician, telephone, door-to-door, or culture or serologic surveys—may be necessary to find cases. Regardless of the method, you must establish some system(s) of case finding during the investigation and perhaps afterwards (see Chapter 3).

Simply knowing the number of cases does not provide adequate information. Control and prevention measures depend upon knowing the source and mode of spread of an agent as well as the characteristics of ill patients. Therefore, case finding should include collecting pertinent information likely to provide clues or leads to the natural history of the epidemic and, particularly, relevant characteristics of the ill. First, collect basic information about each patient's age, gender, residence, occupation, and date of onset, for example, to define the basic descriptive aspects of the epidemic. Next, get pertinent signs, symptoms, and laboratory data. If the disease under investigation is usually water- or food-borne, ask questions about exposure to various water and food sources; if transmitted by person-to-person contact, ask about the frequency, duration, and nature of personal contacts. If the nature of the disease is not known or cannot be comfortably presumed, you will need to ask a variety of questions covering all possible aspects of disease transmission and risk. Also be mentally prepared for the possibility of having to apply a second questionnaire if the first analysis does not help.

## Orient the Data in Terms of Time, Place, and Person

Now the team should have a reasonably accurate number of cases to view descriptively. So it is time to characterize the epidemic in terms of when patients became ill, where they lived or became ill, and what special attributes the patients had (see Chapter 9 for greater detail). You may want to wait until the epidemic is over or until all likely cases have been reported before performing such an analysis. Don't. The earlier you develop ideas of why the epidemic started, the more pertinent data you can collect. The addition of a proportionately small number of cases later on will usually not affect the analysis or recommendations.

### Time

Characterize the cases by plotting a graph that shows the number of cases (y axis) over the time of onset of illness using an appropriate time interval (x axis) (Fig. 5–1). This "epidemic curve" gives a considerably deep appreciation for the magnitude of the outbreak, its possible mode of spread, and the possible duration of the epidemic—much more than would a simple "line-listing" of cases. One can often infer a remarkable amount of information from a simple picture of times of onset of disease. If the incubation period of the disease is known, relatively firm inferences can be made regarding the likelihood of a point source exposure, person-to-person spread, or a mixture of the two. And just the opposite: if you know when the exposure occurred, you may be able to determine the incubation period. This is particularly important if you do not know what the disease is. Also, if the epidemic is still in progress and you have a good idea of the disease,

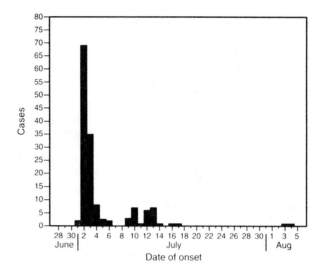

**Figure 5-1.** Cases of Pontiac fever, by date of onset—Michigan, June 28–August 5, 1968. [*Source:* Glick et al., 1978.[2]]

you may be able to predict how many more cases are likely to occur. Finally, an epidemic curve provides an excellent "prop" for ready communication to nonepidemiologists, administrators, and the like who need to grasp in some fashion the nature and magnitude of the epidemic.

The epidemic curve in Figure 5–1 shows cases of Pontiac fever (subsequently confirmed as Legionnaires' disease) that occurred in Pontiac, Michigan, July and August 1968, by day of onset.[2] The epidemic was explosive in onset, suggesting (*1*) a virtually simultaneous point-source exposure of many persons; (*2*) a disease with a short incubation period because of the very tight clustering of cases over a very narrow time frame); and (*3*) a continuing exposure spanning several weeks—all of which were subsequently confirmed.

### Place

Sometimes diseases occur or are acquired in unique locations in the community, which, if you can visualize, may provide major clues or evidence regarding the source of the agent and/or the nature of exposure. Water supplies, milk distribution routes, sewage disposal outflows, prevailing wind currents, air-flow patterns in buildings, and ecological habitats of vectors may play important roles in disseminating microbial or environmental pathogens and determining who is at risk of acquiring disease. If one plots cases geographically, a distribution pattern may appear that approximates these known sources and routes of potential exposure. This, in turn, may help identify the vehicle or mode of transmission.

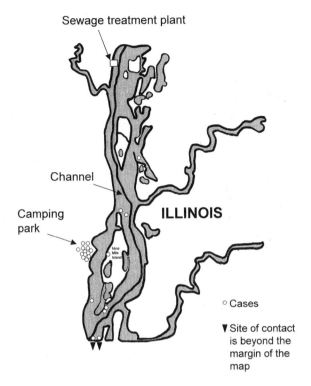

**Figure 5–2.**  Culture-positive cases of Shigella, by sites along the Mississippi River where each case swam within three days of onset of illness. [*Source:* Rosenberg et al., 1976.³]

Figure 5–2 illustrates the usefulness of a "spot map" in the investigation of an outbreak of shigellosis in Dubuque, Iowa, in 1974.³ Early analysis showed that cases were not clustered by place of residence. A history of drinking water gave no useful clue to a possible source and mode of transmission. However, it was later learned that many cases had been exposed to water by recent swimming in a camping park located on the Mississippi River. Figure 5–2 shows the river sites where 22 culture-positive cases swam within three days of onset of illness, strongly suggesting a common source of exposure. Ultimately, the epidemiologists incriminated Mississippi River water by documenting gross contamination by the city's sewage treatment plant five miles upstream and by isolating *Shigella sonnei* from a sample of river water taken from the camping park beach area.

## Person

Lastly, you must examine the characteristics of the patients themselves in terms of a variety of attributes, such as age, gender, race, occupation, or virtually any other characteristic that may be useful in portraying the uniqueness of the case population. If a singular or special attribute emerges, this frequently suggests a strong lead as to the group at risk and even an idea of the specific exposure. Some diseases primarily affect certain age groups or races; frequently, occupation is the key attribute of people with certain diseases. The list of human characteristics—really potential risks and exposures—is nearly endless. However, the more you know about the disease in question (the agent's reservoir, mode(s) of spread, persons usually at greatest risk), the more specific and pertinent information you should seek to determine whether any of these risks or exposures predispose to illness.

## Determine Who Is at Risk of Becoming Ill

You now know the number of ill people, when and where they were when they became ill, what their general characteristics are, and, usually, have a firm diagnosis or a good "working" diagnosis. These data frequently provide enough information to determine with reasonable assurance how and why the epidemic started. For example, a time, place, and person description of the epidemic will strongly suggest that only people in a particular community supplied by a specific water system were at risk of getting sick, or that only certain students in a school or workers in a single factory became ill. Perhaps it was only a group of people who attended a local restaurant who reported illness. However, no matter how obvious it might appear that only a single group of persons was at risk, one should look carefully at the entire community to be sure there are not other affected persons.

Sometimes it is very difficult to know who is at risk, particularly in epidemics that cover large geographic areas and involve many age groups with initially no obvious unique characteristics. Under these circumstances the team may have to do a survey of some kind to get more specific information about the ill persons and some idea of who is at risk.

## Develop a Hypothesis That Explains the Specific Exposure That Caused Disease and Test This Hypothesis by Appropriate Statistical Methods

This next step, the first real epidemiologic analysis of the field investigation, is often the most difficult one to perform. By now you should have an excellent grasp of the epidemic and an overall feel for the most likely source and mode of transmission. However, the exposure that caused disease must be determined.

A simple example was the 1989 investigation of an epidemic of nausea, vomiting, and diarrhea among 20 people who ate at a single pizzeria in McKeesport, Pennsylvania.[4] Since the disease was most likely acquired by eating something (because of the signs and symptoms) and because no other cluster of similar disease had occurred elsewhere in the community, the epidemiologists focused attention only on those who bought food from the pizzeria. The logical hypothesis then was that the exposure necessary to develop nausea, vomiting, and diarrhea was consumption of some food(s) contaminated with a microbial or chemical agent. Therefore, those who bought and ate food from the pizzeria on the presumed day of exposure were given a questionnaire asking what beverages and kinds of foods and pizza they had eaten; that is, what foods had they been exposed to. Early analysis showed that 100% of the ill persons (cases) had eaten mushrooms on pizza. Because so many ill people had eaten these pizzas, one might quickly assume it was the contaminated food. Yet the 100% simply represents how popular the mushroom pizza was among the ill attendees. Alone, the 100% does not give adequate valid support to the hypothesis that exposure to the pizza (i.e., eating the mushroom-topped pizza) caused illness. What had to be done was to determine the food histories of the well pizza eaters (controls) and compare their histories to the ill persons. When this comparison was done, the food histories were very similar between the two groups except for one food, the mushroom pizzas: only 33% of the well attendees ate the mushroom-topped pizza. The hypothesis, then, was that the difference in exposure rates—100% among the ill and 33% among the well—was because the mushroom pizza was contaminated. When these rates were tested statistically, it showed that, assuming that eating the particular pizza had no relation to getting ill, such a difference would occur less than one time in 10,000 such instances. Therefore, the statistical evidence as well as other information (isolation of *S. aureus* from cans of mushrooms) supported the hypothesis that eating the mushroom pizza was the exposure that caused the outbreak.

Again, this phase of the investigation clearly will pose the greatest challenge. Field epidemiologists must review the findings carefully; weigh the clinical, laboratory, and epidemiologic features of the disease; and hypothesize possible exposures that could plausibly cause disease. In other words, you must seek from the patients' histories exposures that could conceivably predispose them to illness. If exposure histories for ill and well are not significantly different, a new hypothesis must be developed. This will require imagination, perseverance, and sometimes resurveying those at risk to obtain more pertinent information.

## Compare the Hypothesis with the Established Facts

At this time in the investigation, epidemiologic and statistical inferences have provided the most probable exposure responsible for the epidemic. Yet you must "square" the hypothesis with the clinical, laboratory, and other epidemiologic facts of the investigation. In other words, do the proposed exposure, mode of spread, and population affected fit well with the known facts of the disease? For example, if, in the gastroenteritis outbreak referred to above, the analysis incriminated a food of high protein and low acid content that supports growth of staphylococcal organisms and production of enterotoxin (as is the case with mushrooms), the hypothesis fits well with our understanding of staphylococcal food poisoning. However, if the analysis incriminated coffee or water—highly unlikely sources of staphylococcal enterotoxin—you must then reassess the findings, perhaps secure more information, reconsider the clinical diagnosis, and certainly pose and test new hypotheses. Unfortunately, on rare occasions this reassessment is necessary, and you should be prepared.

The following investigations illustrate the uses of simple descriptive and analytic epidemiology, how some analyses may not prove helpful, how posing new hypotheses may be necessary, how the facts must fit logically, and how important persistence is in arriving at a defensible conclusion.

Thirty-four cases of perinatal listeriosis and seven cases of adult disease occurred between March 1 and September 1, 1981, in several maritime provinces of Canada.[5] These cases represented a manifold increase over the number of cases diagnosed in previous years, suggesting some common exposure. Although *L. monocytogenes* is a common cause of abortion and nervous system disease in cattle, sheep, and goats, the source of human infection has been obscure. Cases could not be linked together by person-to-person contact; they shared no common water source; and food exposures, as determined from a general food history, were not different between cases and controls. However, a second, more detailed food history and subsequent intensive interrogation of cases and controls revealed that there was a statistically significant difference between cases and controls regarding exposure to coleslaw. Even though this food had never been previously incriminated as a source of listeria, it was the only food item positively associated with disease and essentially the only lead the investigators had at the time. Armed with this clue, the team subsequently found a specimen of coleslaw in the refrigerator of one of the patients that grew out the same serotype of listeria isolated from the epidemic cases. No other food items in the refrigerator were positive for listeria.

The coleslaw had been prepared by a regional manufacturer who had obtained cabbages and carrots from several wholesale dealers and many local farmers. Although environmental cultures from the coleslaw plant failed to reveal listeria organisms, two unopened packages of coleslaw from the plant subsequently grew *L. monocytogenes* of the same epidemic serotype. A review of the sources of the vegetable ingredients was made, and a single farmer was identified who had grown cabbages and also maintained a flock of sheep. Two of his sheep had previously died of listeriosis in 1979 and 1981. Also, he was in the habit of using sheep manure to fertilize his cabbage.

This information does not prove this farm was the source of the listeria organisms that caused the epidemic. However, the hypothesis that coleslaw was the source and the statistical test that supported this hypothesis provided the necessary impetus to continue the investigation. And, ultimately, a single, highly likely source of the bacteria was discovered. These findings strongly suggest listeriosis is a zoonotic infection transmitted from infected animals via contaminated vegetables to humans.

In January and February 1980, an epidemic of 85 cases of salmonellosis in Ohio prompted an extensive field investigation by Taylor et al.[6] All cases were caused by an uncommon serotype of salmonella, S. muenchen. This finding plus the fact that all cases were among teenagers and young adults strongly suggested a common source of exposure. Knowing that the natural reservoirs for almost all serotypes are poultry, chicken eggs, and other domestic farm animals and that the majority of salmonella epidemics can be traced to eating meat or poultry products or having contact with these animals, Taylor and colleagues questioned the cases and appropriate controls. Their questions included food histories and contact with farm animals. Not too surprisingly, the investigators found that significantly more cases than controls gave a history of eating ham. On the surface this evidence strongly incriminated ham as the vehicle of infection. However, in trying to define the source of the contaminated ham, Taylor learned that the ham eaten by the patients came from five different distributors. How likely is it that one uncommon serotype would come from five different distributors who, in turn, secured their ham from different producers? The logic was overwhelming: despite a reasonable food source of the salmonella and persuasive statistics, the ham was not the source of the salmonella, and more questioning had to be done.

At this same time, another, identical, epidemic of salmonella was reported in Michigan. Having more cases to work with and focusing on possible unique characteristics of the teenage/young adult population, the team asked many more questions of cases and controls, including questions about the use of drugs. To their great surprise, they found a highly significant association between illness and smoking marijuana. Although this association seemed as implausible as that with ham, samples of marijuana smoked by the cases were culture positive for S. muenchen, strongly incriminating the marijuana as the vehicle of infection.

## Plan a More Systematic Study

The actual field investigation and analyses have now been completed, requiring only a written report (see below). However, because there may be a need to find more cases, to define better the extent of the epidemic, or to evaluate a new laboratory method or case-finding technique, you may want to perform more detailed and carefully executed studies. With the pressure of the investigation somewhat removed, consider surveying the population at risk in a variety of ways to help improve the quality of data and answer particular questions.

Perhaps the most important reasons to perform such studies are to improve the sensitivity and specificity of the case definition and establish more accurately the true number of persons at risk; that is, to improve the quality of numerators and denominators. For example, serosurveys coupled with a more complete clinical history can often sharpen the accuracy of the case count and define more clearly those truly at risk of developing disease. Moreover, repeated interviews of patients with confirmed disease may allow for rough quantification of degrees of exposure or dose responses—useful information in understanding the pathogenesis of certain diseases.

## Prepare a Written Report

Frequently, your final responsibility is to prepare a written report to document the investigation, the findings, and the recommendations (see Chapter 12). There are several important reasons why a report should be written and written as soon as possible:

### A Document for Action

Sometimes control and prevention efforts will only be taken when a report of all relevant findings has been written. This can and should place a heavy, but necessary, burden on the field team to complete its work quickly. Even if all possible cases have not yet been found or some laboratory results are still pending, reasonable written assumptions and recommendations can usually be made without fear of retraction or subsequent major change.

### A Record of Performance

In this day of input and output measurements, program planning, program justifications, and performance evaluations, there is often no better record of accomplishment than a well-written report of a completed field investigation. The number of investigations performed and the time and resources expended not only document the magnitude of health problems, changes in disease trends, and the results of control and prevention efforts, but also serve as concrete evidence of program justification and needs.

### A Document for Potential Medical/Legal Issues

Presumably, epidemiologists investigate epidemics with objective, unbiased, and scientific purposes and similarly prepare written reports of their findings and conclusions objectively, honestly, and fairly. Such information may prove absolutely invaluable to consumers, practicing physicians, or local and state health department officials in any legal action regarding health responsibilities and jurisdictions (see Chapter 14). In the long run, the health of the public is best served by simple, careful, honest documentation of events and findings made available to all for interpretation and comment.

## Enhancement of the Quality of the Investigation

Although not fully understood and rarely referred to, the actual process of writing and viewing data in written form often generates new and different thought processes and associations in one's mind (see Chapter 12). The discipline of committing to paper the clinical, laboratory, and epidemiologic findings of an epidemic investigation almost always will bring to light a better understanding of the natural unfolding of events and their importance in terms of the natural history and development of the epidemic. The actual process of creating scientific prose, summarizing data, and creating tables and figures representing the known established facts forces you to view the entire series of events in a balanced, rational, and explainable way. This process is considerably more demanding than preparing an oral report to give to the local health department the day of departure from the field. Occasionally, previously unrecognized associations will emerge from a careful, step-by-step written analysis that may be critically important in the final interpretation and recommendations. The exercise of writing what was done and what was found will sometimes uncover facts and events that were more or less assumed to be true, but not specifically sought for during the investigation. This, in turn, may stimulate further inquiry and fact finding in order to verify these assumptions.

## An Instrument for Teaching Epidemiology

There would hardly be disagreement among epidemiologists that the exercise of writing the results of an investigation constitutes an essential building block in learning epidemiology. Much the way a lawyer prepares a brief, the epidemiologist should know how to organize and present in logical sequence the important and pertinent findings of an investigation, their quality and validity, and the scientific inferences that can be made by their written presentation. The simple, direct, and orderly array of facts and inferences will not only reflect the quality of the investigation itself but also the writer's basic understanding and knowledge of the epidemiologic method.

## Execute Control and Prevention Measures

It is not the purpose of this chapter to discuss this aspect of a field investigation. Nevertheless, the underlying purposes of all epidemic investigations are to control and/or prevent further disease.

## SUMMARY

The field investigation is a direct application of the epidemiologic method, very often with an implied and relatively circumscribed timetable. This forces field epidemiologists to: (*1*) establish workable case finding techniques; (*2*) collect data rapidly but carefully; and (*3*) describe cases in a general sense regarding the time and place of occurrence and those primarily affected. Usually, you will know the agent and its sources and modes of transmission, which will allow you to identify the source and mode of spread rapidly. However, when the clinical disease is obscure and/or the origin of the agent ill-defined, you may be hard-pressed to create a hypothesis that will not only identify the critical exposure and show statistical significance but will also logically explain the occurrence of the epidemic. Although you will not be able to prove, scientifically, causation in the strictest sense, in most instances the careful development of epidemiologic inferences, coupled with persuasive clinical and laboratory data, will almost always provide convincing evidence as to why the epidemic occurred. Lastly, a written report sharpens your communication and epidemiologic skills and provides the health community with permanent documentation of the investigation.

## REFERENCES

1. Centers for Disease Control and Prevention (1977). Unpublished data.
2. Glick, T.H., Gregg, M.B., Berman, B., et al. (1978). Pontiac fever. An epidemic of unknown etiology in a health department. I. Clinical and epidemiological aspects. *Am J Epidemiol* 107, 149–60.
3. Rosenberg, M.D., Hazlet, K.K., Schaefer, J., et al. (1976). Shigellosis from swimming. *JAMA* 236, 1849–52.
4. Centers for Disease Control (1989). Multiple outbreaks of staphylococcal food poisoning caused by canned mushrooms. *MMWR* 38, 417–18.
5. Schlech, W.F. III, Lavigne, P.M., Bortobussi, R.A., et al. (1983). Epidemic listeriosis—evidence for transmission by food. *N Engl J Med* 308, 203–6.
6. Taylor, D.N., Wachsmith, K., Shangkuan, Y., et al. (1982). Salmonellosis associated marijuana. A multistate outbreak traced by plasmid fingerprinting. *N Engl J Med* 306, 1249–53.

# 6

# SURVEYS AND SAMPLING

Joan M. Herold

A survey is a canvassing of people for the purpose of collecting information. Surveys are done when there is a question to be answered, and there is no existing data source to provide the needed information. A survey is a lot of work and should never be conducted when the information can be obtained more readily elsewhere. Therefore, it is important to investigate thoroughly the availability of existing data before undertaking a survey. A good place to start is to contact a national statistical office, census bureau, ministry of health, or other governmental organizations that would have knowledge of large data collection efforts and the availability of existing data.

Surveys can be classified in a number of ways. One distinction is between a census, or a complete population survey, in which every element in the target population is included, and a sample survey, in which only a portion of the target population is selected. A census or complete population survey is extremely expensive and is rarely used to collect detailed information from a large population. Even the United States census does not collect detailed information from the total population. Instead it asks fewer than 10 questions of the total population and collects the more detailed census information from a sample of households. Large health-related surveys are also sample surveys. Only when the target population is small should you consider doing a complete population survey.

## STEPS IN CARRYING OUT A SURVEY

1. Write a protocol.
2. Select a survey mode.
3. Develop a questionnaire.
4. Design and select the sample.
5. Train interviewers (or prepare for mail-out).
6. Collect data (fieldwork).
7. Enter data into a computer, edit, and process the data.
8. Analyze the data.
9. Write a survey report.

## Writing a Protocol

Perhaps more than any other type of data collection, a survey cannot be undertaken without a protocol or detailed plan. The various steps in survey design are all interconnected and, therefore, must be thought out carefully prior to beginning any steps of the survey itself. For example, the budget influences the choice of the survey mode, sample design, sample size, and length of questionnaire. The analysis plan affects the format of questions, sample design, and sample size. The sample size influences the mode, analysis, and interpretation of results. The mode dictates the length and format of the questionnaire. A protocol allows all these interrelationships to be considered—and they *must* be considered—before actually choosing a mode, designing a questionnaire, or selecting a sample. The protocol should include: Study Objectives; Methodology, including a list of information to be sought from the survey, survey design, sampling plan, and data editing plan; Analysis Plan, including the computer software necessary to analyze the data; Logistics for implementing the survey, including personnel and equipment needed; Budget; and Time Line. Once all these steps have been thoroughly thought through, you are ready to begin work on the survey.

## Selecting a Survey Mode

Surveys can be classified by their mode of data collection. There are mail and Internet surveys, telephone surveys, and face-to-face interview surveys. Prior to developing a questionnaire and choosing a sample, the survey mode must be decided. Each of these modes has its advantages and disadvantages.

Mail, or self-administered, surveys are seldom used to collect information from the general public because names and addresses usually are not available, and the response rate tends to be low. However, the method may be highly effective with members of particular groups, such as members of an HMO or members of a professional association. The principal advantages of mail surveys are that they may obtain more thoughtful responses, and they are the least expensive to implement. The biggest disadvantage of the mail survey is that it typically obtains a much lower response rate than a telephone or face-to-face interview. A response rate of 50% is not unusual for a mail survey. Questionnaires that are distributed and returned by computer share many of the advantages and disadvantages of the mail survey, including the principal disadvantage of a low response rate. Moreover, a computer survey is not a good choice for a general population survey in most countries because of the selectivity of persons who use or own computers. Sometimes survey data are obtained with self-administered questionnaires that are not mailed or sent over the Internet but are provided to respondents in person, such as at a clinic or at a group gathering. If sufficient time is allowed for response to the questionnaire, this method will have most of the advantages of a mail survey without the principal disadvantage of a low response rate.

Telephone interviewing is an efficient survey method and has become quite popular in the United States. Investigations of epidemics frequently rely on telephone surveys because they are quick, inexpensive, and sensitive (i.e., they quickly reveal whether a problem truly exists). Under good conditions, the response rate for a telephone survey is better than a mail survey but not as high as that of a face-to-face interview. Unfortunately, cooperation with telephone surveys by the public has recently begun to decline, particularly in large cities, as a result of the proliferation of telephone usage for surveys, polls, sales, and the solicitation of donations. Also, populations with and without telephones may differ, creating a possible important bias.

A face-to-face interview is often the preferred or only feasible method of survey data collection. Among its many advantages, the most important is its high response rate (80%–95%). It also has the advantage of permitting the collection of more complex and more sensitive information than a mail or telephone survey. It can tolerate a much longer time for questionnaire administration, thus allowing for more information to be collected. The principal disadvantage of the face-to-face interview is the cost: interviewers' salaries, their transportation, and, at times, their meals and housing have to be considered. Furthermore, it takes longer to locate respondents for face-to-face interviews, which extends the time that interviewers' salaries, transport, room, and meals must be covered. A second disadvantage is the potential for interviewer bias (also a risk in telephone surveys), but we will see later in this chapter that this can be considerably controlled with proper selection and training of interviewers.

Surveys may combine these various modes. The telephone may be used to "screen" for eligible respondents and then to make appointments for face-to-face interviews. Additionally, mixed mode surveys may use a less expensive method to start, then switch to a method that yields a higher response rate for those who fail to respond to the initial method. The most popular of the mixed mode surveys is the combined mail and telephone mode. Caution is advised, however, in the use of mixed mode surveys. Questionnaire construction is usually different for different survey modes, and this difference creates a measurement problem with mixed mode approaches. Moreover, potential biases vary depending on the mode, and this can cause problems in interpreting the results. Therefore, it is highly recommended that you seek the assistance of a survey expert if you choose to use a mixed mode approach.

## Developing a Questionnaire

### Writing Questions

The first step in developing a questionnaire is to define the research question and to list the information that you wish to obtain. A list of information or variables that you want will help you create the questions that will give that information, as well as help you avoid writing unnecessary questions. You will also need to know the type of analysis you plan to use and the mode of data collection. Your analysis plan will determine the form of responses to questions. For example, if you plan to work with proportions, you will want to collect categorical responses. On the other hand, if you can work with means, you may collect scaled responses. It is also possible that you want to do a content analysis on qualitative data, in which case you may seek open-ended responses (see below). The mode of data collection (mail/Internet, telephone, or face-to-face interview) will affect how the question is written, what response categories are shown, the length of the questionnaire, and the overall format of the questionnaire. Here are some general rules on question writing and questionnaire format.

The question format can be of three types:

1. Structured or closed-ended questions. These are questions that have predetermined response categories to choose from. The respondent is told what the response options are and is asked to choose from among the options. Multiple-choice and true/false questions are examples of this format. The structured format is easiest to implement for large samples, for self-administered questionnaires with hand-written responses, and when the range of response possibilities is known. A fundamental rule for writing structured questions is that the response options must be mutually exclusive and exhaustive. To meet the "exhaustive" criterion, it is often necessary to include a response option labeled "Other (specify)_____" in order to allow for responses that were not thought of by the question writer.

2. Unstructured or open-ended questions. This format allows the respondent to answer in his or her own words. The unstructured question is useful when the researcher does not know what the range of response options might be. It may also provide a more accurate response, as it prevents the respondent from guessing or misinterpreting a response category that the researcher has constructed. However, coding and analysis of answers to open-ended questions can be very difficult and time consuming. Open-ended questions, therefore, are to be avoided in large-scale surveys and by researchers inexperienced with coding or interpreting qualitative data.

3. Precoded open-ended questions. Open-ended questions that are precoded are often used in interviewer-assisted surveys. These questions do not provide answer options to the respondent, but have options written in the questionnaire for the interviewer to circle or check that correspond to the respondent's stated answer. Many precoded open-ended questions will also require the "Other (specify)_____" option mentioned above for structured questions.

The interviewer must always be aware that errors in response—both voluntary and involuntary, due to misunderstanding, misrepresentation, or faulty memory—can and will occur. To obtain the most accurate information from a respondent, several things should be taken into account: (*1*) questions should be written as unambiguously as possible; (*2*) the vocabulary used in question construction should be consistent with the vocabulary of the respondents; (*3*) if interviewers are involved, they must be trained to avoid influencing the respondent and to read the question exactly as written so that every interviewee responds to exactly the same question wording; (*4*) use as many questions as possible from previously used questionnaires developed for your target population; (*5*) field test the questionnaire to ensure that respondents understand the questions and concepts in the same way that the researcher does.

## Questionnaire Format

The order of questions in the questionnaire varies depending on the mode of data collection. A questionnaire administered by an interviewer should have some easy and non-threatening questions to start. Often demographic questions are asked first to give the respondent an opportunity to get comfortable with the interviewer prior to being asked more difficult or sensitive questions. On the other hand, a mail/Internet survey should get right to the point, with questions specific to the principal purpose of the survey at the beginning of the questionnaire. In this way the respondent's attention is immediately engaged, and he or she is more likely to complete and return the questionnaire.

Threatening or embarrassing questions should be kept to a minimum and placed toward the end of the questionnaire. If the respondent chooses not to answer these questions, you will at least have obtained other information asked earlier in the questionnaire that you can use in analysis.

Avoid asking questions that are not applicable to a particular respondent. This is done by using filter questions and skip patterns that direct the respondent to skip over questions that do not pertain to him or her. It is possible to lose the interest and thoughtfulness of respondents if they feel you are asking irrelevant questions. Skip patterns may be used frequently in a questionnaire administered by an interviewer. They are to be used sparingly in a self-administered questionnaire.

Avoid offering the respondent a "don't know" option. A questionnaire that is developed for a personal interview may have "don't know" categories for all questions in the questionnaire, with instructions to the interviewer not to read these options. A questionnaire that is developed for self-administration, on the other hand, should keep "don't know" options to a minimum.

Use transition sentences to prepare the respondent for a new topic. Remember that the data you collect are only as good as your respondent's interpretation and memory. Transition sentences allow the respondents to adjust their minds for a shift in subject matter.

Above all, the questionnaire must be well spaced, clearly typed or printed, and easy to follow. The placement of response categories for questions should be consistent throughout the questionnaire. They should be listed vertically and not horizontally, so they are easily seen. Keep in mind that the easier it is for the eye to identify the response options, the quicker will be the completion of the questionnaire, the fewer will be the errors in selecting a response category, and the fewer will be the errors in reading the response category when entering the data into the computer.

The questionnaire will need to be reviewed numerous times, by both content experts and editors. A questionnaire with many errors will produce data with many errors.

Finally, a cover page is usually advisable for interviewer-administered questionnaires. The cover page to a questionnaire will have a place for the interviewer to code the final status of the interview—"completed"; "unable to locate household or respondent"; "refused"; and other useful categories. It may also have a place for the interviewer to record date and time of attempts to reach the respondent, which is helpful in scheduling revisits. Most important, the cover page will also contain information that will allow the interviewer to identify the correct member of the sample. It may contain an address or name or telephone number of the potential interviewee along with other identifying information. The purpose of having identifying information on its own page is so that the page can later be removed from the questionnaire after fieldwork and data entry are completed. In this way, the respondent cannot be linked to the answers he or she has provided.

### The Pretest

A newly developed questionnaire that has not been used previously in a population *must* be pretested. A pretest is a form of pilot study to check on the validity and reliability of the individual questions and the instrument as a whole. In a pretest, the final questionnaire is administered, using the mode that will be used in the actual survey, to a small (usually purposive) sample taken from the same population that the final sample is drawn from. It is very important, however, that the respondents for the pretest *not* be included in the final sample. Thus the pretest is usually not conducted until after the final sample has been drawn. Depending on the length and complexity of the questionnaire, the sample size for a pretest can vary from 25 to 100 individuals. The pretest should reveal any problem respondents may have in understanding the questions and whether or not there are any difficulties in following the questionnaire. If the pretest is of sufficient size, it may also be used to identify questions that may be removed from the questionnaire because of lack of variability in responses to those items. The pretest of the questionnaire also affords an opportunity to test other aspects of survey procedures, such as ability to locate respondents, willingness of prospective respondents to consent to the interview, the duration of the interview, and so forth.

## Selecting a Sample

### To Sample or Not to Sample

Seldom do public health budgets have the resources for complete population surveys. Therefore, sampling methods are used to obtain information from a smaller number than the total population. When a large population is involved, well-designed sampling will usually provide better data than a census-type survey. Given an always limited budget, a few reliable, well-trained interviewers working on a properly selected sample of the population can obtain more accurate information than would be possible for a larger team of less–well-trained field staff trying to interview all members of a population. Sampling *does* introduce sampling error, which is inherent to the sampling process. However, with available resources concentrated on a sample of a large population, the reduction in interviewer, nonresponse, and other errors that would come about from resources spread too thin will more than compensate for the introduction of sampling error.

Proper sampling techniques can provide a measure of the amount of error produced by the sampling process. Any estimate made from a sample is subject to error, but sampling errors have the favorable characteristic of being controllable through the size and design of the sample. Sampling errors, even for small samples, are often the least of the errors present in a survey. (See below for a listing of other sources of error.)

Nevertheless, it is important to keep in mind that, for a small, geographically concentrated population, it may be possible to do a complete or census-type survey. For example, an outbreak in a small village or at a church supper may be best studied by surveying everyone in those small populations and thus completely avoiding sampling error.

## Types of Samples

Sampling error cannot be calculated for all samples. Our ability to calculate sampling error depends on the type of sampling employed. There are two broad types of sampling used in sample surveys: probability sampling and nonprobability sampling. Probability sampling uses statistical theory in the design of the sample and, consequently, permits the calculation of sampling error. Probability sampling is the selection of a sample such that every member in the population has a known and nonzero probability of being included. This type of sampling is unbiased and enables you to draw valid conclusions about the population from which your sample is drawn. Nonprobability sampling is not based on statistical theory. It is a type of sampling that is inherently biased and does not permit the calculation of sampling error. Nonprobability samples include purposive samples, convenience samples, and the like.

Purposive (or judgment) sampling is the selection of a sample based on someone's judgment and knowledge of the subject matter. This type of sampling is biased and generally used only when there is no time to define a probability sample. An example might be the selection of community leaders in a refugee camp in such a way as to try to get maximum representation of the various ethnic groups residing there when the target population are all refugees in the camp. The community leaders would then be asked questions about the members of their community.

Convenience sampling is the use of a sample that is near at hand. Such a sample is inherently biased by the fact that it includes only persons that happen to be out and about or taking a specific route or engaged in a specific activity at the time of the survey. Route samples, street-corner political surveys, or a sample based on persons coming into a clinic are convenience samples when the target population is the resident population of a given area.

On occasions when the goal of a study is not to make statistical estimates about a population but rather to explore ideas and opinions of people about a new topic that may not be ready for a quantitative investigation, convenience samples may be very useful. They can provide ideas about people's thoughts and opinions and can be used to generate hypotheses for further study. But any study that wishes to produce statistics about the total population must use probability sampling.

## Probability Sampling

As stated before, a probability sample is one in which every member of the population has a known and nonzero probability of being selected into the sample. A special case of the probability sample is the random sample, where each member of the population has an equal chance of being selected. The vast majority of the statistical tests we use carry with them the assumption that the sample has been randomly selected. While the selection of a random sample may not always be feasible, if we know the probability of selection of every member of the population, we can make adjustments to the data (through computer programs) to account for the differences between our probability sample and a strictly random sample. If we do not meet the criteria of a probability sample, we cannot draw conclusions about the population using standard significance tests and confidence intervals.

To draw a random sample you need to have a list of all members of the population from which the sample is to be drawn. This list is called a *sampling frame*. It is important that this frame be current and accurate. For example, when drawing a sample of college students, you will want a list of current students and not a list of those attending the college a year ago. When drawing a sample of housing units in a town, you will not want to use a list of housing units identified at the previous census eight years ago. We often fail to realize that our sample is only as good as the sampling frame from which it is selected. It is, therefore, very important to obtain an updated sampling frame that lists all elements of the population as close to the survey date as possible. If none is available, it is up to you, the survey implementer, to add to your budget the personnel and materials necessary to produce a current sampling frame. If you have to create a sampling frame for your sample, pay close attention to cluster sampling, described below.

### Probability Sample Designs

*Simple random sampling* gives every member of the population an equal chance of being included in the sample. It requires a listing of every member of the population. Once all members of the population are assigned a number, a table of random numbers may be used to select individuals for the sample. Simple random sampling is theoretically simple, but often unrealistic in practice, because it can be expensive and may present logistical difficulties such as geographic dispersion of the study sample. Since no control of the distribution of the sample is exercised in this case, the variables in some samples may be poorly distributed (not biased, but unrepresentative). Therefore, simple random sampling is not always desirable. The principle of simple random sampling, however, is the basis of all good sampling techniques and can be utilized in each of the following more specialized designs.

*Systematic sampling* is often used when elements (e.g., individuals or households) can be ordered or listed in some manner. Rather than selecting all elements randomly, one determines a selection interval ($n$), by dividing the total population listed by the sample size. The sampler then chooses a random starting point on the population list, and selects every $n$th person (the length of the selection interval). Good geographic or strata distribution can be assured if the population is listed according to geographic area or other stratifying characteristic. It is an easy method to apply and a popular one among public health professionals.

In *stratified sampling*, the target population is divided into suitable, non-overlapping subpopulations or strata. Each stratum should be homogeneous within and heterogeneous between other strata. A random sample can then be selected within each stratum. In this way, each stratum is more accurately represented, and since members are more alike within each stratum, the overall sampling error is reduced. Separate estimates can be obtained from each stratum, and an overall estimate can be obtained for the entire population defined by the strata. The sample selection for each stratum is further defined by whether it is proportionate or disproportionate across strata. *Proportionate stratified sampling* uses the same *sampling fraction* that is calculated for the total population (sample size divided by the total population size) for selecting a sample from each stratum. *Disproportionate stratified sampling* uses different sampling fractions across strata in an attempt to get sufficient numbers of elements to make separate statistical estimates for each stratum. Disproportionate sampling is the method used when "oversampling" of a particular stratum is done. This method frequently is used to get sufficient representation of minority ethnic groups and to enable independent estimates of characteristics by ethnicity. While disproportionate stratified sampling allows for sufficient sample size within each stratum to make stratum-specific estimates with relatively equal precision, it requires the extra step of weighting the data when estimates are made for the total population, or all strata combined.

*Cluster sampling* is of particular value to save resources in surveys of human populations when the population is geographically dispersed or when a sampling frame for the elements of the population you wish to study is not available. In this type of sampling, the units first sampled are not the individual elements we are ultimately interested in, but, rather, clusters or aggregates of those elements. For example, in sampling the population of a rural area that is widely dispersed and difficult to reach, a sample of villages may be selected, and then all of the households in the sampled villages may be included in the survey. It is apparent that such a sample involves less traveling than a simple random sample of households throughout the rural area. Another typical example is in a study of schoolchildren, when a list of all children attending schools in an area is not available. One would then use a list of schools, and select a sample of schools from the list. In this case, schools are the sampling unit or clusters. Once the sample of schools has been selected, all of the students in the sampled schools may be surveyed. This type of sampling almost always loses some degree of precision. To maintain the same degree of precision as in simple random sampling, one would have to approximately double the sample size that would be calculated for a simple random sample.

*Multistage sampling* involves sampling at different levels of population groupings. It is most often used in surveys where cluster sampling is necessary. In the cases given in the previous paragraph, for example, if one were to sample the households in the selected villages, or sample the children in the selected schools, there would be two levels of sampling involved, and they would demonstrate a two-stage sample design. The first stage would be the selection of a sample of villages or schools, and the second stage would be the selection of a sample of households or students. Both of these examples, however, may be converted to three-stage designs. If, in the example of the population of rural areas, we were first to select a sample of villages (clusters), then select a sample of households (clusters) in each selected village, and finally select one adult (final sampling unit) in each of the sampled households, we would have a three-stage sample design. With respect to the children attending school, our first stage would be the selection of schools (clusters), the second stage might be the selection of a sample of classes or grades (clusters) in the selected schools, and the third stage would be the selection of a sample of students (final sampling unit) in the classes. Again, we would have a three-stage design. An obvious advantage in the school example is that you need only a listing of schools, classes within the selected schools, and students in the selected classes. You have bypassed the need for a list of all children attending school!

Most national surveys involve multistage sampling, with geographically defined clusters being the first stage or the primary sampling unit. This is, in part, because of the prohibitive cost of dispersing interviewers across a broad geographic area, but more important, it is due to many countries' not having a list of all members of their population. The United States is an example. The United States does not have a list of all members of its population. Instead it has a list of census tracts. To conduct a sample survey for the U.S. population, one would have to first select census tracts from a list provided by the Census Bureau, then update the sampling frame for the selected tracts by mapping out the number and location of housing units in those tracts (unless that had been done with a recent census or survey), then select housing units from the updated frame, and finally select people living in the selected housing units.

## Sample Size

Ideally, the sample size chosen for a survey should be based on how reliable the final estimates must be. In practice, usually a trade-off is made between the ideal sample size and the expected cost of the survey. The size of the sample must be sufficient to accomplish the purpose but should not be larger than necessary, because it will draw resources from other aspects of the survey process.

Sample size is determined by the desired confidence level and precision of your estimates and the variability of the characteristic being measured for the population. The formula for calculating the sample size needed to estimate a proportion is:

$$n = z^2 \, pq/d^2$$

where,

> $n$ = the sample size
> $z$ = the standard normal deviate (1.96 for a 95% confidence level)
> $d$ = the level of accuracy desired, or sampling error (often set at .05)
> $p$ = the proportion of the population having the characteristic being measured (if proportion is unknown, set $p$ = .50, which is maximum variability)
> $q$ = the proportion of the population that does not have the characteristic (i.e., $1-p$)

If the total population from which the sample is to be drawn is less than 10,000, then the size of the population must also be taken into account. Thus, for a population of size 10,000 or greater, $n$, above, is the final sample size; for populations less than 10,000, the following adjustment must be made:

$$nf = n/1 + (n/N)$$

where,

> $nf$ = the final sample size, when population is less than 10,000
> $n$ = the sample size for populations of 10,000 or more
> $N$ = the size of the total population from which the sample is drawn

The above formulas may be easily modified when the estimates of interest are means rather than proportions. As stated, these formulas are the basic ones for simple random sampling. However, we know that in reality we often use stratified or multistage sampling methods. Adjustments to these formulas are necessary for these more complex designs or for more complex analysis than estimating proportions and means. Under such circumstances it is best to consult a statistician. If one is not easily available, some rules of thumb that may come in handy are: (*1*) for cluster designs, you will want to double the calculated sample size for a simple random sample; (*2*) for disproportionate stratified samples, you will want to calculate a sample size for each stratum.

Once a sample size is calculated, it must be appraised to see whether it is consistent with the resources available to conduct the survey. This appraisal demands an estimation of the personnel, materials, and time required to pursue the proposed sample size. It often becomes apparent that the calculated sample size has to be reduced. The usual loss is through increasing sampling error and losing precision in your estimates. If this happens, you are faced with the decision of whether to proceed with reduced precision or whether to abandon efforts until more resources can be found. On the positive side, however, is that if you conduct the survey and find less variability in your characteristics of interest than you estimated for your sample size calculations, your precision will be improved.

## Preparing for Fieldwork

This section focuses on procedures relevant to face-to-face surveys. In field epidemiology, this is the mode you are likely to use, and the training of interviewers is the paramount feature for putting this type of survey into motion. You have spent time and effort in developing a good questionnaire and a representative sample of your target population, but your work can be all for naught with a casually selected and poorly trained group of interviewers. Remember, the interviewers are collecting your data!

You will want interviewers who are most likely to elicit honest responses from the respondents. You do not want high-ranking people whose status may influence the respondent to respond favorably (and untruthfully) to questions. Instead, choose interviewers who interact well with people and who are empathetic and unthreatening to the respondent. For certain situations, it may be preferable to have interviewers with similar social or demographic characteristics to the respondents, such as gender, age, or ethnicity.

Interviewers should be thoroughly trained in the following matters:

1. How to find the correct households or sample points. Detailed instructions on the importance of keeping to the sample design and how to locate the selected households or persons must be given. Often maps of survey areas are involved, and interviewers must be well trained in how to read the maps.
2. How to approach the respondent to assure they agree to be interviewed. This includes introducing oneself, specifying the value of the survey, and the authority behind the survey.
3. How to inform the respondent of the anonymity and confidentiality of their participation. The fact that the respondent's identification will be eliminated from the data, if this is the case, is important to convey.
4. How to introduce a consent form, if applicable, and obtain a signature (see Chapter 14).

5. How to administer the questionnaire so that question wording is not changed from one interview to the next. This is best done by strong instructions to read the question and to resist the temptation of stating the question in the interviewer's own words.

6. How to define the terms used in the questionnaire, so that all respondents receive the same explanation of terms.

7. How to deal with new situations. It is important for the interviewer to consult with a supervisor about any new situations that arise in the field, especially those involving errors in the questionnaire or the interview procedure. Decisions in such situations should be made by, or communicated to, a field supervisor, so that determinations can be standardized across all interviewers.

8. How to administer the questionnaire. Sufficient practice sessions are needed to ensure adherence to skip patterns and other issues related to filling out the questionnaire, as well as to other procedures listed above.

9. How to dress for interviewing so the respondent feels at ease in the presence of the interviewer.

10. How to review the completed questionnaire after the interview has taken place to check for accuracy, consistency, and completeness in the field. At this point, there still is the opportunity for the interviewer to return to the respondent if there are any errors that must be corrected. For large-scale surveys, it is best to have supervisors in the field with the interviewers, one of whose tasks would be to review questionnaires.

11. The importance of the information they are gathering, to adhering to the sample design, to finding the respondent, to minimizing refusals, and of their contribution to the overall survey effort. The few additional hours required to explain to the interviewers the use of the data, the work that has gone into the survey thus far, and the value of the representative sample, is time well spent.

Interviewer training should comprise both classroom and field training. It is critical that interviewers not practice on members of the actual sample. A day or two of supervised practice interviews in the field can do much to assure quality data collection when the real fieldwork begins.

It is also recommended that a reference manual or interviewer's manual be developed that contains all the interviewer instructions for the fieldwork, including how to locate the sample points, definitions, and such.

Preparation for fieldwork also includes instruction on revisits to households or other places where respondents are to be found, in order to keep to a minimum the number of members of the sample that are not located.

When fieldwork is about to begin, the following supplies will be needed for the interviewers:

1. Sufficient supplies of questionnaires, pencils, and pencil sharpeners. (Pencils are easier to use because of erasures that are often needed during the interview.)
2. Any cards or pictures that may accompany the questionnaire.
3. Identification of the interviewer via a letter and/or an ID card.
4. A clipboard to make it easier to fill out the questionnaire.
5. A copy of the reference manual.
6. Maps or instructions on how to locate the respondents.

## Response Rate

A response rate needs to be calculated at the end of every survey. The response rate is simply the number of completed questionnaires divided by the number of people in your original sample. Often survey directors will report other rates, using a smaller denominator, such as the number of people from the original sample who were actually located, or the number of people who answered their telephone, or the number of mailed questionnaires that actually reached a correct address. These rates are not true response rates. They are simply ways of avoiding having to report a response rate that may not have been as high as desired. Note that nonresponse is not simply a function of the number of refusals obtained, but also the number of sample points that were never located. Therefore, the response rate reflects not only the compliance of the population contacted, but also the skill of the survey personnel in finding the members of the selected sample.

## Entering and Editing the Data

Depending on the duration of fieldwork, the collected data may be entered into a computer while data collection is taking place or at the completion of data collection.

Data entry is a stage of survey work when many errors can occur. In the past, the standard way of checking for data entry error was to require double entry. Double entry simply means the data are entered twice, by different enterers. Then the two sets of data are compared (by computer), and if disagreement in the data is found between the two data sets, the original questionnaire is consulted and the incorrect code is corrected. Double data entry is both costly and time-consuming. Fortunately, there is less need for it today because of the proliferation of data entry/edit programs.

As can be deduced from the previous paragraph, in the recent past, data entry and data editing were two separate activities. Today, there are numerous computer programs that accomplish editing of data entry error concurrent with data entry. One such program is *Epi Info* (see Chapter 7). These programs usually reproduce the questions from the questionnaire on the computer screen and allow movement from one question to the next only if an acceptable entry is made. An acceptable entry may be defined by allowable codes or by following the appropriate skip pattern. An example of allowable codes may be an age range of 15 to 49 for a reproductive health survey. If the data entry person attempts to enter a 52 as the response for age, the computer will not accept it. Or, if there are five response categories for educational level, coded 1 to 5, the computer will only accept an entry in the 1 to 5 range. If the computer entry person mistakenly enters a 6, the computer will not move on to the next question until it is corrected. Such a data entry/edit program can identify the majority of data entry errors and consequently obviate the need for double data entry. In the absence of an entry/edit program, double data entry may be called for.

The data entry/edit program, however, does not identify all errors, and it cannot correct all errors. A mis-keyed code that falls within the range of acceptable codes will not be caught. Furthermore, any errors that are in the questionnaire, and not due to data entry, cannot be corrected by the data entry person. The latter errors can only be corrected by the interviewer and often not without returning to the individual respondent. This usually is only done if data entry is timed close to the original interview.

Once sufficient data have been entered into the computer, other edits can be done. Consistency checks that may not have been easily programmed into the data entry/edit program may be written and run on the data (see Chapter 7). And when all the data have been entered, a set of frequencies for all the items in the questionnaire should be produced for further scrutiny for previously undetected errors.

After all the data have been entered and edited and there is no possibility of returning to the field, the cover sheets with identifying information on the respondents should be destroyed, as well as any other material (such as lists) that can identify participants in the survey. The questionnaires themselves should be kept—at least through the initial stages of analysis. Consistency errors may still be discovered during the analysis phase, and it is always helpful to be able to return to the original questionnaires.

## Analyzing the Data

Principles of data analysis are described elsewhere in this book (see Chapter 10). The analysis consideration unique to survey data, however, is the importance of using the appropriate statistical techniques to adjust for the sample design and to calculate sampling errors. As mentioned earlier, when disproportionate stratified sampling is used, weights must be calculated and used when producing any statistics, including percentages, for the total sample. Most popular statistical packages, such as *Statistical Analysis System* (*SAS*), *Epi Info*, and *Statistical Programs for the Social Sciences* (*SPSS*) accommodate weights very nicely for producing descriptive statistics. When calculating sampling error, statistical significance, and confidence intervals, however, for any sample design other than simple random or systematic sampling, it will be necessary to use a statistical package that can adjust for the design effect. The most common package with this ability is *Survey Data Analysis* (*SUDAAN*), but others are available as well.

## Reporting the Results

As in all epidemiologic work, the survey should be described in a written report. The report should include the survey's objectives, methods, results, and your interpretation of the findings. The report serves two purposes: (*1*) to document the methods used to conduct the survey; and (*2*) to communicate to decision makers, such as policy makers, funding sources, and program managers, the findings of the survey. Thus, you should keep in mind that you are writing for two very distinct audiences. A detailed description of your methods is of paramount importance to demonstrate to other researchers and users of the data that your data collection was sound and your results are reliable. (Be sure to include the response rate!) Your description of findings, on the other hand, must be clear and appropriate for decision makers who may be neither epidemiologists nor statisticians. Percentages and means may be the best way to communicate to this audience. Bear in mind that the findings must be presented in a way that is understandable to non-researchers.

## SOURCES OF ERROR

All along the route of survey implementation there are places for error to contaminate the data. While it is not possible to eliminate all error, you must be cognizant of potential error, must attempt to keep it at a minimum, and when all else fails, be prepared to define the bias that error may cause in the data. When conducting a survey, the following broad areas for error must be foremost in your mind as the survey planner and implementer.

1. Coverage error. Coverage error occurs when the population from which the sample is drawn is not equivalent to the target population. This usually results from outdated or poorly constructed sampling frames. It can also

occur from incorrect information included in the sampling frame, such as incorrect addresses; or from an incomplete frame, such as only those households with computers or telephones when the target population is the total population. Attention must be given to the quality of the sampling frame and its close equivalence to the target population before a sample is drawn. If coverage error is not discovered until after the survey is implemented, you should report the bias caused by coverage error and its effect on interpretation of findings.

2. Sampling error. Sampling error is the least problematic in field surveys in that it is quantifiable and unbiased. As stated earlier, sampling error is linked to both the design and size of the sample. All sample surveys have sampling error.

3. Measurement error. Measurement error may be the most difficult to avoid. It often goes undetected and is nonquantifiable. Measurement error arises from various sources in the data collection process and is the error that makes a single respondent's answer incomparable to another's. Questions that are not clear or not interpreted in the same way by all respondents may not be measuring what you intend to measure for all respondents. Interviewers who are not consistent in the way they present questions or in the definitions they provide to respondents will create error, in that different respondents will have a different understanding of the question. Questions that are embarrassing or threatening or interviewers who are authority figures can evoke untruthful responses from interviewees. Questions that ask about events in the past may lead to recall bias that varies directly with the length of time that has passed since the event occurred.

4. Error due to nonresponse. This may be the most serious and most easily avoidable error in performing field surveys. Ask yourself, "What is the value of a carefully selected sample, designed to be representative of the population, when a response rate of 50% is obtained?" If only 50% of your sample has responded, you are very likely to have lost the representative properties of your sample design. Nonresponse can be attributed to two major factors: (1) failure of the interviewer to locate the respondent; and (2) failure of the respondent to consent to the interview. Both of the factors are controllable to a large degree by good selection and training of interviewers. At least three revisits should be made to households or other locations before assigning the status of "unable to locate respondent" to the interview. Often five to six revisits are recommended. As for "refused to participate," when surveying during a field investigation, you should not expect the level of refusal rate you would likely see in political, marketing, or other types of surveys. If you explain the health value of the

survey to the prospective respondents, it is usually not difficult to obtain their consent. A face-to-face survey, the mode that typically obtains the highest response rate, should never result in a response rate lower than 70%. An 80% to 90% response rate is not unusual for a face-to-face public health survey. In the case of a response rate lower than 80%, you are obliged to consider whether nonresponse has created a bias in the data and the direction of that bias. Keep in mind that respondents who are easily located may have different characteristics than those who are never at home. Persons who refuse to participate in the survey are likely to be less compliant in other areas, including health behaviors, than those who readily consent to be interviewed. A low response rate does more damage in rendering a survey's results questionable than merely reducing the sample size, since often there is no valid way of scientifically inferring all the characteristics of the nonrespondent population.

5. Data processing error. In the past, data entry was another significant source of error in surveys. But today the use of data entry/edit programs has reduced data entry error substantially. Another source of processing error still needs attention: that of coding. In surveys with reasonably large sample sizes that have open-ended questions in the questionnaire, it will be necessary to code these responses in order to manage them. The coding of open-ended responses should never be left to an unsupervised assistant. Coding takes skill and often the experience of a veteran investigator.

## SHORTCUTS TO AVOID

Conducting a successful survey entails scores of activities, each of which must be carefully planned and controlled. Taking shortcuts can invalidate the results or cause them to be seriously misleading. Four of the shortcuts that occur too often are:

1. Failure to use probability sampling procedures. One way to greatly reduce the usefulness of an otherwise well-conceived survey is to use a convenience sample rather than one based on probability design. It may be easy and cheap, for example, to get some needed information by selecting a sample of patients attending a public clinic one afternoon. However, this sampling procedure could give incorrect results if you attempt to generalize them to all clinic attendees.

2. Failure to pretest to the questionnaire. No qualified investigator will accept your results if they are based on newly formulated questions that have not

been pretested. The pretest not only demonstrates whether or not the target population understands the questions in the same way as the person who created them but also offers an opportunity to identify errors in the questionnaire.

3. Failure to train the interviewers thoroughly. Interviewers not only need to learn to conduct the interviews in a standardized fashion but they must also be taught the importance of *locating* the correct respondent and *persuading* that person to be interviewed. A week or two of interviewer training is not unreasonable for a large-scale survey.

4. Failure to use adequate quality control procedures. You should build into your survey necessary checks on its different facets at all stages—review of sample selection procedures, supervision of interviewing, random checks that interviews have actually taken place, and oversight of editing and coding decisions, among other things. Insisting on proper standards in recruitment and training of survey personnel helps a great deal, but equally important are proper review, verification, and evaluation to ensure that the execution of the survey corresponds to its design. Without proper quality control of all steps in the survey process, errors can occur that can be irreversible, costly, and have damaging results.

## REFERENCES AND FURTHER READINGS

### Survey Methods

1. Abramson, J.H. (1974). *Survey Methods in Community Medicine*. Churchill Livingstone, Edinburgh and London.
2. Couper, M.P., Baker, R.P., Bethlehem, J.,et al. (1998). *Computer Assisted Survey Information Collection*. John Wiley and Sons, New York.
3. Dillman, D.A. (1978). *Mail and Telephone Surveys: The Total Design Method*. John Wiley and Sons, New York.
4. Dillman, D. (2002). *Mail and Internet Surveys: The Tailored Design Method*. John Wiley and Sons, New York.
5. Fowler, F.J. (2002). *Survey Research Methods*, 3rd ed., Sage Publications, Thousand Oaks, Calif.
6. Groves, R.M., Fowler, F.J., Couper, M.P., et al. (2004). *Survey Methodology*. John Wiley and Sons, Hoboken, N.J.
7. Lessler, J., Kalsbeek, W. (1992). *Nonsampling Error in Surveys*. John Wiley and Sons, New York.
8. Rossi, P.H., Wright, J.D., Anderson, A.B. (1983). *Handbook of Survey Research*. Academic Press, Orlando, Fla.
9. Salant, P., Dillman, D.A. (1994). *How to Conduct Your Own Survey*. John Wiley and Sons, New York.

## Questionnaire Design and Interviewing

1. Beimer, P., Groves, R.M., Lyberg, L.E., et al. (1991). *Measurement Errors in Surveys.* John Wiley and Sons, New York.
2. Belson, W.A. (1981). *The Design and Understanding of Survey Questions.* Gower, Aldershot, England.
3. Converse, J., Presser, S. (1986). *Survey Questions.* Sage Publications, Beverly Hills, Calif.
4. Fowler, F.J., Mangione, T.W. (1990). *Standardized Survey Interviewing: Minimizing Interviewer Related Error.* Sage Publications, Newbury Park, Calif.
5. Groves, R.M., Dillman, D.A., Eltinge, J., et al. (2002). *Survey Nonresponse.* John Wiley and Sons, New York
6. Sudman, S., Bradburn, N.M. (1982). *Asking Questions: A Practical Guide to Questionnaire Design.* Jossey-Bass, San Francisco.
7. Sudman, S., Bradburn, N., Schwartz, N. (1996). *Thinking about Answers: The Application of Cognitive Processes to Survey Methodology.* Jossey-Bass, San Francisco.

## Sampling

1. Cochran, W.G. (1977). *Sampling Techniques*, 3rd ed., John Wiley and Sons, New York.
2. Kish, L. (1965). *Survey Sampling.* John Wiley and Sons, New York.
3. Levy, P.S., Lemeshow, S. (1980). *Sampling for Health Professionals.* Lifetime Learning Publications, Belmont, Calif.
4. Lohr, S. (1999). *Sampling: design and analysis.* Duxbury Press, Pacific Grove, Calif.
5. World Health Organization (1986). *Sample Size Determination.* World Health Organization, Geneva.

# 7

# USING A COMPUTER FOR FIELD INVESTIGATIONS

Andrew G. Dean and Consuelo M. Beck-Sagué

Computers are increasingly important tools for epidemiologic field investigations. Epidemiologists routinely use computers in field investigations along with questionnaires, statistics, laboratory tests, and other essential epidemiologic tools.

Computers, whether laptop, desktop, or palmtop, are machines, and, like most machines, require an investment of technical skill and setup time that must be balanced against the anticipated increase in quantity and quality of output.

Computers are most useful for:

- Tasks that are clearly defined and that will be done many times in the same way
- Rapid computation or counting involving large numbers of similar records
- Tasks matching the capabilities of existing software
- Numerically intensive calculations
- Accurate retention of details
- Investigators who have used the same system before

Manual processing is still indicated for:

- One-time or occasional tasks
- Small numbers of records

- Complex or changing tasks requiring human judgment, perhaps prior to computer entry
- Operators who are not familiar with computer use
- Situations where staffing for manual tasks is easier to obtain than computers or knowledgeable operators

Tasks that may be usefully performed on a computer during an outbreak investigation include searching for information, sample size calculation, questionnaire design, data entry, importing or exporting files in various formats, tabulation of results, statistical calculations, graphing, mapping, presentation graphics, and computer communication.

## MICROCOMPUTERS

Progress in the miniaturization of computers has been nearly miraculous in the past three decades, and a description of microcomputer hardware is sure to be outdated as soon as it is printed. At present a portable computer and a printer can be carried to the field in a briefcase and operated either from batteries or standard electrical power. Palmtop computers that fit in a pocket and do not require a keyboard are becoming popular, although they are still limited compared with laptop models. A laptop or desktop computer may have a hard disk capable of storing millions of records. Portable modems make it technically possible to send files, access bibliographical databases, or search the Internet from any area with cable or telephone Internet service, although some countries place restrictions on modem use. Wireless connections are rapidly becoming available in some areas, and useful work can be performed from "Internet cafés" if private connections are not available.

The most common type of microcomputer is the Intel-compatible computer with a Microsoft Windows® operating system. There are more than 500 million copies of Microsoft Windows in the world, at least 22% of which are pirated.[1] Since microcomputers running some form of Microsoft Windows are ubiquitous and also permit fairly easy development of software, most epidemiologic software is available for these models. Macintosh and Linux computers require different software, but browsers in all three systems can access the Internet for searching, communication, and calculation. Windows programs can be run within or beside the other operating systems using Windows emulators or "dual boot" systems. Documents and spreadsheets can be created, edited, and shared on the Internet using only a browser, thus allowing those with different types of computer operating systems to participate.

Laptop computers are more expensive than desktop models of the same capacity but are fairly rugged and light enough to carry, and most models easily adapt to international electrical variations. Because they have built-in batteries, they are easy to use during power outages.

The overall issues in choosing a computer include compatibility with other computers in the home office and field environment; availability of epidemiologic and statistical software; and the usual factors of cost, capacity, speed, durability, and repair service. As the age of computer communication progresses, the types of connections and provisions for security and virus checking assume greater importance.

## SOFTWARE

The type of software available for epidemiologic investigation is more important than the brand of computer or operating system. During a field investigation, software may be needed for word processing, data entry, database management, data analysis and statistics, communications, bibliographical searching, and miscellaneous functions such as scheduling and note-taking. Commercial programs are available for word processing, scheduling, note-taking, graphing, and other functions that are common business applications. Data entry and database management can be done with commercial programs such as Microsoft Access, but these programs do not offer statistics for epidemiology, and setting up databases and manipulating records may require more attention than investigators are able to spare in a busy field situation. Commercial database software can also be quite expensive if multiple copies are required. Statistical software is available commercially, the most popular general-purpose programs being Statistical Analysis System (SAS, www.sas.com), and Statistical Programs for the Social Sciences (SPSS, www.spss.com). They perform a wide variety of statistical procedures for those familiar with the statistics and with programming in SAS or SPSS. Since their commands are different from those of the database programs, the use of both statistics and database programs requires learning two "languages." SAS and SPSS both offer facilities for data entry, and thus may be used without a database program, although data entry usually cannot be controlled to the extent that it can in a database program.

Epidemiologic fieldwork often requires statistics for categorical (coded or yes/no) data rather than continuous data. Mantel-Haenszel analysis of stratified data is important, and logistic regression may be desirable after preliminary Mantel-Haenszel analysis. It is important that entry, checking, coding, and editing of data be easy to perform. Setting up a new questionnaire is almost always required in a field investigation, and this should be easy to do in the software that is chosen.

The Centers for Disease Control and Prevention (CDC) and the World Health Organization (WHO) have developed a program called Epi Info for use in epidemiologic investigations that attempts to provide the best compromise between ease of use and flexibility. It is in the public domain, and versions for both DOS and Windows may be downloaded from the CDC website, copied for use by others, or translated. In this chapter, we use Epi Info to illustrate many of the tasks to be performed with computers in the field. Other free and inexpensive software for use in epidemiology can be found by searching the Internet. A recent search turned up links to free calculators for purposes as diverse as estimating caloric intake, civil engineering, producing random numbers, and doing specialized statistics, many of which could be useful in epidemiology.

Whatever software you choose, it is important that you be familiar with its use and limitations before leaving for the field. A tense field situation with high stakes and an insistent press leaves little time for learning about software or devising programs to solve new problems. The analysis does not have to be sophisticated, but it should be correct with regard to the totals obtained and the elementary statistics. Logistic regression analysis can be refined later, but the basic data must return from the field intact, properly backed up, and well documented.

## THE WORKING AND TRAVELING ENVIRONMENT

To minimize problems in the field, hardware, software, and operator skills should be practiced as much as possible before leaving the home office. A "dress rehearsal" should be conducted before leaving to be sure that all necessary elements are available.

Magnetic disks must be treated like fine phonograph records and protected from fingerprints, scratches, coffee, magnets, sharp bending, and denting by firm objects like ballpoint pens. They will not be harmed by a reasonable number of passes through a modern airport X-ray machine, but metal detectors and motor-driven moving belts do generate magnetic fields that could be harmful to diskettes. Diskettes should be protected from both heat and intense cold. They should never be left in a parked car in warm weather. If possible, a portable Compact Disk (CD-ROM) writer should be used to make permanent backups of data, as optical media, particularly the CD-R or write-once CD-ROMs, are not affected by magnetic fields and are more resistant to physical abuse than floppy disks. They can be damaged by fingerprints or scratches, however. Extra copies can be made and mailed home by more than one route in case of loss or theft of luggage. CD-ROM drives are delicate, however, and should be treated gently.

When traveling, it is important to be sure that the type of power at your destination (120 vs. 240 volts) and connecting plug are known and compatible with the equipment being used. Portable computers may be run from car batteries in remote locations with appropriate adapters. Whenever possible, the computer should be protected from voltage surges with a voltage spike protector. Increasingly, uninterruptible power supplies (UPSs) are affordable, and will protect against power interruptions for long enough to allow you to save current work and shut down the computer. The device used must be designed for local voltage levels, as voltage spike protectors designed for 110 volts perish with a puff of smoke when plugged into 220 volts. Battery power is much less subject to voltage variations.

Some countries require prior clearance to bring a computer in or out. Others have restrictions on the use of modem communications. It is important to check on such regulations with appropriate embassies, scientific colleagues, or customs officials.

In the field, your work space should be shielded from direct sun and protected from dust. The power cord for a desktop computer can be fastened to the outlet with tape or other means so that power will not be accidentally interrupted.

Organization of a portable computer's hard disk can contribute greatly to ease of use. Some investigators recommend creating a new directory for each investigation, keeping all files pertaining to that investigation in the same directory. The 1.4 megabyte floppy diskette has become a universal standard, but for files larger than one diskette, it is important to have software such as PKZIP or WinZip, which compresses files and automatically spans more than one diskette. A number of higher-capacity removable-storage devices such as zip and flash drives or external hard disk drives are available, but with the more proprietary formats, it is important that more than one compatible drive be available, and that both generating and receiving machines use the same drive format. Files can be transferred via Local Area Network (LAN) connections or the Internet if these options are available.

Sending backup files to the home office can provide protection against loss of data through theft or loss of luggage during a trip. A colleague should be asked to verify that the files arrived intact, however, as various e-mail systems may refuse to transmit an attachment, or worse yet, simply remove an attachment that they sense could carry a program with malignant intent (as Hotmail does with MDB—Microsoft Access files—used by Epi Info). There are Internet file storage facilities (search for "file storage") that are less stringent in their requirements, and that may be used for transmission, and sometimes "zipping" or compressing the file will solve the problem.

When transmitting files over the Internet or other networks, it is important to protect their confidential contents. This can be done by encrypting the files with a program such as Epi Info's EpiLock, which offers 128-bit or better encryption. One can also reduce the risk of disclosing personal material by omitting names and personal identifiers as much as possible in files to be transmitted or stored.

## WORD PROCESSING

Word processing is used for producing questionnaires, plans, and reports, and for recording miscellaneous observations during the investigation. A word processing package previously used by the investigator is preferable, since it takes time to adjust to a new package.

If collaborators in the investigation use different software for word processing, a common format such as "Rich Text Format" (RTF) files can be used, but compatibility should be tested in both types of software, as even standard formats are sometimes version-dependent. Plain text or ASCII files can be used as the lowest common denominator if necessary. Sending files or text by e-mail can also bridge compatibility gaps.

## DESIGNING A QUESTIONNAIRE FOR COMPUTER USE

A questionnaire is a tool or template for structuring data collection so that items to be tabulated by computer or by hand are all of the same type. An item called AGE, for example, will contain data expressing age in a uniform way, perhaps as a number representing years. A good questionnaire, like a computer program or written essay, begins with an outline of major topics to be addressed. Theoretically, it is even more desirable to begin with the type of output desired and work backward to define the necessary input elements. In practice, an iterative approach to consider both input and output is often used until a satisfactory "design" is achieved.

Often the objective is to explore correlations between an illness or injury and one or more exposures or risk factors. The large topics in an outline could then be:

- A unique identifier for each record or questionnaire copy
- Identifiers and follow-up information
- Demographic information (age, sex, etc.)
- Outcome (disease or injury) as determined by the case definition
- Exposures
- Possible confounders

The desired outputs might include:

- Graph of case onset over time (Time)
- Map of cases by residence and/or workplace (Place)
- Tables of exposure by outcome (Person)

If the database design begins with a questionnaire, a series of questions is identified within each major section. These are usually given names that can also serve as field or variable names in the computer file-names, like First Name, Social Security Number, Diarrhea, and Potato Salad. Each of these can be developed into a question understandable to the subject or to the interviewer. Some, like Diarrhea, may require several questions (onset date and time, frequency, consistency, etc.) that may be summarized in a final yes/no conclusion for meeting the investigator's case definition of diarrhea.

In designing a questionnaire, it is useful to know what computer program will be used to enter and analyze the data. If Epi Info is used, the following computer terms will be useful in describing data entry and analysis.

A *field* or *variable* is one data item, such as first name or age. Usually Field is used to describe the blank in which data items are entered and Variable refers to the field name that may be manipulated later during analysis. A *record* is usually the information from one respondent to a questionnaire. Many records are stored together in a *file* or *table*. Epi Info for DOS data files end in **.rec** as in **data01.rec** and contain both data and a description of the questionnaire.

Epi Info for Windows records are stored in tables in Microsoft Access (.MDB) files. "Views" in Epi Info for Windows are separate tables containing a description of the questionnaire to be displayed on the screen. A file may be recalled for analysis or data entry, stored on floppy or hard disks, or copied from one disk to another. A file compression program such as WinZip can be used to compress files too big to fit on a single diskette, or a CD-ROM writer can be used to store larger files. The EpiLock program can be used to encrypt the file so that only those knowing the correct password can decrypt it.

In Epi Info, a field has a prompt or text question and a space for entering data. In Epi Info for DOS, the questions are typed into a text questionnaire in a word processor. In Epi Info for Windows, the MakeView program guides the design of a questionnaire through dialogues that appear after right-clicking a location on the screen. For each field, the dialogue requires a prompt and a field type, such as Text, Number, or Date. A variable name is created automatically after a question or prompt is supplied, but can be edited if desired.

Almost all data entry programs accept data of the specified type (e.g., numeric) and reject other entries (e.g., "Jones" in a numeric field). Many have sophisticated methods for evaluating entries and taking appropriate action to prevent erroneous entries. In Epi Info, for example, setting field properties or inserting commands in the Check Code scripting language for data entry allows specification of minima, maxima, legal codes, skip patterns, automatic coding, and copying of data from the preceding record. In Check Code command blocks, the user can set up more complex checks to issue an error message if a particular date precedes another date or a diagnostic code conflicts with the person's age or gender. Check Code can also be written to do mathematics or to call another program to perform complex calculations and put the results in other parts of the data entry form.

Complex checking on data entry has a cost in terms of setup time and skill required. During an outbreak investigation with Epi Info, most epidemiologists would insert a few checks, such as ranges or legal codes, and would tell the program to skip questions shown to be irrelevant by previous answers (e.g., skip the section on symptoms if the person was not ill). If several different people will be entering the data, it may be worth spending extra time to set up checks for consistency and acceptability, but this may be less necessary if one person enters all the data and the number of records is small enough to allow manual checking after entry.

In some situations, it is preferable to enter data directly into the computer rather than using paper forms first. Direct entry has been used in door-to-door survey work and for abstracting records in medical record rooms. In most outbreak investigations, however, a paper form will be used for interviews and the results will be transferred to a computer later, perhaps in a health department office or in a motel room with a portable or laptop computer. In the future it is likely that palmtop hand-held computers will expand the possibilities for direct data entry in the field.

There are several styles of questionnaire images that may be used on the computer screen. The first is a telegraphic or "keypuncher's" form. It consists of field names and data entry blanks only, arranged on the screen to allow the fastest possible entry by a person thoroughly acquainted with both the paper and the screen forms. Such a questionnaire might begin as follows:

Idnum ____
Name _____
Age __
Sex (M/F) __
County _____
Disease _____
Chicken (Y/N) ___
Ham (Y/N) ___
Beef (Y/N) ___

In spreadsheet format, such as used in Microsoft Excel or OpenOffice.org's spreadsheet facility:

Idnum Name Age Sex (M/F) County Disease Chicken (Y/N) Ham (Y/N)
Beef (Y/N)

The third style is an extended format offered by Epi Info that resembles the paper form as closely as possible, complete with headings, questions, instructions to the user, and blanks. With slight editing, the same form may be used in an actual interview. This format is most useful if there are relatively few questionnaires, if there are several people entering the data who do not have time to become "experts" on the data format (entering 100 questionnaires might produce an "expert"), or if those entering data will be frequently interrupted.

In Epi Info, either format may be used, according to the investigator's preference. With either form, the screen prompts can be more extensive than the brief name chosen for the variable to be manipulated during data analysis.

In using Epi Info and other programs, it is important to know how the program handles missing values before finalizing the questionnaire. Epi Info allows a missing value to be entered by pressing the <Enter> key to leave the field blank. Some programs record missing values as zero for numeric fields. In these programs the questions must be designed so that there is no confusion between a true code or value of zero and a missing value where this distinction is important. Zero glasses of water consumed and "unknown" glasses of water consumed, for example, are quite different, so a special code (often 9 or 99) should be assigned for the case of "unknown." Such codes are unnecessary in Epi Info and most current data entry programs, since missing data are stored as values distinct from zero.

In some investigations, particularly in research settings, it is useful to assign additional codes (e.g., 8's) to distinguish answers cited as "unknown" by the subject, those considered less accurate or unknown by the interviewer, and those somehow omitted during data entry. These extra codes can complicate the analysis considerably and should be assigned only after careful thought about the format of the table that will show the results. "Somebody might ask about it later" is not sufficient reason to burden the investigation with a series of extra codes unless they contribute meaningfully to the analysis. In a field investigation it is often sufficient to use only one kind of missing value, since the modest number of cases and rough-and-ready data-collection process may not permit analysis of bias that may have arisen due to more than one type of missing data.

To provide proper analysis of questions, codes should be assigned during data entry. Merely typing in the names of counties or diseases can result in a profusion of synonyms and misspellings that is impossible to analyze. Either numeric or text codes may be used. When producing tables during analysis, codes indicating the actual values are more useful than numeric codes, although numeric codes can be recoded to produce useful labels during analysis. Generally "Y" and "N" are less likely to produce errors in data entry than "0" and "1", and "URI" is more meaningful than "7002" for Upper Respiratory Infection.

A key issue in setting up data entry forms involves multiple-choice questions. The question:

How many glasses of water do you drink per day (choose one)?

0. None
1. 1–2
3. 3–4
5. 5 or more
9. Don't know
Water #

has five mutually exclusive answers including a blank entry, and the entire question, therefore, has a single answer. A one-digit numeric field called WATER is enough to record the answer.

Another type of question is:

What symptoms have you had in the past month?

1. Diarrhea
2. Fever
3. Chills

Note that all three symptoms might have been present. Each part of what looks like a single question requires a yes/no answer, and this question should be set up as follows:

What symptoms have you had in the past month?

Diarrhea <Y>
Fever <Y>
Chills <Y>

The same would be true of a list of foods possibly eaten at a meal. Each item is really a separate question, since the answers are not mutually exclusive. In the Analysis program in Epi Info, the first question is summarized with the command FREQ WATER, to display the codes for each level and the number of times each code is represented.

The symptom question is more complicated, however. By asking for a frequency distribution of the variable Diarrhea (FREQ DIARRHEA, in Epi Info), it is a simple matter to ascertain the number of persons with and without diarrhea. But discovering how many symptoms each person had takes more complex programming—complex enough so that it may be easier to add another summary question below the list of symptoms, such as "Number of symptoms," if this is important for the analysis. The person entering data can quickly scan the paper form, count symptoms, and enter this number rather than requiring the investigator to do extra programming during the analysis stage. The trade-off between intelligent data consolidation during data entry and having the computer do the work is evident at many points during the design of computer entry forms and paper questionnaires. If you will be using both, consider simplifying as much as possible the data transferred to the computer from the paper form. Names, addresses, and other follow-up information may be omitted, and complex case definitions may be summarized with a single yes/no question. Field investigation usually results in scores or hundreds of questionnaires, and the human mind and eye may be a simpler processing alternative for some kinds of questions than having a busy investigator with modest computer skills try to write a program to condense the data electronically.

In the end, the investigator must decide what to collect, how much of a completed questionnaire to process by hand, and in what form to code it for computer use. Although experience plays a major role, pilot testing can be a good substitute. A pilot test might consist of entering data from five or six instances of a questionnaire (preferably from people who will not be included in the final study). These are then processed to produce a model for the final analysis, saving the program that results. This procedure will often reveal gaps, inconsistencies, or ambiguities in the questionnaire and point out questions that do not contribute to the analysis, and is almost guaranteed to improve the final questionnaire design. Before finalizing the design, the investigator should examine each question with the additional questions, "What do I really want to know? " and "How am I going to process this variable?"

## DATA ENTRY AND VALIDATION

Usually paper questionnaires from the field are far from ready for analysis after data entry. They contain misspellings, synonyms, abbreviations, upper/lower case mixtures, marginal notes, and missing data. Data entry is an opportunity for partial "cleaning" of the data set. It must be done with scrupulous dedication to preventing bias—the kind that could insert data favorable to a hypothesis or eliminate items detrimental to it. Since field investigations seldom have the luxury of "blind" coders and data entry personnel, only strict and literal attention to accuracy can prevent bias.

It is a good idea to alternate case and control forms during data entry to avoid bias from the small decisions and adaptations that occur during the course of entering forms. If there is more than one data entry person, each should enter the same ratio of case to control forms.

In most data entry systems, including Epi Info, a cursor on the screen indicates where entry will occur. The cursor jumps automatically from field to field. When an entry is made, the item is checked for correct type (numeric, date, etc.) and additional checks programmed into the check file are performed. If a problem is encountered, the program indicates this and waits for correction before going on to the next field. At the end of each questionnaire, the record is saved automatically or by answering an explicit question such as "Save data to disk? (Y/N)". In Epi Info, a power failure (or someone tripping over the power cord) will not result in loss of records already saved, although the partial record being entered may have to be reentered. If other programs do not have this feature, save your work frequently. It is a good idea to mark each paper questionnaire as data entry is completed to avoid accidental reentry.

When all records have been entered, the entries should be carefully validated to be sure that they represent the source documents accurately. One person can read the data entered aloud while the other verifies that the entries represent the source document accurately.

Further checking may be done by performing frequencies on each field. FREQ * will accomplish this in Epi Info. Examining the results will often disclose outliers such as "*Gf!" that crept in during a moment of distraction. These may be edited in the data entry program before beginning the actual analysis.

Some investigators prefer to have the same set of questionnaires entered in duplicate by two different operators in separate files. The two files are then compared, and differences are reconciled by a person authorized to make data entry decisions. Programs for making the comparison are included with Epi Info.

At intervals during data entry and after it is completed, backup copies should be made and stored in a secure place away from the original computer. Placing encrypted copies in a file storage facility on the Internet will offer additional security.

## ANALYSIS OF DATA IN FIELD EPIDEMIOLOGY

Analysis of a descriptive study or survey usually begins with a simple frequency for each variable (in Epi Info, FREQ *). Then, for a study with two or more groups, such as cases and controls, ill and well, exposed and unexposed, you would want to compare the two groups. For categorical (coded) data the TABLES command in Epi Info, for example TABLES * ILL, will produce cross-tabulations of each variable by illness status (Y/N), with appropriate statistics for each.

Often in a case-control or cross-sectional study, a histogram or epidemic curve is needed. In Epi Info, the case group would first be selected before doing the histogram, for example, SELECT CASE = "Y." The histogram might be performed with: HISTOGRAM ONSETDATE. Continuous variables such as age or diastolic blood pressure are analyzed with the MEANS command, for example, MEANS SBP ILL if SBP is systolic blood pressure and ILL is case status.

In most analytic programs it is necessary to use names of variables to do an analysis. Unlike algebraic notation, computer programs usually allow a descriptive name for each field. In some programs the length of these names is limited to, for example, 8 or 10 characters. If transfer of data from one program to another is contemplated, be sure that variable names truncated to the length allowed in the most restrictive program are unique. For example, "ADDRESSLINE1" and "ADDRESSLINE2" might both emerge as ADDRESSLIN in a program with variable names limited to 10 characters. "ADDRESS1" and "ADDRESS2" would survive truncation to eight characters, however. Many programs will object to names beginning with a number.

After doing frequencies for each field, you will have an idea of how many records are in each group, and how many missing values there are for each field. If missing values are displayed, many of the tables may be three-by-three rather than two-by-two tables, and the statistics that result are not as complete as those that accompany two-by-two tables. Some packages allow you to suppress missing values (in Epi Info, with the SET command). Repeating the analysis after giving this command will omit the missing values and focus the analysis solely on records that have data for the tables and frequencies being produced. Two-by-two tables in Epi Info are automatically accompanied by chi-square tests, odds ratios, risk ratios, confidence limits, and Fisher and mid-P exact tests.

Often one or more "significant" findings may be indicated by $p$ values less than 0.05 or confidence limits that exclude 1.0 for odds ratios or risk ratios. Further analysis to consider confounding variables is indicated, at least for frequent confounders such as age and sex. This is done by stratifying the table of interest (say SALAD by ILL), producing a separate table for each value of the confounder.

In Epi Info, the crude table is produced by TABLES SALAD ILL and stratification by sex by TABLES SALAD ILL SEX to produce separate tables for males and females. The Mantel-Haenszel summary chi-square and $p$-value for the stratified result may be compared with the results of the crude analysis. If the odds ratios in the two or more strata are similar, interaction is not present, and a difference in the crude and Mantel-Haenszel odds ratios may be taken as an indication that sex was a confounder. Other potential confounders such as age, socioeconomic status, etc., can be evaluated similarly, either one by one or in combination (TABLES SALAD ILL SEX RACE).

Stratification does not work well for small data sets if there are many strata, and variables such as age may need to be recoded to produce fewer strata, such as

CHILD and ADULT, rather than a number of age groups. Examples of data manipulation, including automation of a complex case definition, are included in the *Epi Info for DOS* manual in a chapter on epidemic investigation.

At this point the analysis may be complete enough for field purposes, if confounding has been identified and eliminated through stratification, and interaction has been addressed (perhaps recording the results for more than one stratum rather than the overall results, as in "For people up to the age of 18, the effect was_____ . . .; those over 18 did not react the same way."). The significant findings must be evaluated from a biomedical point of view and distributed to interested parties.

Graphing important findings may be helpful in visualizing or explaining results, particularly those pertaining to temporal variables. Epi Info offers bar, histogram, pie, scatter, and line graphs. Two variables are required for scatter graphs, and one variable for other formats. A second variable can be represented by plotting a separate graph for each of its values, as in showing date of onset in separate histograms for males and females, for example.

In cases where there are several significant risk factors or several confounders, logistic regression may be helpful. Logistic regression is offered as part of Epi Info, and a number of other programs are available for this purpose after exporting data from Epi Info.

## GEOGRAPHIC INFORMATION SYSTEMS AND THE ANALYSIS OF "PLACE"

In some outbreaks, the place of residence, work, visitation, food or water consumption, or aerosol inhalation is important in the analysis. Geographic Information Systems (GIS) are used to link database information with maps or other graphics to provide opportunities for spatial analysis. Locations can be recorded in variables such as city, state, mail code, or census tract. Exact locations can also be recorded as longitude and latitude, obtained through geocoding or from field measurements with a hand-held geographic position sensor (GPS). *Geocoding* means obtaining exact longitude and latitude coordinates from street addresses or other location information. It is done through the use of special geocoding databases or services available commercially or provided on the Internet.

One or more geographic variables must match the geographic information in the "map," called a *boundary file* in Epi Info 6 and Epi Map for DOS, and a *shape file* in Epi Info/EpiMap for Windows. City names must be spelled the same way in both data sets, for example, or point coordinates must be in the same units, such as latitude/longitude in decimal degrees. The GIS software combines the map image with the database to show locations as colors, patterns, dots, or other symbols that represent spatial information. An entire science has developed around the analysis of geographic information, but the basic operations can be performed in Epi Info for Windows with the Epi Map program, and refined if necessary in dedicated GIS software. S.B. Eng describes the use of dot maps in investigating an outbreak.[2] Epi Info uses software produced by the makers of ArcView (Environmental Systems Research Institute, Inc., www.esri.com) so that maps can be displayed by either system.

## OBTAINING AND USING EXISTING COMPUTERIZED DATA

Sometimes useful computerized information already exists at the site of an investigation. For example, hospital computer systems may have laboratory values, diagnostic information, or operative schedules; a water treatment plant may have results of water analysis. Such files may contain more information than is relevant and may be in a variety of file formats. Selection of relevant information can be done by the person managing the data system. If you specify a time period or category of record to be selected, it may be relatively easy for the data manager to create a file containing only the desired items, perhaps with only certain fields represented.

The file format is also important. Most computerized database and statistics programs, including Epi Info, will accept an ASCII file in fixed-field format. This means that only the first 128 standard characters are included, and each line represents a different record. A field is distinguished by its position on the line and either occupies a fixed number of characters or is terminated by a comma or other delimiter. It is important to obtain a list of the fields, their types and length, and the delimiter(s) used.

Epi Info for DOS will analyze files in the DBASE format directly and will import files in the Lotus 1-2-3, comma-delimited, DBASE, and fixed-field ASCII formats with a program called Import. The Analysis program in Epi Info will read and analyze files in more than 20 different formats and can write files in these same formats, allowing for extremely flexible data conversion.

Whenever external files of any kind are copied, the source disk should first be checked for computer viruses with a suitable program, no matter how reputable the supplier of the data. Reference data such as telephone lists or the Epi Info manual may be carried to the field as files on CD-ROMs or the computer's hard disk, so that heavier paper copies are not needed.

## COMPUTER COMMUNICATIONS

A computer equipped with a wireless connection, an Ethernet connection to a local network, or a modem can be used to send files of any type to another computer or the Internet. In many parts of the world, Internet access is available for modest charges in Internet cafés. If available, the Internet provides not only facilities for e-mail but also access to searches, guidelines, textbooks, calculators, reference data, and information (of variable quality) on almost any conceivable subject. J. Woodall provides a review of the use of computer networking in investigating disease outbreaks, with particular reference to biological and toxic weapon use.[3]

It is not always easy to connect a portable computer to a telephone line, as many businesses and hotels have digital telephones that do not work with standard types of modems. Hotels increasingly have made special provisions for wireless (Wi-Fi) connections or fast Internet by cable connection, and asking about these facilities in advance is a good idea before traveling to a field site.

## OBTAINING INFORMATION FROM THE WORLD ELECTRONIC AND PRINT LITERATURE WHILE IN THE FIELD

Unless the investigator is a specialist in the type of problem being investigated, bibliographic searching may be of great importance. The MEDLARS database of the National Library of Medicine is the most comprehensive source of medical and public health information. It contains references and often abstracts describing millions of articles in thousands of biomedical journals. Searches can be performed free of charge at the National Library of Medicine portal http://gateway.nlm.nih.gov/gw/Cmd or at other sites that allow MEDLARS searches.

The website www.google.com provides free-text searching, returning first the references most heavily cited by others, thus filtering out much of the chaff from billions of possibilities. Other search engines, such as www.yahoo.com, provide classification hierarchies that may be better for reviewing a systematic field of knowledge. In either case, the Internet is becoming more and more a reflection of the state of the world and of both episodic and cumulative information that cannot be ignored. A quick search of the Internet is often a practical way to obtain a grasp on a new field, such as air handling, plumbing, laws, lay medical advice, organizations dealing with relevant problems, and even telephone numbers or methods of locating people.

Most computer products are supported by websites, including Epi Info, and it is possible to download a free copy of Epi Info, or an update, from www.cdc.gov/epiinfo/. Many hardware companies such as printer manufacturers provide free downloads of current drivers for their products. Many statistical calculators can be accessed from www.openepi.com and the links it provides to other sites. Maps in great detail are available for downloading, and Epi Info contains an on-line reference chapter with links to hundreds of sites that provide resources for mapping.

## OBTAINING TECHNICAL ASSISTANCE DURING A FIELD INVESTIGATION

Occasionally a computer problem arises in the field that requires more expertise than the investigator possesses. Computer breakdowns, unfamiliar file formats, access to special printers or other equipment, and difficulties with telephone connections may all require assistance. Technical expertise is available in most communities from a variety of sources. If calling your home base support staff does not solve a problem, a search of local health departments, technical schools, computer stores, and computer clubs may lead to a person with the necessary knowledge or piece of equipment. The Internet and e-mail provide sources of information that can be accessed at any hour of the day or night because of the differences in time zones. Googling for information with words from error messages or your own description of the problem frequently turns up others who have met and conquered the problem.

## COMPUTER VIRUSES AND DATA BACKUP

There is little satisfaction in having written a book whose only manuscript was lost in a fire. Similarly, proper backup of computer data is essential. Whatever can go wrong should be expected to do so—perhaps more than once. In the past few years computer viruses have been added to the list of things that can go wrong, but they are only an additional cause for careful backup procedures that already were necessary to protect against hard disk crashes, power outages, theft, and late-night human errors.

Computer viruses are becoming more and more prevalent. They cause a variety of problems, but the most serious destroy all data on disks used in a particular computer. They may be acquired from a source outside a previously uninfected computer, either by copying files or through communication with another system.

Commercial programs are available to detect and often remove these viruses, and one of these should be used to check all disks inserted into the computer before copying any files, processing data, or running programs. A suitable virus protection program should be active at all times in a computer, and special care should be taken to check diskettes that may have been in other computers and become infected. Portable computers are attractive to thieves, and their hard disks—like all hard disks—may "crash," making data difficult or impossible to recover. More than one floppy disk or CD-ROM copy of all data should be made on a regular basis, and the backups should be carefully stored in places separate from the computer itself, to rule out the possibility of complete loss from theft, carelessness, or fire. Several well-verified disks, traveling by different routes, mailed home, and/or stored with different people are the best backup system. New backups should be made at intervals, perhaps every hour or two during data entry. It is also useful to have CD-ROM copies of important software in case a hard disk must be replaced in the field. As described in a previous section, Internet file storage facilities can be used for off-site backup if the files are first encrypted to protect confidentiality.

Generally in a field investigation it is practical to give new names to each new set of backup files so previous files are not written over. If anything goes wrong with a current file or disk, the previous set of files may provide a good copy of most of the data set. Although good commercial programs are available for backing up hard disks, they are usually not necessary in field investigations, since the data files are usually small. The files may simply be copied to external storage media, maintaining several such carefully labeled disks to be used in sequence.

When things go wrong, a frequent reaction is to make the problem worse through panic. If difficulties in recovering files are experienced, first obtain technical help in diagnosing the problem. If you decide to restore files from the backup disks, be sure that the WRITE-PROTECT function (see previous section) is set on these disks to avoid having the backups destroyed by a virus or faulty procedure. If files have been accidentally erased on the hard disk, it is important to avoid entering further records or copying files until an attempt has been made to recover the lost files. Programs such as Norton Utilities can restore erased files and repair many corrupted files if they have not been written over by further manipulations.

## DATA CONFIDENTIALITY AND LEGAL ISSUES

Maintaining confidentiality of data on a portable computer is similar to protecting a stack of questionnaires. The best protection is through maintaining careful physical custody of any disks containing data, including the internal hard disk of the computer. With small data sets, files can be kept on floppy disks so the hard disk does not contain confidential data. In many investigations, names and addresses are not needed in data files, and such data should not be entered unless it is absolutely necessary. Arbitrary identification numbers are adequate for most computerized data sets. Frequently names and other identifiers may be left with the local health department and only code-identified data transported to a more central site. Encryption programs or compression programs with password protection should be used to protect data in case CD-ROMs or diskettes are stolen, lost in the mail, or the computer itself is stolen. A program for 128-bit encryption is provided with Epi Info as the utility EpiLock. If the password used for encryption is lost, however, the encrypted file cannot be recovered, so adequate password management is essential.

Occasionally outbreaks lead to legal proceedings for negligence or even homicide. Records of the investigation may be subpoenaed or otherwise required for legal purposes. This possibility and scientific documentation make it important to keep good records of the investigation and to store them in such a way that they can be accessed by appropriate parties even if the investigator moves on to another job. Analytic programs may be written with comments explaining important steps, which also facilitates reuse of the programs in another investigation.

Computer disks should be carefully labeled, and after the investigation stored in an organized way so others can access the files. Paper copies of the data may be made for permanent documentation and ease of filing, since computer disks lose their magnetic data after a few years and for archival purposes should be copied to new disks annually or stored on CD-ROMs.

## THE FUTURE OF COMPUTERS IN EPIDEMIOLOGIC FIELD INVESTIGATION

Future computers for field investigation will be smaller, lighter, and more powerful. Soon both voice and handwritten input will be practical. Medical and other records will be computerized to a greater extent, offering opportunities for capturing relevant information in detail for the investigator with the skills and tools to convert data from diverse formats. Eventually, perhaps, better programs will alleviate some of the compatibility problems between various types of software, but the competitive marketplace will ensure that other types of incompatibility arise. Palmtop computers will extend direct data collection to environments such as earthquake sites, the bedside, or other field locations, and digital cameras will find more use in documentation.

The Internet has begun the process of providing access to the entire world from a portable computer as though all the world's resources resided on a single hard disk ("in the cloud"). Current Internet sites offer storage of files, document and spreadsheet sharing, statistical calculations, and many other functions that are independent of computer brand or operating system and accessible anywhere there is an Internet connection. Search capabilities are used, not only for bibliographical purposes, but through access to news articles, as a way of monitoring (for example) influenza activity. Actual investigations may be carried out via the Internet, as many have already been conducted or aided by e-mail communication.[4] There is a growing field of computer forensics dealing with the investigation of computer crime, computer viruses, and corporate malfeasance.

Like most aspects of field investigation, computer use will continue to require ingenuity and adaptation. Those who have acquired the skills for using a portable computer, however, will find that the rewards in quantity and quality of epidemiologic work accomplished make it an indispensable companion in field investigation, and that the communication and information access offered by the Internet are becoming more and more central to the epidemiologic process.

## REFERENCES

*Note*: References to Internet addresses supplied in the text may change but can usually be recovered by searching for the topic of interest or a trade name with an Internet search engine.

1. PC Plus: http://www.pcplus.co.uk/news/home_news/microsoft_windows_22_of_copies_ are_bogus. Accessed April 10, 2008.
2. Eng, S.B., Werker, D.H., King, A.S., et al. (1999). Computer-generated dot maps as an epidemiologic tool investigating an outbreak of toxoplasmosis. *Emerg Infect Dis* 5(6), 815–9.
3. Woodall, J. (1998). The role of computer networking in investigating unusual disease outbreaks and allegations of biological and toxin weapons use. *Crit Rev Microbiol* 24(3), 255–72.
4. Kuusi, M., Nuorti, J.P., Maunula, L., et al. (2004). Internet use and epidemiologic investigation of gastroenteritis outbreak. *Emerg Infect Dis* [serial online] 2004 Mar, Accessed April 10, 2008. Available from: http://www.cdc.gov/ncidod/EID/vol10no2/02-0607.htm

## FURTHER READING

Beck-Sague, C., Jarvis, W.R., Martone, W.J. (1997). Outbreak investigations. *Infect Control Hosp Epidemiol* 18, 138–45.
Dean, A.G., Arner, T.G., Sangam, S., et al. (2002). Epi Info 2002, a database and statistics program for public health professionals for use on Windows 95, 98, NT, 2000, ME, and XP computers. Centers for Disease Control and Prevention, Atlanta. (Can be downloaded from www.cdc.gov/epiinfo/).
Dean, A.G., Dean, J.A., Burton, A.H., et al. (1991). Epi Info: a general-purpose microcomputer program for public health information systems. *Am J Prev Med* 7(3), 178–82.
Epidemiologic Case Studies. Available from: http://www.cdc.gov/epiinfo/tutorials/ and http://www.epiinformatics.com/.
Gerstman, B.B. (2000). Data analysis with Epi Info. http://www.sjsu.edu/faculty/gerstman/ EpiInfo/.
Zubieta, J.C., Skinner, R., Dean, A.G. (2003). Initiating informatics and GIS support for a field investigation of bioterrorism: the New Jersey anthrax experience. *Int J Health Geogr* 2, 8. Published online 2003 November 16. http://www.ij-healthgeographics.com/content/ 2/1/8. Accessed April 10, 2008.

# 8

# DESIGNING STUDIES IN THE FIELD

Richard C. Dicker

Many clusters and even outbreaks of disease are investigated by local health department staff by focusing on information about the cases, sometimes with supplemental laboratory and environmental information. For some outbreaks, this approach is sufficient to identify the source and/or determine whether others remain at risk. Sometimes, however, this approach is insufficient. After all, the fact that an exposure is shared by many cases does not necessarily mean that that exposure is the source. For example, all of the football players on a professional team who developed methicillin-resistant *Staphylococcus aureus* skin infections breathed the air in the stadium, but air is not likely to be the source. Sometimes the cases have numerous different exposures in common, as is typical in an outbreak of gastroenteritis associated with a banquet or pot-luck dinner. Or perhaps many of the cases report a particular exposure, but investigators are uncertain just how common that exposure is in that population. Perhaps residents are concerned that the number of cases of cancer in a community is "too many." In these situations, an epidemiologic study (also called an analytic study) of some sort is called for.

The objective of most epidemiologic studies is to determine whether a particular exposure (or which exposure) is associated with the disease of interest. The way epidemiologic studies accomplish this objective is by enrolling and comparing two groups—an index group and a comparison group. The first group is either a group of ill persons or a group of people with a particular exposure. If the index group comprises ill persons ("cases" or "case-patients"), then the comparison group comprises those who did not become ill ("controls"). If the index group comprises exposed persons, then the comparison group is made up of people who were not exposed. In this way the epidemiologic study is like a biostatistical test that compares *observed* and *expected* values—the ill or exposed group provides the observed data, while the healthy or unexposed comparison group provides the baseline or expected data. When the data from these two groups are similar; i.e., exposure among cases or disease incidence among exposed persons is about what one would expect, then one can conclude that exposure and disease are unrelated. If however, exposure or disease incidence is substantially higher than expected, then one would conclude that exposure is indeed associated with disease, and further study and/or public health action is warranted.

The gold standard for an epidemiologic study is an experimental study. In public health, experimental studies usually take the form of randomized clinical or community trials. For example, a randomized clinical trial may be conducted in which children are randomly assigned to either the experimental vaccine or the placebo group to assess whether the vaccine reduces the incidence of disease. Or people with a particular disease may be enrolled and randomly assigned to a new antibiotic or "usual care" group. However, in practice, only a few field epidemiologists conduct such experimental studies. For the types of problems that health departments commonly face, epidemiologists do not randomly assign people to eat the undercooked ground beef or not, or have sexual intercourse with someone infected with human immunodeficiency virus or not. Almost always, the exposures have already occurred through genetics, circumstance, or choice.

As a result, almost all studies conducted by field epidemiologists are observational studies, in which the epidemiologists document rather than determine exposures.

The two most common types of observational studies conducted by field epidemiologists are cohort studies and case control studies. Conceptually, a *cohort study*, like an experimental study, begins with exposure and looks for differences in disease incidence among different exposure groups. In a *case control study*, enrollment is based on the presence ("case") or absence ("control") of disease, and the frequency of exposures is compared between the cases and controls. Each type of study has its strengths and limitations, but each has an important place in field investigations.

This chapter provides an overview of these two study designs, emphasizing methodological considerations in the field. For more in-depth discussion of the theory and other features of study design, the reader is referred to other epidemiology texts.[1-3]

## DEFINING EXPOSURE GROUPS

Because both cohort and case control studies are used to quantify the relationship between exposure and disease, defining what is meant by "exposure" and "disease" is critical. In general, the term *exposure* is used quite broadly, meaning demographic characteristics, genetic or immunologic makeup, behaviors, environmental exposures, and other factors that might influence one's risk of disease.

Since precise exposure information is essential for accurately estimating an exposure's effect on disease, exposure measures should be as objective and standard as possible. For an exposure that is a relatively discrete event or characteristic, developing a measure of exposure can be conceptually straightforward—for example, whether a person ate the Greek salad at Restaurant A during the last week or whether a person has received influenza vaccine this year. While these exposures may be straightforward in theory, they may be subject to interpretation in practice. Should the husband who ate one olive from his wife's Greek salad be labeled as "exposed" or "unexposed"? Whatever decision is made should be documented and applied consistently.

In addition, many exposures are subject to the whims of memory. Memory aids, such as Restaurant A's menu, and exposure documentation, such as a vaccination card or evidence of vaccination in the patient's medical record, may help in these situations.

Some exposures can be further characterized by dose or duration, such as the number of glasses of apple cider or number of years working in a coal mine. A pathogen may require a minimum (threshold) level of exposure to cause disease and may be more likely to cause disease with increasing exposures. The disease may require prolonged exposure or have a long latency or incubation period. These relationships may be missed by characterizing exposure simply as "yes" or "no." Similarly, the vehicle of infection, for example, may be a component or ingredient of other measured exposures. One could then create a composite measure, such as whether a person ate any item with mayonnaise as an ingredient.

Some exposures are subtle or difficult to quantify. Surrogate measures may be used (census track or level of education as a surrogate for socioeconomic status, which in turn may be a surrogate for access to health care, adequacy of housing, nutritional status, etc.), but should be interpreted with caution.

## DEFINING OUTCOMES ("CASE DEFINITION")

A *case definition* is a set of standard criteria for deciding whether an individual should be classified as having the health condition of interest. Employment of a case definition ensures uniformity of case classification because every case must meet the same criteria. In addition, for an epidemiologic study, a well-conceived case definition helps reduce bias from misclassification of the outcome by ensuring that those classified as cases truly have the disease of interest.

A case definition consists of clinical criteria and, particularly in the setting of an outbreak investigation, certain restrictions on time, place, and person. The clinical criteria may include confirmatory laboratory tests, if available, or combinations of symptoms, signs, and other findings. In general the criteria should be kept simple and objective—for example, the presence of elevated antibody titers, three or more loose bowel movements per day, illness severe enough to require hospitalization, or primary hospital discharge diagnosis of ICD-10 code J09–J18. The case definition may be restricted by time (e.g., to persons with onset of illness within the past two months), by place (e.g., to employees at a particular manufacturing plant or to residents of a town), and by person (e.g., to persons who had previously tested negative for chlamydia or to children at least nine months old). Whatever the criteria, they must be applied consistently and without bias to all persons under investigation to ensure that persons with illness are characterized consistently over time, locale, and clinical practice.

In general, the case definition for an epidemiologic study should not include the exposure of interest. The purpose of the epidemiologic study is to determine whether the exposure is associated with the disease. If exposure is included in the case definition, all cases will have been exposed, so that exposure will appear to be associated with disease even if, in actuality, it is not.

A case definition can have degrees of certainty, such as a suspected case (usually based on clinical and sometimes epidemiologic criteria) versus a confirmed case (based on laboratory confirmation). For example, during an outbreak of measles, a person with fever and rash is categorized as having a suspected, probable, or confirmed case of measles, depending on the absence or presence of laboratory and epidemiologic evidence. Sometimes a case is temporarily classified as suspected or probable while awaiting laboratory results. Depending on the lab results, the case will be reclassified as either confirmed or "not a case." In the midst of a large outbreak of a disease caused by a known agent, some cases may be permanently classified as suspected or probable because investigators may feel that running laboratory tests on every patient with a consistent clinical picture and a history of exposure (e.g., varicella) is unnecessary or even wasteful. Use of positive laboratory culture results for a case definition in the absence of symptoms should be weighed carefully. On one hand, organisms can sometimes be present without causing disease. On the other hand, infection can by asymptomatic, and persons with asymptomatic infections, if identified, should be considered cases, not controls.

The case definition may also vary depending on the purpose. For case finding in a local area, the case definition should be relatively sensitive or inclusive to capture as many potential cases as possible. However, for enrolling persons into an epidemiologic study to identify risk factors, a relatively specific or narrow case definition will minimize misclassification and bias.

For an epidemiologic study, a definition for controls can be just as important as the definition for cases. Controls should be persons who do not have the disease in question. The difficulty arises with people who have mild or asymptomatic cases of the disease. If these people are enrolled as controls, then the control group includes people who are really cases. This misclassification is a type of bias, resulting in less difference in exposure between the cases and the controls than there ought to be. To the extent possible, mild and asymptomatic cases should not be included as controls, although testing of such persons is uncommon. Nonetheless, when testing of the control group is possible, doing so may be helpful in reducing bias. For example, in a study of a cluster of thyrotoxicosis, a surprise finding was that 75% of asymptomatic family members of cases also had elevated thyroid function test results.[4] Had these family members been enrolled as controls, the epidemiologic study would not have identified a difference in exposure between cases and controls, and the association with consumption of locally produced ground beef that inadvertently included bits of thyroid gland would have been missed.

## COHORT STUDIES

In concept, a cohort study, like an experimental study, begins with a group of persons without the disease under study but with different exposure experiences, and follows them over time to find out if they develop disease or a health condition of interest. In a cohort study, though, each person's exposure status is merely recorded rather than assigned randomly by the investigator. Then the occurrence of disease among persons with different exposures is compared to assess whether the exposures are associated with increased risk of disease.

A cohort study sometimes begins by enrolling everyone in a population regardless of exposure status, then characterizing each person's exposure status after enrollment. Alternatively, a sample rather than the whole population could be enrolled. The enrollees are then followed over time for occurrence of the disease(s) of interest. Incidence of disease by exposure status is compared. The unexposed or lowest-exposure group serves as the comparison group, providing an estimate of the baseline or expect amount of disease. If the incidence of disease is substantially different in the exposed group than in the unexposed group, the exposure is said to be associated with disease.

The type of cohort just described, with participants being enrolled then followed prospectively over time to document occurrence of the outcome of interest, is called a *prospective* or *follow-up* study. In a prospective cohort study, enrollment takes place before the occurrence of disease. In fact, any potential subject who is found to have the disease at enrollment should be excluded. Thus each subsequently identified case is an *incident* case. Incidence may be quantified as the number of cases divided by the sum of time each person was followed (*incidence rate*), or as the number of cases divided by the number of persons being followed (*attack rate* or *risk* or *incidence proportion*).

The length of follow-up can vary considerably. Many epidemiologic studies conducted by public health departments are done in response to a current public health concern, so the duration of the studies tends to be relatively brief. On the other hand, research and academic institutions are more likely to conduct studies of cancer, cardiovascular disease, and other chronic diseases; their follow-up may last for years and even decades. Of course, maintaining follow-up that is as complete as possible and comparable for each exposure group is a major challenge for prospective studies. Examples of well-conducted prospective cohort studies that have spanned many years include the Framingham Study, a study of cardiovascular disease among over 5,000 residents of Framingham, Massachusetts,[5] and the Nurses' Health Studies, a pair of studies of the effects of oral contraceptives, diet, and lifestyle risk factors among over 100,000 nurses.[6]

Note that, for a prospective study, disease should not have already occurred. Therefore, in field epidemiology, a prospective study is only likely to be conducted after a known exposure has occurred and the illness of concern has a long incubation or latency period. Examples include the follow-up studies of survivors of the atomic bomb dropped on Hiroshima in 1945,[7] and of the attack on the World Trade Center on September 11, 2001.[8]

While many cohort studies enroll all members of a group and then determine exposure, cohort studies can also begin with the enrollment of persons based on their exposure status. In this type of cohort study, two or more groups defined by their exposure status are enrolled. For example, to determine whether U.S. military service in Vietnam in the 1960s and 1970s would be associated with greater long-term mortality than expected, investigators enrolled and followed one ("exposed") group of 9,324 U.S. Army veterans who served in Vietnam and a comparable ("unexposed") group of 8,989 Vietnam-era Army veterans who served in Korea, Germany, or the United States.[9, 10]

As noted earlier, in a prospective study, anyone who already has the disease at the time the study begins is excluded from the study. However, many times, a number of people from some well-defined population—persons who attended a banquet, students at a school, workers in a particular industry—have gotten sick, and the responsible public health agency must conduct a study to determine what caused the illness. Under those circumstances, the agency may decide to conduct a *retrospective cohort study*, a study in which all members of a group are enrolled after disease has already occurred. Investigators then elicit exposure histories, and calculate and compare disease incidence for different exposures.

Consider, for example, the archetypal outbreak of gastroenteritis after a church picnic. Typically, investigators can obtain a list of attendees; solicit information on attendees' food exposures and subsequent illness, if any; calculate attack rates for those who did or did not eat each food; and compare those attack rates to identify the food associated with the greatest increase in risk. This *retrospective* cohort type of study is the technique of choice for an acute outbreak in a well-defined population, particularly one for which a roster of names and contact information such as telephone numbers are available. Examples include not only the church picnic for which membership lists are available but also weddings, company banquets, cruise ships, nursing homes, and schools. Retrospective cohort studies can also be used in a noninfectious disease context and are popular in occupational epidemiology. For example, a list of persons exposed to a work-site hazard years ago or over many years (e.g., welders) and a comparable group not exposed (e.g., non-welders from the same manufacturing plants) are constructed from available employment records, and the morbidity or mortality of the two groups is determined and compared.[11] However, when illness has occurred but the population from which the cases came is not well circumscribed, a retrospective cohort study is not a practical approach. The most expedient and scientifically sound way to address that situation is to use a case control study (see Appendix).

## CASE CONTROL STUDIES

In field epidemiology, a case control study is usually conducted when a cohort study is impractical, particularly when the population from which the cases came is not well defined. Whereas a cohort study proceeds conceptually from exposure to disease, a case control study begins conceptually with disease and looks backward at prior exposures. Specifically, in a case control study, a group of people with the disease of interest (cases or case-patients) and an appropriate group of people without disease (controls) are enrolled, and their prior exposures are ascertained. The case group represents the "observed" level of exposure, while the control group is needed to provide the "expected level" of exposure. Differences in exposure between the two groups indicate that the disease is associated with the exposure.

### Selection of Subjects

The case control study begins with the identification of cases and the selection of controls. In a typical case control study under field conditions, cases are identified through surveillance and additional case-finding efforts. An appropriate control group that represents the population the cases came from can then be determined and enrolled.

The cases in a case control study must meet the case definition; that is, they must have the disease in question. The case definition must be independent of the exposure(s) under study. Ideally, the cases will be limited to new or incident cases rather than prevalent cases, so that the study does not confuse factors associated with disease occurrence with those associated with survival. Whereas the case definition used for case-finding is often broad and inclusive enough to capture as many cases as possible, the case definition for a case control study should be relatively narrow or specific. A specific case definition ensures that enrollees in the case group truly have the disease in question, thus minimizing selection bias from misclassifying non-cases as cases.

A comparable group of controls must be identified and enrolled. While this statement is simple, debates about the selection of controls can be among the most complex in epidemiology.[1, 12] The controls should not have the disease in question and, like the cases, should be chosen independently of exposure. As a general rule, the controls should be representative of the population from which the cases arose, so that if a control had developed the disease, he or she would have been included as a case in the study. Suppose the cases are persons with community-acquired pneumonia admitted to a single hospital during the past month. The controls should be persons who would have been admitted to the same hospital if they had developed the disease during the same period. This condition helps ensure comparability between cases and controls, since persons admitted to a different hospital might reflect a different population with a variety of different host characteristics and other exposures that may affect their risk of disease. Commonly, controls for hospital-based cases are selected from the group of patients admitted to the same hospital, but with diagnoses other than the case-defining illness. Similarly, cases diagnosed in the outpatient setting are often compared to controls from the same clinical practices. Non-hospitalized cases scattered throughout a community should be compared with community-based controls.

Controls should be free of the disease under study. This underscores the importance of both the case definition and the control definition in distinguishing persons who have the disease from those who do not. In some studies, controls are required to have laboratory or other confirmation that they are disease-free. In other studies, lack of symptoms and signs of illness are presumed to indicate absence of disease. However, the stricter the definition of the controls, the less opportunity for misclassification and bias from enrolling someone with mild or asymptomatic disease as a control.

Consider the thyrotoxicosis outbreak mentioned earlier, with about 75% of asymptomatic family members with elevated thyroid function tests because they ate the same contaminated ground beef as the cases.[4] Had the investigators not tested the family members, and had the family members thus been included in the control group, they would have had exposures similar to the cases, making the exposure–disease association virtually impossible to identify.

In general, controls should be at risk for the disease. While this can be challenged on academic grounds, the assertion has face validity and needs little justification. For example, in a case control study of risk factors for uterine cancer, most epidemiologists would not include men in the control group. While men might adequately represent the distribution of A-B-O blood groups in the population, they surely would represent an inappropriate estimate of the "expected" levels of sexual activity, contraceptive choices, and the like.

Sometimes the choice of a control group is so vexing that investigators decide to use more than one type of control group. For example, in a study where the cases are persons hospitalized with West Nile encephalitis, investigators might choose to use both a hospital-based control group (since only a minority of persons with West Nile infection require hospitalization and are the cases most easily found) and a community-based control group. If the two control groups provide similar results and conclusions about risk factors for West Nile infection, then the credibility of the findings is increased. On the other hand, if the two control groups yield conflicting results, then interpretation becomes more difficult.

## Sources of Controls

Controls come from a variety of sources, each with potential strengths and weaknesses. As noted previously, two of the guiding principles in selecting a control group are that they represent the population the cases came from, and that they will provide a good estimate of the level of exposure one would expect in that population. Some common sources of controls include persons served by the same health-care institutions or providers as the cases; members of the same institution or organization; relatives, friends, or neighbors; or a random sample of the community from which the cases came.

For outbreaks in hospitals or nursing homes, the source of controls is usually other patients or residents of the facility. For example, in the investigation of postoperative surgical site infections the epidemiologist might select as controls persons who had similar surgery but who did not develop postoperative infections. The advantages of using such controls are that they come from the same catchment area as the cases, have similar access to medical care, have comparable medical records, have time on their hands, and are usually cooperative. The disadvantage is that they may have conditions that are associated either positively or negatively with the disease or risk factors of interest. For example, hospitalized patients are more likely to be current or former smokers than the general population.

Depending on the disease and risk factors under study, the best strategy might be to select controls with only a limited number of diagnoses known to be independent of the exposures and disease, or, alternatively, to select controls with as broad a range of diagnoses as possible, so that no one diagnosis has undue influence.

In other settings with a well-defined or easily enumerated population, controls generally come from lists of persons in that population who did not become ill. For example, controls for an outbreak of nausea, lightheadedness, and fainting among seventh graders at a middle school might be seventh grade students at the same school who did not experience those symptoms. Similarly, on a cruise ship, controls might be selected as a random sample of well passengers or perhaps cabin mates of cases who ate together but remained well. These population-based controls have advantages similar to those listed for hospital-based controls, but without the disadvantage of having another disease.

When an outbreak occurs in a community at large, a control group comprising randomly selected residents from that community is appropriate. However, you are not likely to have an available list of all persons from which to choose. Therefore, you must enlist controls either by telephoning a randomly or systematically selected set of telephone numbers, or by mailings to residents, or by conducting a door-to-door neighborhood survey. Several case control studies have now been conducted using Internet-based controls in technologically adept settings such as a college. Each approach has its relative strengths and weaknesses and associated potential biases. For example, both telephone dialing and door-to-door canvassing are labor-intensive and are best done in the evenings when people are likely to be home. Even so, the public has become wary of telephone solicitations and even more so of strangers, however well intentioned, knocking on their doors. Mailings require far less labor but have notoriously low response rates, and those who respond may be a skewed rather than representative group.

When an investigation is not limited to a specific location but, for instance, involves multiple states or the entire country, the selection of an appropriate control group is not as straightforward. In such circumstances, epidemiologists have successfully used friends, relatives, or neighbors as controls. Typically, you interview a case, then ask for the names and telephone numbers of a certain number of friends to call as possible controls. For example, to investigate a multistate outbreak of *Salmonella* Newport infection linked to mango consumption, investigators asked each case-patient to name two friends or co-workers of the same age group and ethnicity as possible controls.[13] One advantage is that the friends of an ill person are usually quite willing to participate, knowing that their cooperation may help solve the puzzle. On the other hand, they may have exposure experiences quite similar to those of the cases, such as similar personal habits and preferences. The consequence of enrolling controls who are too similar to the cases is "overmatching," resulting in less difference in cases and controls than there ought to be and decreased ability to document exposure–disease associations. To reduce the possibility of overmatching, the investigators of the *Salmonella*-mango outbreak further specified that the two named friends or co-workers could not live or share meals with the case-patients.[13]

## Sampling Methods for Selecting Controls

A variety of approaches can be used to select controls, depending on the hypotheses to be evaluated, the urgency of the investigation, the resources available, and the setting.

### Using all non-ill persons in the same population

Occasionally, an outbreak occurs in a well-defined, relatively small population. Examples include a food-borne outbreak among people who attended a wedding or an outbreak of respiratory disease among residents of a nursing home All persons with the disease under study could be called cases, and all persons who did not become ill could be called controls. However, enrollment of everyone in the population is actually a complete cohort and should be analyzed as a cohort study—calculating and comparing rates of disease among exposed and unexposed groups—rather than as a case control study.

### Random or systematic sampling

For community outbreaks, controls are often selected at random by a method called *random-digit dialing*—dialing random telephone numbers with the same area code, exchanges, and sometimes the next two digits as the cases, then choosing the remaining digits at random. However, with increasing use of cell phones, answering machines, and caller-ID screening, it has become more challenging for random-digit dialing to find suitable and willing control participants.

For investigations in settings where a roster is available, controls can be selected by either random or systematic sampling. For random sampling, a table or computer-generated list of random numbers should be used to select individuals. For systematic sampling, every *n*th (e.g., every tenth or thirtieth or other appropriate interval) person on the list is selected. To identify controls for the investigation of intussusception following receipt of oral rotavirus vaccine, investigators randomized a list of infants born at the same hospital on the same day as each case-patient, and prioritized the first four infants on the randomized list for enrollment as controls.[14]

### Pair matching

*Pair matching* is the selection of one or more controls for each case who have the same or similar specified characteristics as that case. For example, if the criteria for pair matching were same gender, school, and grade as the case, and the control-to-case ratio were one-to-one, then a female ninth-grade case at Lincoln High School would need to be matched to a female Lincoln High School ninth-grade control. Although the term *pair matching* implies one case and one control, the term may also refer to two, three, or more, or even a variable number of controls matched to each case.

In field epidemiology, pair matching is used in two circumstances—to control for potential confounding, or for logistical ease. In the first circumstance, one or more factors may be suspected to confound the relationship between exposure and disease; that is, the factor may be linked to the exposure and, independently, be a risk factor for the disease. To help eliminate the intertwining of the effect of the confounder with the effect of the other exposures of interest, the epidemiologist may choose to match on the confounder. The result is that the cases and controls are the same in terms of the confounding factor, and, when analyzed properly, any apparent association between the exposure and the disease cannot be due to confounding by the matching factor. Note that matching in the design of the study—that is, choosing controls matched to the cases—requires the use of matched analysis methods (see Chapter 10).

A second reason for pair matching is simple expedience. As noted earlier, sometimes the quickest and most convenient method of selecting controls is to ask the cases for the names of friends, or to walk next door to a neighbor's home. This is pair matching because Jane's friend or neighbor in Seattle is not the friend or neighbor of Mary in Chicago. While such pair matching may be done for expedience, the net result is that cases and controls generally do wind up being matched for such difficult-to-measure factors such as socioeconomic status, cultural influence, exposure to local advertising, and the like. Note that if these friend or neighbor controls are too similar to the cases in terms of exposure ("overmatching"), the study's ability to find an association between exposure and disease by documenting differences in exposure among cases and controls is diminished.

## Frequency matching

*Frequency matching*, also called *category matching*, is an alternative to pair matching. Frequency matching involves the selection of controls in proportion to the distribution of certain characteristics of the cases. For example, if 70% of the cases were ninth graders, 20% were eighth graders, and 10% were seventh graders, then the same proportion of controls would be selected from those grades. Frequency matching works best when all the cases have been identified before control selection begins.

In general, matching has several advantages. Matching is conceptually simple. It can save time and resources, as noted above with friend controls, and it can control for confounding by numerous social factors that are difficult to quantify and, hence, otherwise difficult to control for in an analysis. Finally, if the matching factor would have been a strong confounder, then matching improves the precision or power of the analysis.

However, matching has important disadvantages as well. First and foremost, if you match on a factor, you can no longer evaluate its effect on disease in your study, because you have made the controls and cases alike on that factor. For example, if infants with nosocomial infections in a neonatal intensive care unit were matched by birth weight to newborn controls, then investigators would not be able to study birth weight itself as a risk factor for infection. Therefore, match only on factors that you do not need to evaluate. Second, if too many or too rigid matching criteria are used, controls that meet these criteria will be hard to find, and cases without matched controls will have to be excluded from the study. This happens when, for example, siblings are used as controls—cases without siblings have no eligible controls and cannot be included in the study.

## Size of Control Group

The size of the control group may be determined by circumstances, resources, or power considerations. Circumstance—for example, the number of eligible controls—sometimes is a limiting factor. At other times, time and resources may limit the number of controls that can be enrolled. However, when the size of the population from which the cases arose is large and resources are adequate, power calculations can be performed to determine the optimal number of controls needed to identify an important association. Most case control studies use a control-to-case ratio of either 1:1, 2:1, or 3:1. In general, little power is gained with control-to-case ratios in excess of 3:1 or 4:1. While uncommon, the number of eligible and enrolled cases can exceed the number of eligible or available controls.

## COMPARISONS OF COHORT AND CASE CONTROL STUDIES

Some outbreaks occur in settings that are amenable to either a retrospective cohort or case control study design. Others are better suited to one study type or the other. The advantages and disadvantages of these two approaches are listed in Table 8–1.

## Risk Measurement

One of the most important advantages of the cohort design is that disease risk (attack rate) of disease can be measured directly. This information is particularly important if the exposure is at the discretion of the individual. Only a cohort study can fill in the blank of "What is my risk of developing [name of disease]

**Table 8–1.** Features of Case-Control and Retrospective Cohort Studies

| FEATURE | CASE-CONTROL STUDY | RETROSPECTIVE COHORT STUDY |
|---|---|---|
| Sample size | Smaller | Larger |
| Costs | Less | More because of size |
| Study time | Short | Short |
| Rare disease | Efficient | Inefficient |
| Rare exposure | Inefficient | Efficient |
| Multiple exposures | Can examine | Often can examine |
| Multiple outcomes | Cannot examine | Can examine |
| Natural history | Cannot ascertain | Can ascertain |
| Disease risk | Cannot measure | Can measure |
| Recall bias | Potential problem | Potential problem |
| Loss to follow-up | Not an issue | Potential problem |
| Selection bias | Potential problem | Potential problem |
| Population not well circumscribed | Advantageous | Difficult |

if I choose to [be exposed]?" The case control study, with a set number of cases and an arbitrary number of controls, does not permit calculation of disease risk for a given exposure group.

## Rare Exposure

Cohort studies are better suited than case control studies for examining health effects following a relatively rare exposure. With a cohort approach, all persons with the exposure can be enrolled and monitored, as well as a sample of comparable persons who were not exposed. This rationale explains the popularity of retrospective cohort studies in occupational epidemiology, where a group of workers with an exposure common among that group but relatively rare in the community at large can be followed over time.

## Rare Disease

Case control studies are the design of choice for sporadic occurrences or an outbreak of an otherwise rare disease in a population. You can enroll all cases and an appropriate number of controls, and evaluate differences in their exposures to look for association between exposure and disease. In contrast, a cohort study would have to enroll an extremely large number of persons to have enough cases who develop the rare disease of interest.

## POTENTIAL PITFALLS IN THE DESIGN AND CONDUCT OF EPIDEMIOLOGIC STUDIES

Designing and conducting a good epidemiologic study in the field is not easy. In designing a study many choices must be made. Many of these choices have no "right" answer but involve trade-offs or compromises between theory and practical issues such as time constraints and resources (see Chapter 11). Other choices involve deciding between two less-than-perfect options, such as two different control groups with different potential flaws. Some of the pitfalls that result from less-than-ideal study design and conduct are described below.

### Selection Bias

*Selection bias* is a systematic error in choosing the study groups to be enrolled (e.g., cases and controls in a case control study, exposed and unexposed groups in a cohort study) or in the enrollment of study participants that results in a mistaken estimate of an exposure–disease association. Consider, for example, an infectious disease with low pathogenicity; i.e., one with many asymptomatic cases. If a case control study was conducted but controls were not tested for evidence of asymptomatic infection, then at least some of the controls could have the infection under study. The exposures among these controls who are really cases would be the same as the cases. Thus the prevalence of exposure in the control group would be more similar to that in the case group than it should be, resulting in an underestimate of the exposure–disease relationship. Alternatively, use of an overly broad case definition, such as one that includes possible and probable as well as confirmed cases, can also result in selection bias and underestimation of the association by including non-cases in the case group. Another type of selection bias is *diagnostic bias*, in which knowledge of the exposure–disease hypothesis may prompt a clinician to make a diagnosis. For example, if physicians are more likely to make a diagnosis of deep venous thrombosis if they know that the patient has just returned from a long flight overseas, then subsequent studies of deep venous thrombosis will show an association with airline flight! A third source of selection bias is *nonresponse bias*, in which persons who choose to participate may differ in important ways from persons who choose not to participate or cannot be found. In occupational epidemiology, a well-known source of selection bias is called the *healthy worker effect*. This effect is based on the observation that workers who remain on the job are, in general, healthier and fitter than the population at large, and comparisons between workers and the general population may not be appropriate. The list of types of selection bias is lengthy, so investigators must be careful to use an objective and consistent case definition; select controls that represent the population from which the cases arose, using objective and consistent control criteria; and work hard to promote high response rates among all groups.

## Information Bias

*Information bias* is a systematic error in the collection of data from or about the participants who are already in the study that results in a mistaken estimate of an exposure's effect on the risk of disease. One of the most common types of information bias is *recall bias*, in which one group is more likely than the other to remember and report an exposure. For example, persons who developed severe diarrhea are very likely to have thought about all the preceding meals and foods they have eaten, while healthy controls are not. *Interviewer bias* occurs when interviewers are more probing about exposures when interviewing cases than controls. In some cultures, another source of information bias is from respondents trying to "please" the interviewer by providing answers that they think the interviewer wants to hear rather than providing accurate information. To minimize information bias, good studies use standard and pretested questionnaires or data collection forms, and interviewers or abstractors who are trained in the objective use of the forms. In general, participants should not be told of the study's specific hypotheses. Memory aids, such as calendars, menus, or photographs of medications, can often aid participants' recall.

## Confounding

*Confounding* is the distortion of an exposure–disease association by a third factor that is related to both exposure and disease. Consider, for example, a study of an investigational cancer drug versus "usual treatment." Suppose that most people who received the drug had early-stage disease, and most people who received the usual treatment had later-stage disease. Then even if the investigational drug had no beneficial effect, it might look efficacious because its effect was intertwined with that of the disease stage. For a factor to be a confounder it must be an independent risk factor for the disease, and it must be unequally distributed between the exposure groups. Since age is independently associated with almost every health condition imaginable, age automatically fulfills one of the two criteria for confounding, so it must always be considered a potential confounder. In outbreak investigations, confounding can occur when two foods are eaten together (or any two exposures go hand-in-hand), but only one is the culprit. Nonetheless, basic analysis will identify both foods as associated with disease. In observational studies, confounding can be addressed through restriction, matching, stratified analysis, or modeling. *Restriction* means, simply, that the study population is limited to a narrowly defined population. In the investigational drug example above, if the study had been limited to persons with early-stage disease, the disease stage could not confound the results. Similarly, if age is a suspected confounder, the study could be limited to a narrow age range. Matching in the study design has been addressed previously in this chapter. Matching in the analysis, as well as stratified analysis and modeling, are addressed in Chapter 10.

## Small Sample Size

Sample size and power calculations can provide estimates of the number of subjects needed to find an association that is statistically significant and that would be judged to be important. In general, sample size and power calculations are based on the magnitude of association worth detecting, the prevalence of exposure or the risk of disease, and the ratio of the two groups i.e., the ratio of controls to cases. In practice, the size of a study is sometimes limited by the number of cases, time, and resources available. While the two most popular measures of effect—risk ratio and odds ratio—are not influenced by the size of the study, their measures of precision—confidence intervals—and measures of statistical significance, such as chi-square tests and $p$ values, are all affected by study size (see Chapter 10). Many investigators have wished for a larger study after calculating a large and potentially important risk ratio or odds ratio that fails to reach statistical significance and has a wide confidence interval. Would a larger study confirm that the association is statistically different from the null, or would it show that the apparent association was indeed just chance variation from the null? Often, you will never know. Determination of an adequate sample size in advance could avoid this situation (see Chapter 10).

## SUMMARY

Cohort and case control studies are the two types of analytic studies used most commonly by field epidemiologists. They are effective mechanisms for evaluating—quantifying and testing—hypotheses suggested in earlier phases of the investigation. Cohort studies, which are oriented conceptually from exposure to disease, are appropriate in settings in which an entire population is well defined and available for enrollment, such as invited guests at a wedding reception. Cohort studies are also appropriate when well-defined groups can be enrolled by exposure status, such as employees working in different parts of a manufacturing plant.

Case control studies, on the other hand, are quite useful when the population is less clearly defined. Case control studies, oriented from disease to exposure, identify persons with disease ("cases") through, say, surveillance, and a comparable group of persons without disease ("controls"), then the exposure experiences of the two groups are compared. While conceptually straightforward, the design of a good epidemiologic study requires many decisions, including who would make up an appropriate comparison group, how many controls per case to enroll, whether or not to match, and how best to avoid potential biases.

## REFERENCES

1. Rothman, K.J., Greenland S. (1998). *Modern Epidemiology*, 2nd ed., Little, Brown, Boston.
2. Kelsey, J.L., Whittemore, A.S., Evans, A.E., et al. (1997). *Methods in Observational Epidemiology*, 2nd ed., Oxford University Press, New York.
3. Koepsell, T.D., Weiss, N.S. (2003). *Epidemiologic Methods: Studying the Occurrence of Illness*, Oxford University Press, New York.
4. Hedberg, C.W., Fishbein, D.B., Janssen, R.S., et al. (1987). An outbreak of thyrotoxicosis caused by the consumption of bovine thyroid gland in ground beef. *N Engl J Med* 316, 993–8.
5. Kannel, W.B. (2000). The Framingham study: its 50-year legacy and future promise. *J Atheroscler Thromb* 6, 60–6.
6. Colditz, G.A., Manson, J.E., Hankinson, S.E. (1997). The Nurses' Health Study: 20-year contribution to the understanding of health among women. *J Womens Health* 6, 49–62.
7. Shimuzu, Y., Mabuchi, K., Preston, D.L., et al. (1996). Mortality study of atomic-bomb survivors: implications for assessment of radiation accidents. *World Health Stat Q* 49, 25–9.
8. Brackbill, R.M., Thorpe, L.E., DiGrande, L., et al. (2006). Surveillance for World Trade Center disaster health effects among survivors of collapsed and damaged buildings. *MMWR Surveill Summ* 55, 1–18.
9. Boehmer, T.K., Flanders, W.D., McGeehin, M.A., et al. (2004). Post-service mortality in Vietnam veterans: 30-year follow-up. *Arch Intern Med* 164, 1908–16.
10. Boyle, C.A., DeCoufle, P. (1987). Post-service mortality among Vietnam veterans: The Centers for Disease Control Vietnam Experience Study. *JAMA* 257, 790–5.
11. Steenland, K. (2002). Ten-year update on mortality among mild-steel welders. *Scand J Work Environ Health* 28, 163–7.
12 Wacholder, S., McLaughlin, J.K., Silverman, D.T., et al. (1992). Selection of controls in case control studies: I. Principles. *Am J Epidemiol* 135, 1019–28.
13. Sivapalasingam, S., Barrett, E., Kimura, A., et al. (2003). A multistate outbreak of *Salmonella enterica* serotype Newport infection linked to mango consumption: impact of water-dip disinfection technology. *Clin Infect Dis* 37, 1585–90.
14. Murphy, T.M., Gargiullo, P.M., Massoudi, M.S., et al. (2001). Intussusception among infants given an oral rotavirus vaccine. *N Engl J Med* 344, 564–72.

# 9

# DESCRIBING THE FINDINGS: DESCRIPTIVE EPIDEMIOLOGY

Robert E. Fontaine
Richard A. Goodman*

As a field epidemiologist, one of the first things you will do will be to collect, or be presented with, data from outbreak investigations, surveillance systems, vital statistics, or other sources of information—all for appropriate analysis. One of the fundamental tasks will be to orient and organize these data to construct useful and relevant presentations and interpretations. This task is called *descriptive epidemiology*. Descriptive epidemiology answers the following questions about disease occurrence: How much? When? Where? and Among Whom? The first dimension, "How much?" is expressed as counts or rates, while the last three dimensions are usually referred to as *time*, *place*, and *person*. Time, place, and person have universally standardized units of measurement (e.g., years, longitude and latitude, county, or age group) that can be applied both to the cases or events under study and to the underlying population. Once the data are organized and appropriately displayed, the practice of descriptive epidemiology then involves interpretation of these patterns that should allow the epidemiologist to construct ideas that explain why illness or adverse health events occurred. In some situations the descriptive epidemiology may be sufficient to initiate control measures. In others the descriptive findings will provide a basis for analytic studies (see Chapters 7, 8, and 11).

In epidemics and other health-related events, the causative agents and exposures to these agents are usually not distributed randomly with regard to the time, place, and person, but instead usually assume a unique profile that reflects the underlying epidemiologic process. In descriptive epidemiology these patterns are contrasted with the expected patterns or norms to generate ideas or hypotheses about the possible modes of exposure or risk factors. Through this process of organization, inspection, and interpretation of data, descriptive epidemiology serves several purposes. It:

- Provides a systematic method for dissecting a health problem into its component parts.
- Ensures that you are fully versed in the basic dimensions of a health problem.
- Helps identify populations at increased risk of the health problem under investigation.
- Provides immediate information that may be given to decision makers, the media, the public, and others regarding the progress of investigations and the relative probabilities of different causative factors.
- Enables generation of testable hypotheses about the etiology, mode of exposure, effectiveness of control measures, and other aspects of the health problem.
- Helps validate the eventual incrimination of causes or risk factors. Whether you use analytic epidemiology, microbiology, or experimental studies, these methods must explain the observed patterns by time, place, and person.

## ORGANIZING AND COUNTING CASES

The simplest way to determine the extent of a health problem is to count cases of disease, deaths, or other health events. Cases are customarily organized in a line-listing format (as shown in Table 9–1[1] or in Table A–2 in the Appendix at the end of the book). Whether on paper or index cards, or as a computerized database, this arrangement facilitates sorting to reorganize and count cases by relevant charac-teristics. For example, the line listing in Table 9–1 has been sorted by days between vaccination and onset to reveal the pattern of this important time relationship.

Cases may be either *incident cases* or *prevalent cases*. Incident cases or health events are changes in the status of an individual—from well to ill, from uninfected to infected, from alive to dead. Prevalent cases represent the existing status of an individual—well, ill, uninfected, infected, alive, deceased. Incident cases are determined by following individuals over time and counting those who change their status. If the change in status is overt, a population may be followed and incident cases identified through public health surveillance or other health information systems. On the other hand, prevalent cases are determined by taking

**Table 9-1.**   Reported Cases of Intussusception among Recipients of Tetravalent Rhesus-based Rotavirus Vaccine (RRV-TV) Rotashield), by State—United States, 1998–1999[a]

| STATE | AGE[b] | SEX | DAYS[c] | DOSE |
|---|---|---|---|---|
| New York | 2 | M | 3 | 1 |
| California | 3 | M | 3 | 1 |
| Pennsylvania | 6 | M | 3 | 1 |
| Pennsylvania | 2 | M | 4 | 1 |
| Colorado | 4 | F | 4 | 1 |
| California | 7 | M | 4 | 2 |
| Kansas | 2 | F | 5 | 1 |
| Colorado | 3 | M | 5 | 1 |
| New York | 3 | F | 5 | 1 |
| North Carolina | 4 | F | 5 | 1 |
| Missouri | 11 | M | 5 | 1 |
| Pennsylvania | 3 | F | 7 | 1 |
| California | 4 | F | 14 | 2 |
| Pennsylvania | 2 | M | 29 | 1 |
| California | 5 | M | 59 | 1 |

a. Use of trade names and commercial sources is for identification only and does not imply endorsement by CDC or the Department of Health and Human Services.
b. Age in months
c. Days from vaccine dose to onset.
[*Source:* MMWR, 48 (27), 577.]

a measurement on individuals usually at one point in time. For diseases or conditions with a fairly long duration (years or decades) and negligible mortality, incident cases may be estimated by taking periodic measurements of the prevalent state of the individuals. Incident cases must be counted over a specified time period. Figure 9–1 shows time lines representing 10 illnesses among 20 individuals over 16 months.[2] Between October 1, 1990, and September 30, 1991, four had onset of disease and are, therefore, incident cases of illness during the year period. At a specific point in time, April 1, 1991, there are seven persons with disease, and, therefore, they are prevalent cases. It is always critical to know if data sources you use are providing incident or prevalent cases. Similarly, you should not mix incident with prevalent cases in epidemiologic comparisons or analyses.

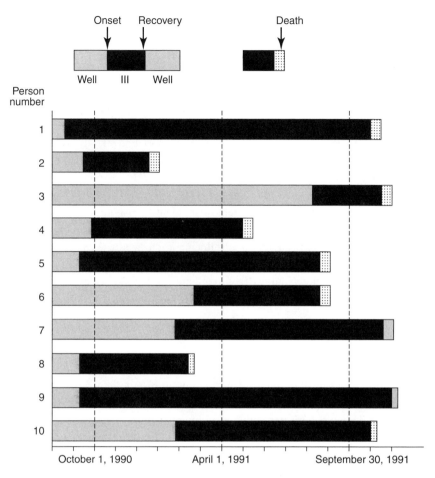

**Figure 9–1.**  Ten episodes of an illness in a population of 20 [*Source:* CDC, 1992.[2]]

## RATES

Once counted, either incident or prevalent cases may be compared to their historical norm, expressed as an expected value or distribution. For instance, we might expect, based on the experience in the previous five years, that 175 incident cases of hepatitis A would be seen in the current year for a specific urban area. If double that number were actually observed, we might conclude that the area is experiencing an increase in transmission of hepatitis A. However, these simple case counts are valid for epidemiologic comparisons only when they come from a population of the same or nearly the same size. Suppose that in a large urban county twice the number of persons developed hepatitis A than in a small rural county. Is the urban dweller twice as likely to contract hepatitis as the rural dweller? Clearly, the hepatitis A count depends upon the number of persons available to acquire hepatitis A. In this example the excess number may simply reflect the far larger population of the urban area.

Therefore, to make valid comparisons of health events between population groups and to assess the issue of risk, cases must be assessed in light of the size of the population they came from. Rates, then, rather than simple numbers, must be determined by relating case counts to the population under study. Through the use of rates you may determine whether one group is at increased risk of disease and to what degree. From a population perspective, these so-called high-risk groups can be further targeted for special intervention. From an individual perspective, by comparing rates, you may also identify risk factors for disease. Identification of these risk factors may be used by individuals in their day-to-day decision making about behaviors that influence their health. A variety of rates, ratios, and derivatives thereof are used in epidemiology to quantify risk. In descriptive epidemiology only a few elementary rates are widely used: these include incidence, cumulative incidence, prevalence, specific rates, and adjusted rates.

## Incidence Rates

All incidence rates involve counts of incident cases over a defined time period in a defined population. The numerator is the number of incident cases in a time period. The denominator is normally the midpoint estimate of the population from which the cases arose. Returning to Figure 9–1, we see that during the year period (October 1990 through September 1991), four incident cases occurred in a population of 20 persons that were present at the beginning of the year. (*Note*: only sick persons are represented. The well persons (10) are not shown.) Two persons died of the disease before the middle of the year, leaving a midpoint population of 18. Thus, we first divide 4 cases by 18 persons at risk, giving 0.22. The next step is to convert this result to a more understandable format by multiplying it times a standard population size. In this example we use 100, resulting in 22 cases per 100 per year. The standard population size is normally in units of 100, 1,000, 10,000, 100,000 or 1,000,000. For routine disease statistics, the population size is established by convention. However, in field investigations with small populations you should try to select a population size that results in rates between 1.0 and 100 as in the example. Clearly, this is an artificial example, since in a natural population births, deaths, immigration, and emigration will affect the midyear population. However, normally, these are estimated from census data. A wide range of standard morbidity and mortality incidence rates is available for routine use in field epidemiology (Table 9–2).[2]

**Table 9-2.** Frequently used Measures of Morbidity

| MEASURE | NUMERATOR (X) | DENOMINATOR (Y) | EXPRESSED PER NUMBER AT RISK ($10^n$) |
|---|---|---|---|
| Incidence Rate | No. of new cases of a specific disease reported during a given time interval | Average population during time interval | Varies: $10^n$ where $n= 2,3,4,5,6$ |
| Attack Rate | No. of new cases of a specified disease reported during an epidemic period | Population at start of the epidemic period | Varies: $10^n$ where $n= 2,3,4,5,6$ |
| Secondary Attack Rate | No. of new cases of a specified disease among contacts of known cases | Size of contact population at risk | Varies: $10^n$ where $n= 2,3,4,5,6$ |
| Point Prevalence | No. of current cases, new and old, of a specified disease at a given point in time | Estimated population at the same point in time | Varies: $10^n$ where $n= 2,3,4,5,6$ |

[*Source:* Table 2.5 *from Principles of Epidemiology: Self-Study Course.*]

## Attack Rates or Cumulative Incidence Rates

Whereas many morbidity and mortality rates use standard time periods, certain situations such as outbreaks, epidemics, or problems in limited populations require counting incident cases over limited periods of time. For these attack rates or cumulative incidence rates, the denominator is the population at risk at the beginning of the time period. Theoretically, persons who are not at risk, for example, because of previous disease or infection, are not included in this denominator. In the example (Fig. 9–1), between October 1, 1990 and September 30, 1991, four incident cases occurred. The population at risk was 20 at the beginning of the period yielding an attack rate of 4/20 or 20% for the 12-month period. If knowledge of preexisting disease were available, you would then also subtract previously affected persons (6) from the denominator. You must be careful, when comparing attack rates to standard morbidity incidence rates, to adjust both rates to the same time period.

## Secondary Attack Rates

A secondary attack rate is a measure of the frequency of new cases of a disease among contacts of cases. A secondary attack rate equals the number of cases among contacts of primary cases during the study period divided by the total number of contacts. To calculate the total number of household contacts, we normally subtract the number of primary cases from the total number of people residing in those households.

For example, seven cases of hepatitis A occurred among 70 children attending a child care center. Each infected child came from a different family. The total number of persons in the seven affected families was 32, including the seven infected children and 25 contacts. One generation period later, five family contacts also developed hepatitis A. The secondary attack rate then is: 5 infected contacts/25 contacts or 20%.[2]

Multiple cases in households or other living groups could also arise from food, water, or factors other than person-to-person transmission. Accordingly, you should determine that the timing between the cases in a household is compatible with secondary transmission. Also, you should always compare rates in these groups to the rates in the general population without presuming that the cases are secondary.

## Person–Time Incidence Rates

A person–time incidence rate directly incorporates time into the denominator. Typically, each person is observed from a set beginning point to an established end point (onset of disease, death, migration out of the group, or into the group). The numerator is still the number of new cases, but the denominator is a little different. The denominator is a sum of the time each person is observed, totaled for all persons. Therefore, the person–time rate equals the number of cases detected during the observation period divided by the time each person was observed, totaled for all persons.

For example, a person enrolled in a study who develops a disease of interest five years later contributes five person-years to the denominator. A person who is disease free is followed for one year, and, subsequently, is lost to follow-up and contributes one person-year plus one-half of the subsequent year (if the follow-up intervals are years) to the denominator.

Person–time rates are often used in cohort (follow-up) studies of diseases with long incubation or latency periods, such as some occupationally related diseases, AIDS, and chronic diseases. In addition, the person–time rates may be very useful in acute outbreaks or special surveillance systems where individuals may spend extremely variable periods of time in the general area of exposure (e.g., in nosocomial infection outbreaks where duration in the hospital may vary markedly between individuals).

## Prevalence Rates

Prevalence rates reflect the proportion of the population that has an existing condition (prevalent cases). Point prevalence means that the measurement on each individual is made at one point in time. In the example (see Fig. 9–1), the seven prevalent cases on April 1 were among 18 (living) individuals, yielding a point prevalence rate of 7/18 = 39%.

Prevalence is determined by two factors:

- Incidence, which converts an individual from an unaffected state to an affected state, and
- Recovery (or death), which converts the affected state to another state.

Since the interval from onset to recovery is the duration of illness, this relationship may be approximated as: prevalence = incidence × duration.

Historically, prevalence has been less utilized than incidence in field epidemiology. However, more recently, a number of conditions measured by prevalence (e.g., blood lead levels, birth defects, and behavioral risk factors) have come under surveillance and, accordingly, been routinely scrutinized by field epidemiologists. In addition, the prevalence rates before, during, and after an outbreak may be compared to make estimations of incidence in situations when incidence cannot be measured directly.

## Ratios and Alternative Denominators

In some situations the population at risk is unknown, costly to determine, or even inappropriate. In these situations you must consider using alternative denominators to estimate risk or compare risks among population groups. These resultant quotients are properly termed *ratios* rather than rates.

Commonly used ratios include an infant mortality rate, a maternal mortality ratio, and a death-to-case ratio (Table 9–3). To assess adverse effects from a vaccine or pharmaceutical you might use total doses distributed, since the actual numbers of individuals who received the product may be difficult to obtain. Similarly, in a food-borne outbreak you might use restaurant receipts or the number of portions of a suspect food served as a denominator rather than the actual number of persons visiting the restaurant or eating a food. Injuries from snowmobile usage have been calculated, both as ratios per registered vehicles and as per crash incident (Fig. 9–2).[3]

## TIME, PLACE, AND PERSON

In the preceding overview we have referred to counts or rates in populations. In order to identify and depict epidemiologically relevant patterns, these counts and rates should be organized by time, place, and person.

**Table 9–3.**   Frequently used Measures of Mortality

| MEASURE | NUMERATOR (X) | DENOMINATOR (Y) | EXPRESSED PER NUMBER AT RISK (10") |
|---|---|---|---|
| Crude Death Rate | Total number of deaths reported during a given time interval | Estimated mid-interval population | 1,000 or 100,000 |
| Cause-Specific Death Rate | No. of deaths assigned to a specific cause during a given time interval | Estimated mid-interval population | 100,000 |
| Proportional Mortality | No. of deaths assigned to a specific cause during a given time interval | Total number of deaths from all causes during the same interval | 100 or 1,000 |
| Death-to-Case Ratio | No. of deaths assigned to a specific disease during a given time interval | No. of new cases of that disease reported during the same time interval | 100 |
| Neonatal Mortality Rate | No. of deaths under 28 days of age during a given time interval | No. of live births during the same time interval | 1000 |
| Postneonatal Mortality Rate | No. of deaths from 28 days to, but not including, 1 year of age, during a given time interval | No. of live births during the same time interval | 1000 |
| Infant Mortality Rate | No. of deaths under 1 year of age during a given time interval | No. of live births reported during the same time interval | 1000 |
| Maternal Mortality Rate | No. of deaths assigned to pregnancy-related causes during a given time interval | No. of live births during the same time interval | 100,000 |

[*Source:* Table 2.8 from *Principles of Epidemiology: Self-Study Course.*]

## Depicting Data by Time

Since all epidemiologic field investigation take place over a certain time frame, the field epidemiologist will need to know how to organize and describe these time patterns in the effort to understand the health event being studied. Rates should be used whenever possible. However, for short time periods in stable populations, you may safely organize only numerator data to identify time patterns.

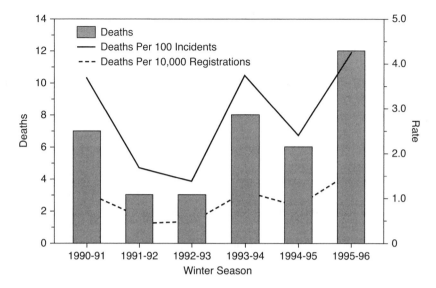

**Figure 9–2.** Number of deaths and death rates per snowmobile-related incident and per snowmobile registration—Maine, 1990–91 through 1995–96 winter seasons. [*Source:* CDC, 1997.³]

Health events may present with several important time characteristics. Most critical are the time of exposure to suspected or known risk factors and the time of onset of health events. Other relevant events should also be placed in temporal sequence to help create an accurate chronological framework for investigating the problem.

The accuracy of this information can vary considerably by situation or disease and may be greater for acute problems that have occurred recently than for those that are chronic. For certain types of problems, the time of precipitating events must be carefully distinguished from the time of occurrence of the outcome (e.g., injury and death).

Events in time may be related to one another. If you know both time of onset and time of known or presumed exposure, you can estimate the incubation or latency period. When the agent is unknown, the time interval between presumed exposure and onset of symptoms is critical in hypothesizing the etiology. If an agent is suspected, then a similar comparison may help to either dispel or reinforce suspicions. For example, the consistent time interval between rotavirus vaccination and onset of intussusception (see Table 9–1) helped build the hypothesis that the vaccine precipitated the disease. Similarly, when the incubation period is known, the time interval of exposure may be estimated and potential exposures during that interval may be identified.

Identification of special events or certain unusual circumstances temporally related to the problem may also help in the formulation of relevant hypotheses. These principles are illustrated in the depiction of the incidence of malaria in the United States as shown for the period from 1930 to 1998, which compares incidence rates to important modifying events (see Fig. 3–1).[4]

Graphic display of time data provides a simple visual depiction of the relative magnitude, past and current trends, potential future course of the problem, and the impact of specified related events. Depending on the health event you are studying, the time period may include years, months, weeks, days, or even hours. For chronic diseases or other conditions, time is usually depicted as a secular trend—the annual rate plotted over many years or decades. For more acute conditions, incident cases or incidence rates are plotted. For an acute disease the ideal point in time to plot is the onset of disease. However, in surveillance systems the date of report is often the only available time information.

## Time line

For small numbers of cases the critical times may be graphed on a simple time line. Points on time lines can represent disease onset or point exposures, while bars may represent time periods of exposure or illness. Using this type of graphic device for an investigation of nosocomial malaria, investigators were able to demonstrate a time–space coincidence of hospitalization of malaria patients with other patients who developed malaria at home after hospital discharge (Fig. 9–3). This data display quickly led investigators to the hypothesis, substantiated through subsequent analytic studies, that malaria was transmitted from patient to patient through syringes used on heparin locks.[5]

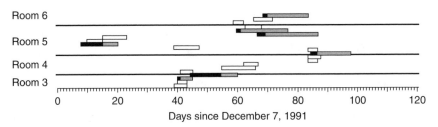

**Figure 9–3.** Duration of hospitalization in days and location by rooms of seven *Plasmodium falciparum* patients and 14 other patients who developed *P. falciparum* infections after discharge from Riyadh Central Hospital, Pediatric Ward 2, Riyadh, Saudi Arabia, December 1991–April 1992. [*Source:* Abulrahi et al., 1997.[5]]

### Epidemic curves

As case numbers increase, a histogram gives a better view of onset times of a health event (see Figure A–1 in the Appendix of this book). If the time period of interest is the duration of an epidemic, this histogram is called an *epidemic curve*. Time intervals by which onsets are grouped are shown on the *x* axis while the corresponding case counts in each interval on the *y* axis.

The choice of the time interval used is critical. Intervals that are too short (like hours for diseases with long incubation periods) will cloud the underlying pattern with random noise and hinder interpretation. Intervals that are too long (like weeks for diseases with short incubation periods) will group many cases into a few intervals and obscure the real pattern. As a general rule, intervals between one-fourth to one-third of an incubation/latency period work best at revealing the time pattern of an epidemic. As case numbers increase, shorter intervals will reveal more detail to the pattern (Fig. 9–4, A, B).[6]

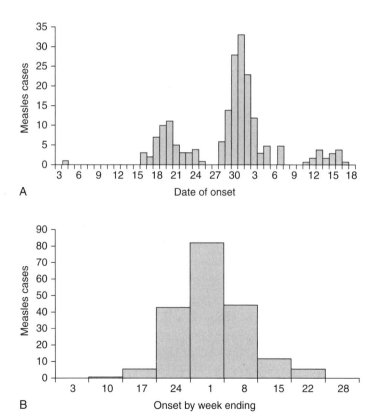

**Figure 9–4.** Measles cases by (A) day or (B) week of rash onset—Saint Louis County, Missouri, and Jersey County, Illinois, April 4–May 17, 1994. [*Source:* CDC, 1994.[6]]

A second point is where to begin and end the *x* axis. You should show when the epidemic started with a sufficient lead period to demonstrate the pre-epidemic background. Similarly, extend the time sufficiently after the last case to convincingly show the end of the epidemic. Usually two incubation periods before and after are necessary, and in some situations more may be necessary. This will also reveal possible source cases, secondary transmission, and other outliers of interest.

Labels, data markers, and reference lines should be used to indicate suspected exposures (Fig. 9–5).[7] These could include case-persons suspected of introducing the disease, introduction of a food, a new procedure, a special event, an environmental change, of any other factor that could be related in time to the outbreak.

As mentioned in Chapter 2, there is a variety of ways diseases are transmitted. The epidemic curves you draw will often reveal these modes of transmission. The following are certain kinds of epidemic situations that can frequently be "diagnosed" by simple, appropriate plotting of cases.

### Point source

An epidemic curve that shows a tight clustering of cases in time (less than 1.5 times the range of the incubation period if the agent is known) with a sharp upslope and a trailing downslope is consistent with a point source (Fig. 9–6).[8] Variations in slopes (e.g., bimodal or a broader-than-expected peak) should suggest ideas about the appearance, persistence, and disappearance of and the differences in exposure to the source.

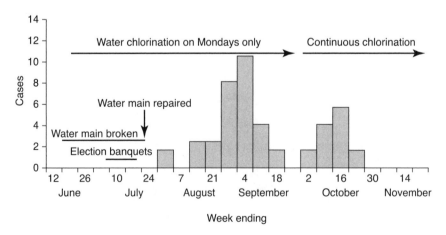

**Figure 9-5.** Cases of jaundice by week of onset, June–October 1999, Jaf'r, Ma'an Governorate, Jordan. [*Source:* Ministry of Health, Jordan, 1999.[7]]

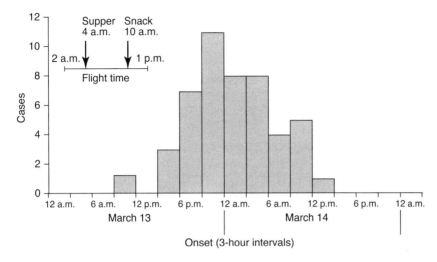

**Figure 9–6.** Cases of Salmonellosis in passengers on a flight from London to the United States, by time of onset, March 13–14, 1984. [*Source:* Tauxe et al., 1987.[8]]

In point source outbreaks, the time of exposure may be approximated by counting back the average incubation period before the peak, the minimum incubation period from the initial cases, and the maximum incubation period from the last cases. These three points should bracket the time of exposure.

### Point source with secondary transmission

Point source outbreaks of some communicable diseases potentially produce substantial numbers of infected individuals who, themselves, may serve as sources of the agent to infect others. Although such transmission often may be through direct personal contact, other vehicles of transmission may also lead to secondary cases. Secondary cases may appear as a prominent wave following a point source by one incubation period, as noted in a hepatitis E outbreak resulting from repairs on a broken water main (Fig. 9–5).[7] With diseases of shorter incubation and lower rates of secondary spread, the secondary wave may appear only as a more prolonged downslope. Although the period between the peak of the primary outbreak and the secondary wave often approximates the incubation period, it is really a combination of the incubation period and the period of infectivity of the primary cases, and is called a *generation period*.[9, 10]

### Continuing common source

Outbreaks may arise from common sources that continue over time. The epidemic curve will rise sharply as with a point source. Rather than rise to a peak, this type of epidemic curve will find a plateau. The downslope may be precipitous if the common source is removed or gradual if it exhausts itself. All three of these features are reflected in an epidemic curve for a salmonellosis outbreak involving cheese distributed to multiple restaurants (Fig. 9–7).[11]

### Propagated

A propagated pattern arises with agents that are communicable between persons either directly or through an intermediate vehicle. This propagated pattern has four principal characteristics:

- It encompasses several generation periods for the agent.
- It begins with a single case or small number of cases and rises with a gradually increasing upslope.
- Often a periodicity equivalent to the generation period for the agent may be obvious during the initial stages of the outbreak.
- After the outbreak peaks, the exhaustion of susceptible hosts usually results in a rapid downslope.

An outbreak of rubella illustrates these features, including an approximately three-week periodicity (Fig. 9–8).[12] Certain behaviors such as drug addiction and mass sociogenic illness may propagate from person to person, but the epidemic curve will not necessarily reflect generation times. Propagation between individuals generally represents a circumscribed, localized occurrence. Epidemic curves

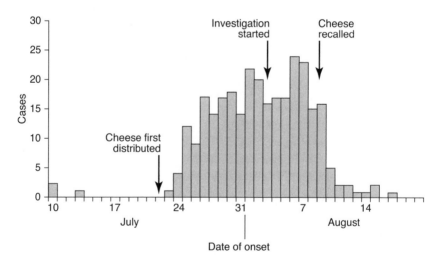

**Figure 9–7.** Cases of *Salmonella heidelberg* infection, by onset, Colorado, July 10–August 17, 1976. [*Source:* Fontaine et al., 1980.[11]]

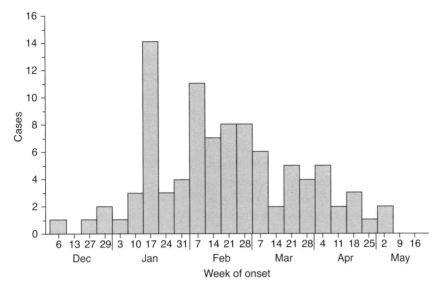

*n=93. Two patients did not have a rash.

**Figure 9-8.**  Confirmed cases of rubella, by week of rash onset—Westchester County, New York, December 1997–May 1998. [*Source:* CDC, 1999.[12]]

for large areas such as states, large cities, or heavily populated counties may not reveal the periodicity or the characteristic rise and fall of a propagated outbreak. For these larger areas it is important to stratify the epidemic curves by smaller subunits.

### Environmental

Epidemic curves from environmentally spread diseases reflect complex interactions between the agent and the environment and the factors that lead to exposure of humans to the environmental source. Outbreaks that arise from environmental sources will usually encompass several generation or incubation periods for the agent. They differ from propagated outbreaks in that they normally do not show the periodicity that approximates the agent's generation time. In addition, a gradually increasing upslope and a rapid downslope are normally seen only with zoonoses where the natural animal host itself is experiencing a propagated outbreak.

The epidemiologist should attempt to include on the epidemic curve a representation of the suspected environmental factor, as is done in Figure 9–9 with rainfall for an outbreak of leptospirosis.[13] In this example, nearly every peak of rainfall precedes a peak in leptospirosis, supporting the hypothesis of the importance of water in transmission.

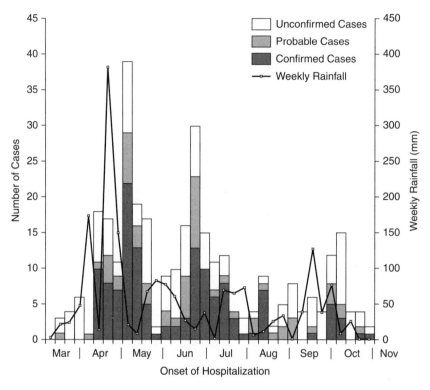

**Figure 9–9.** Cases of leptospirosis by week of hospitalization and rainfall in Salvador, Brazil, March 10–November 2, 1996. [*Source:* Ko et al., 1999.[13]]

### Zoonotic

The epidemic curve for a zoonotic disease in humans will generally represent the variations in prevalence among the reservoir animal population as it is modified by the variability of contact between humans and the reservoir animal. Since zoonoses often grow rapidly among reservoir hosts, the epidemic curve among humans may also appear as a rapid rise. This tendency can be appreciated in the West Nile virus outbreak in New York City (Fig. 9–10).[14]

### Vector-borne

Vector-borne diseases (excluding mechanical transmission) propagate between an arthropod vector and a vertebrate host. Because two incubation periods (an extrinsic one in the vector and an intrinsic one in the human) are involved, the generation times tend to be longer than for person-to-person outbreaks. The early phase of these outbreaks tends to develop more slowly. Three additional biological factors profoundly affect the shape of the epidemic curve.

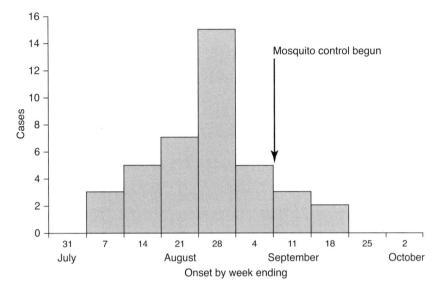

**Figure 9–10.** Number of seropositive cases of West Nile virus, by week of onset—New York City, 1999. [*Source:* CDC, 1999.[14]]

- Arthropod vectors, once infected, characteristically remain so until they perish. This tends to prolong and stabilize vector-borne outbreaks and obscure any underlying propagative periodicity.
- Environmental temperatures exert a marked effect on the development and multiplication of infectious agents in an arthropod.
- Arthropod populations may grow explosively and can "crash" even more rapidly.

These last two factors will lead to irregular peaks during the progression of the outbreak and precipitous decreases.

An outbreak of *Plasmodium falciparum* malaria under highly favorable environmental conditions in Saudi Arabia shows several of these features (Fig. 9–11).[15] The outbreak developed very slowly until after week seven. Although periodic peaks typical of a propagated outbreak are not apparent, a stepwise increase with a three-to-four week period is noticeable. Finally, the outbreak declines abruptly after control of adult vectors.

Many vector-borne diseases are zoonoses in which the agent propagates in a non-human host while humans are a dead-end host. The West Nile virus epidemic in New York in 1999 revealed a rapid rise and a fairly abrupt decrease, perhaps related to a sudden decline in the vector population or exhaustion of the susceptible zoonotic population in late August of that year (see Fig. 9–10).[14]

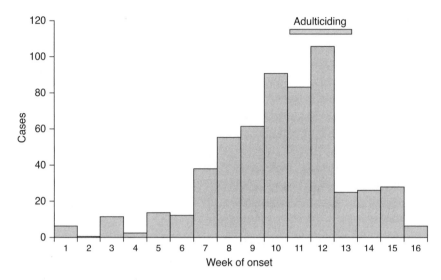

**Figure 9–11.** *Plasmodium falciparum* infections by week of onset of fever, Gelwa, Al-Baha Region, Saudi Arabia, January–April 1996. [*Source:* Ministry of Health, Saudi Arabia, 1996.[15]]

### Relative time

As an alternative to plotting onset by calendar time, plotting the time between suspect exposures and onset may help in understanding the epidemiologic situation. For example, a plot of the time between contact with a case of severe acute respiratory syndrome (SARS) by days since first contact with another SARS case shows an approximation to the incubation period while suggesting person-to-person transmission (Fig 9–12). The data from Table 9–1 could also be plotted as relative time from vaccination to onset.

### Multiple strata display

To assess whether critical epidemiologic times show distinctive internal patterns (e.g., by exposure, method of case detection, place, or personal characteristics) epidemic curves should be stratified. For example, in a continuing common source outbreak of typhoid fever, stratification revealed that confirmed cases both began and ended earlier among hospital staff than among the community or military base personnel (Fig. 9–13).[16] The reason for the time difference was related to the hospital's obtaining water from a commercial well while its own well was under repair. New cases among hospital staff ceased to occur one week after the hospital began using its own well again. The commercial well also sold water through three outlets in the community, and cases decreased in both the community and a nearby military base about one to two weeks after chlorination was enforced.

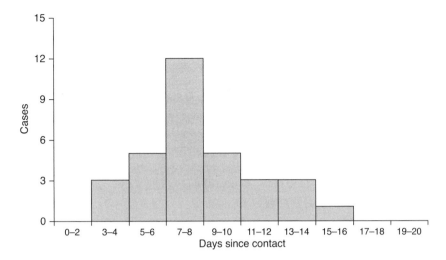

**Figure 9–12.** Days (two-day intervals) between onset of a case of severe acute respiratory syndrome (SARS) and onset of the corresponding source case, Beijing, China, March-April, 2003. [*Source:* S Xie et al., 2003.[18]]

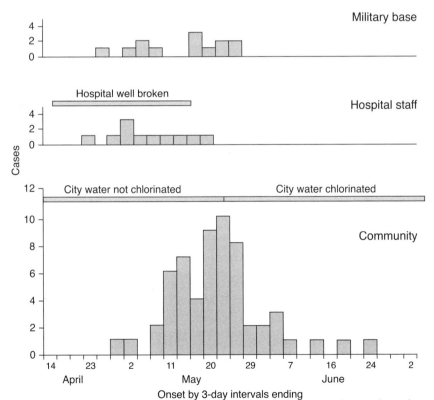

**Figure 9–13.** Cases of typhoid fever by date of onset, Tabuk, Saudi Arabia, April–June 1992. [*Source:* Al-Qawari et al., 1995.[16]]

## Examining rates in time

Whereas case counts over time are usually graphed as a histogram, disease rates over time are usually graphed with a line graph or a frequency polygon (see Appendix 9–1). The $x$ axis represents a period of time of interest: decades, years, months, or days of the week. The $y$ axis represents the rate of the health event. For most conditions, when the rates vary over one or two orders of magnitude, an arithmetic scale is appropriate. For rates which vary more widely and/or when comparisons are to be made, a logarithmic scale for the $y$ axis may be more appropriate.

## Secular trend

For some conditions, including many chronic diseases, the time characteristic of interest is the secular trend—the rate of disease over many years. Review of these secular trends may suggest or indicate key events, improvements in control, sociological phenomena, or other factors that have modified the epidemiology of the condition. Secular trends are most often shown on a line graph along with important modifying factors. The secular trend of malaria from 1930 to 1998 may thus be compared to important events that influenced malaria incidence (see Fig. 3–1).

## Cyclical, seasonal, and other cycles

For many conditions, a description by season, month, day of the week, or even time of day may be revealing. For example, the incidence of varicella appears to be seasonal, since outbreaks tend to occur between March and May (Fig. 9–14).[17] Seasonal patterns also may be summarized in a seasonal or cyclical curve (see Appendix 9–1). These in turn may be stratified by place or person or other features to compare or contrast patterns. For instance, the pattern of seasonality shows distinct differences between villages and *Plasmodium* species in El Salvador (Fig. 9–15).[18]

## Examining Data by Place

Place represents another dimension for organizing and identifying patterns of epidemiologic data. Indeed, careful localization of cases can provide clear insight into an epidemiologic process. As with time, rates are important, but not necessary in every situation.

Information on place may include residence, workplace, school, recreation site, other relevant locales, or even movement between these fixed geographic points. Always distinguish between place of onset, place of known or suspected exposure, and place of case identification: they are often different and have distinct epidemiologic implications. Information on place may range in precision

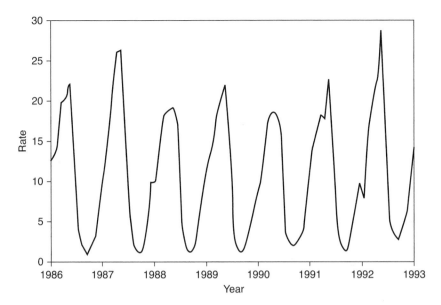

**Figure 9-14.** Rate (reported cases per 100,000 population) of Varicella (Chicken-pox)—United States, 1986–1992. [*Source:* CDC, 1992.[17]]

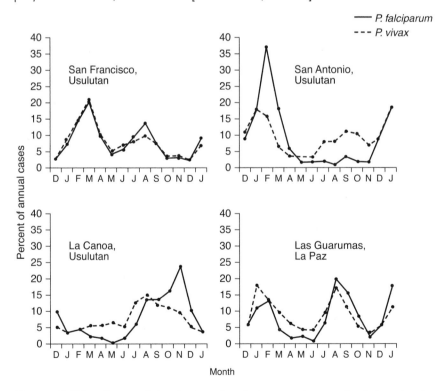

**Figure 9-15.** Seasonal distribution of malaria cases by month of detection by voluntary collaborators in four villages, El Salvador, 1970–1977. [*Source:* Fontaine et al., 1984.[18]]

from the geographic coordinates of a residence or bed in a hospital to simply the state of residence. Since population estimates or censuses are limited to standard geographic areas (e.g., city, census tract, county, state, or country), determination of rates is also restricted to these same areas.

## Maps

Place data are best organized, displayed, and examined on maps. Maps give you the ability to compare rates of disease by place. Maps efficiently display a wealth of underlying detail to compare with disease distribution. Maps allow quick recognition and comparisons relative to tables or other data displays. A simple, comparative display of rates by place on a table or chart may not show a pattern. However, on a map, the same data may show a spatial trend or aggregation of higher rates in one area.

*Spot Maps:* Cases can be plotted on a base map, a detailed picture of the earth's surface (using satellite imagery and hand-held geographic positioning units), a floor plan, or other spatially accurate diagram to create a spot map. Dots, other symbols, onset times, or case identification numbers for indexing with a line-listing may represent cases. The map of a dengue outbreak using numbers to represent the order of days of onset reveals the spread of dengue cases up one street in the direction of the prevailing wind (Fig 9–16).[19] Note that the first identified case is near a clinic, raising suspicions about the original introduction of dengue into the neighborhood.

A spot map of an airplane cabin (Fig. 9–17) shows where passengers who developed tuberculosis infection sat in relation to the source case.[20] Spot maps that do not show spatial aggregation of cases may suggest a widespread environmental source, a distribution system (e.g., for food, water, or other product), or dispersal of individuals to or from a common area. The map of dengue (Fig 9–16) has been supplemented with scaled $x$ and $y$ axes to show the determination of the central point (centroid) by computing the mean of the horizontal (west–east) and of the vertical (south–north) location of each case. Centroids may lie close to, and help you identify, possible common sources.

You may also use spots or other plotting symbols to represent affected houses, towns, or other population units. If the denominator of the population unit is known, spots of different sizes or color intensity may be used to represent rates or ratios.

Spot maps that show only cases have a general weakness. The pattern of cases could represent a distinctive quality of the health event, variability in the underlying population distribution, or a combination of the two. Accordingly, when interpreting spot maps you should keep in mind the population distribution with particular attention to unpopulated (e.g., parks, vacant lots, abandoned warehouses) or densely populated areas.

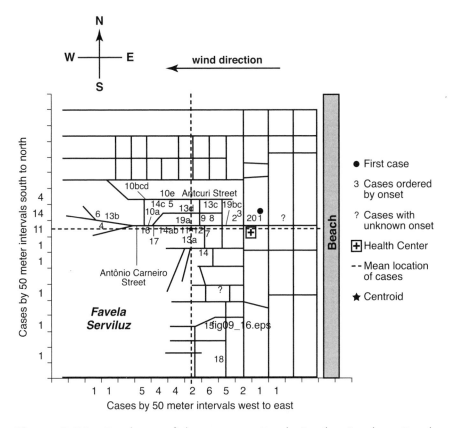

**Figure 9–16.** Distribution of dengue cases, *Favela Serviluz*, Forteleza, Brazil, June-July 1999. [*Source:* Heukelbach et al., 2001.[19]]

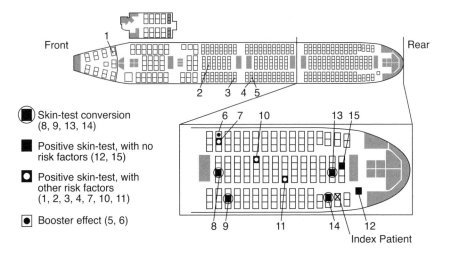

**Figure 9–17.** Diagram of the Boeing 747–100 with seat assignments of the passengers and flight crew on Flight 4 who had positive tuberculin skin tests. [*Source:* Kenyon et al., 1996.[20]]

*Area Maps and Rates:* Rates are normally shown on area (patch or choropleth) maps. The map is divided into population enumeration areas for which rates (or ratios) may be computed. The areas are then ranked according to their respective rates, and the ranking is broken up into intervals and shaded. Area maps are an essential tool in descriptive epidemiology, because they give good representations of spatial distributions of rates and ratios.

To reveal underlying patterns in the data, try to increase the data density on these maps by computing rates for the smallest area possible. For example, the county map of Lyme disease in the United States effectively displays several levels of risk for human infection (Fig. 9–18).[21] You should avoid using area maps to display case counts. Plotting only numerators loses the advantages of both the spot map and the area map. If small numbers of cases must be shown over a wide geographic area, then a spot map showing the relationship of the cases to important geographic features is usually more helpful.

Many other forms of epidemiologic maps are available but are less frequently used in field epidemiology (e.g., cartograms and isarithmic maps). More detail on these may be found in other texts.[22–24]

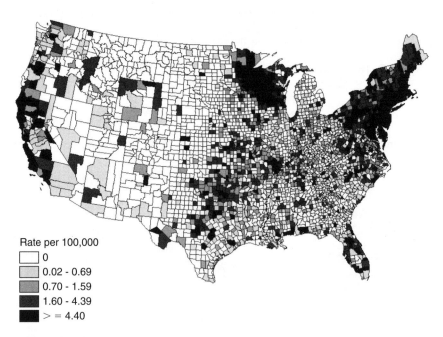

Rate per 100,000
- 0
- 0.02 - 0.69
- 0.70 - 1.59
- 1.60 - 4.39
- > = 4.40

*Categories above zero by quartile.

**Figure 9–18.** Average annual rate of Lyme disease cases per 100,000 per year in the United States, 1992–1998. [*Source:* CDC, 1999.[21]]

## Person

Persons may be characterized by several categories of attributes: demographic characteristics of those affected (including age, race, ethnic group, and gender); socioeconomic status; education; occupation; leisure activities; religion; marital status; contact with other persons or groups; and other personal variables (such as pregnancy, blood type, immunization status, underlying illnesses, or use of medications). The recognition of disease patterns, according to these personal attributes, is the third essential step in descriptive epidemiology.

Information on persons can be examined in either tabular or graphic form. Graphic displays of personal characteristics may be very illuminating when one or more personal characteristics are on an ordinal or continuous scale; for example, age or body mass index. Rates for nominative variables alone, such as gender, ethnicity, race, or other traits, are best presented in tabular format. Two important qualifications apply to the assessment of personal data. First, determination of rates for personal data is far more critical than for time and place. Second, age is one of the strongest independent determinants for many causes of morbidity and mortality and, accordingly, deserves primary consideration.

### Personal contact and network groups

Humans characteristically form social groupings. These groups may be as well defined and compact as a family living together in a home or as diffuse as a group linked together only by common interests or behaviors. Description of diseases by family, other well-defined groups, or as diffuse social networks can often uncover patterns that may assist in developing hypotheses. Data concerning these personal linkages are often obtained during initial, exploratory interviews of reported cases.

The underlying epidemiologic process may produce distributions that range from strong aggregation to randomness or to uniformity in a family or household. Clustered distributions may suggest common exposures of household members, an agent that is transmissible from one family member to another, an environmental exposure from the living quarters themselves, localization of the houses near or within an environmental area of high risk, or even human–vector–human transmission in situations where the vector is not highly mobile. In contrast, random or even distributions among households suggest that the exposure lies outside the family unit or that it is uniformly distributed among all units (e.g., a town water supply).

Since census data provide household sizes and numbers of households, denominator data are available, if necessary, to make comparisons. However, assessment of risk among large numbers of small population groups (i.e., families) leads to highly unstable rates. Several statistical methods are available to assess aggregation by household or similar small groupings of people.

For diseases or behaviors spread through personal association or contact (e. g., measles, sexually transmitted diseases, tuberculosis, addiction, and mass sociogenic illness), data concerning linkages between affected individuals are often revealing. Contact diagrams can reveal important characteristics of these linkages, including closeness and quality of relationships, timing between onsets, and places of contact, and provide a quickly interpretable overview that may reveal key details, such as index cases or outliers (Fig. 9–19).[25]

### Age

The epidemiologist will determine disease rates by age in virtually all field investigations. This may be as simple as finding that a health event is affecting only a limited age group or as complicated as comparing age-specific incidence rates among several groups of people. Remember that age actually represents three different categories of determinants of disease risk.

- The condition of the host and their susceptibility to disease: Individuals of different ages often differ in susceptibility or predisposition to disease. Clearly, age is one of the most important determinants in the expression of chronic diseases, many infectious diseases, and mortality.
- Differing intensities of exposure to causative agents: For example, infants and young children may be at far greater risk of exposure to organisms spread through the fecal–oral route than older individuals.

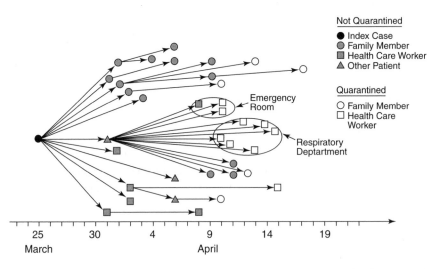

**Figure 9–19.** Contact between SARS cases among a group of relatives and health care workers—Beijing, China 2003. [*Source:* Xie S., 2003.[25]]

- The passage of time: Older individuals will simply have had greater over-all time of exposure or may have been exposed at different periods of time when background exposures to certain agents were greater. A disease with a long latent period, such as tuberculosis, may reflect exposures several decades in the past.

In an analysis of farm tractor–related fatalities in Georgia, age group–specific fatality rates, derived by using two different denominator groups, draw attention to potential risk factors affecting the elderly and to the major difference in risk between farm and non-farm residence (Table 9–4).[26] Since age is a continuous variable, graphic displays of age-specific rates can help compare differences between population groups. A graph, using semi-logarithmic paper, comparing age-specific mortality rates in the United States for 1910, 1950, and 1998 reveals reductions of mortality among persons under 60 years of age (Fig. 9–20).[27–29]

## Age standardization

Because age is a pervasive determinant of disease and because population groups often differ in their age structures, adjustment or standardization by age is a useful tool for comparing rates between population groups. For example, a com-parison of the crude death rates of two Florida counties—Dade and Pinellas coun-ties—for 1960, shows a rate of 15.3/1000 for Dade and 8.9/1000 for Pinellas. Age-specific death rates, however, generally show a higher mortality rate in Dade County. This seemingly contradictory finding can be explained simply by unequal distributions of persons in the various age groups. To "adjust" for these differences you can create a "standard" population by pooling both these two population groups or by using an age distribution from another "representative" population.

**Table 9–4.** Annual Fatality Rates per 100,000 Males in Accidents Associated with Farm Tractors, Georgia, 1971–1981.

| | | FARM RESIDENTS | | ALL RURAL RESIDENTS | |
|---|---|---|---|---|---|
| AGE GROUP (YEARS) | NUMBER OF DEATHS | RATE | STANDARD ERROR | RATE | STANDARD ERROR |
| <20 | 21 | 6.7 | ±1.5 | 0.5 | ±0.1 |
| 20–39 | 32 | 32 | ±4.0 | 1.1 | ±0.2 |
| 40–59 | 65 | 27 | ±3.4 | 3.1 | ±0.4 |
| ≥60 | 80 | 54 | ±6.1 | 6.4 | ±0.1 |
| Total | 198 | 23 | | 1.9 | |

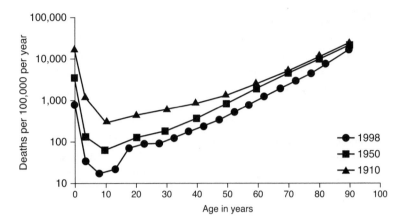

**Figure 9–20.** Age-specific mortality rates per 100,000 per year, United States, 1910, 1950, and 1998. [*Source:* NCHS, 2001.[27–29]]

Finally, you would apply age-specific death rates from each county (or the "representative" population) to those pooled numbers and create new, supposedly age-specific death rates for each county. If you do this, the crude death rates then become 10.9/1000 for Dade County and 10.4/1000 for Pinellas County.[30]

Age-adjusted rates may be used to compare rates among populations from different areas, from the same area at different times, and among any other characteristic such as ethnicity or socioeconomic status. Adjustment produces a summary rate for each population with the effect of age removed. However, at the same time, adjustment hides potentially illuminating patterns in age-specific incidence rates. Accordingly, it is highly advisable to examine age-specific rates in graphic or tabular form before embarking on age standardization.

### Other personal attributes

The use of other personal attributes in descriptive epidemiology is limited only by the availability of denominators for computing rates. Most commonly these include gender, ethnicity, race, education, and socioeconomic level. However, for many priority diseases or conditions, data include risk factors or exposures that do not have readily available denominator data.

## Combinations of Time, Place, and Person

Often comparisons in descriptive epidemiology will require evaluation of two or even all three of the principal epidemiologic variables. These comparisons are best visualized through a series of small, multiple figures. For instance, the progression of a disease in time across a geographic area may be best shown with a series of small maps (Fig. 9–21).[31] When the shape of the epidemic curve must be compared for different localities or different population groups, a series of small epidemic curves offers an efficient method of comparison (see Fig. 9–12). To reveal temporal or spatial variation, a series of small line graphs may be created for comparison (see Fig. 9–14).

## DATA QUALITY

Throughout this chapter we have described epidemiologic data as if they were free of mistakes or artifacts. This is not always true. Interpretation of patterns that arise from poor-quality or haphazardly collected data leads to confusion, loss of valuable time and resources, and, worst of all, invalid conclusions. To assess the quality of descriptive data, you should first try to identify and understand the factors that might be leading you astray. These could include: incomplete data; uneven reporting in time, place, or person; combining prevalent with incident cases; changes or non-uniform application of case definitions; using date of report to represent date of onset; and so forth. Where place is concerned, reports may come from reporting sites that do not correspond to residence or exposure. You should also recognize that some categories of data are inherently more accurate (age) than others (e.g., socioeconomic status). Review the data set, and look for problems such as (for example) terminal digit bias, onset dates that follow diagnosis dates, or age or gender that is incompatible with the disease. Problems with the data may be diverse and are not always or fully under your control. It is important

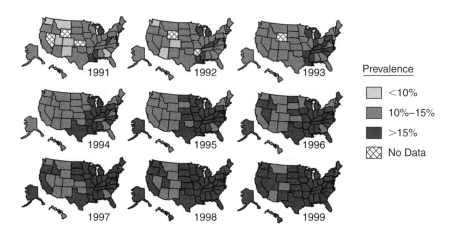

**Figure 9–21.** Prevalence of overweight among adults, Behavioral Risk Factor Surveillance System, United States, 1991–1999. [*Source:* Mokdad et al., 1999.[31]]

to be alert for them, recognize them when they occur, and correct them or take them into account in your interpretation.

## Forming the Hypothesis

Earlier in this chapter we noted that an important use of descriptive epidemiology is to support hypothesis formation. A hypothesis is a testable proposition developed from known facts, data, and information.[9] A hypothesis that is crafted from accurate data and facts will surpass a mere "educated guess." A hypothesis should contain the following elements:

- The population under study
- The cause and applicable co-factors
- The outcome
- A dose–response relationship
- A time–response relationship

Some field investigations will require minimal effort in hypothesis generation. Consider, for example, gastrointestinal illness caused by an agent that must propagate in food and that affects a gathering where only one meal is shared during the incubation period of the causative agent. When, however, a more complicated situation arises (see Chapter 5) you must carefully consider the descriptive epidemiology and additional facts and data. A useful categorization is as follows:

- The distribution by time, place, and person as detailed in this chapter.
- Known facts about the disease and agent including the effect of host factors.
- Known patterns of transmission or risk factors for acquisition of the disease or analogous diseases or conditions.
- Observations about exposures affecting the population under investigation: These can include known facts about the environment, direct observation of key objects or activities, and hypothesis-generating interviews about exposures, habits, or routines.
- Outliers and apparently paradoxical observations: Persons who do not fit the general or expected pattern may have a special, highly specific or unique exposure that serves to support one hypothesis.

After assembling this information, you should then assess each finding to help you to lower the possibility of some potential factors and increase the possibility of other factors. Usually, no single finding will give absolute inclusion or exclusion of a hypothesis. Accordingly, one must weigh the strength, data quality, and specificity of each finding. The sum of the combined evidence will point to the most probable hypothesis.

## SUMMARY

Descriptive epidemiology includes both numbers and rates to document how much of a health condition is present or occurring in a population. It also includes the three critical dimensions for describing health conditions: time, place, and person. *Time* refers to acute changes in disease occurrence, such as an epidemic, and changes over longer time periods, such as seasonal patterns and secular trends. Time data are usually displayed graphically. *Place* refers to geopolitical boundaries, topography, or locations of rooms, buildings, and other structures. Place data are best displayed with maps. *Person* refers to demographic and other personal characteristics of the populations under study. Personal data are usually displayed in tables or graphs. When done well, descriptive epidemiology can characterize the health problem in the community; provide clues that can be turned into testable hypotheses; and promote effective communication with scientific, policy-making, and lay audiences alike.

## APPENDIX 9–1. GRAPHS, MAPS, AND CHARTS IN DESCRIPTIVE EPIDEMIOLOGY:

## GENERAL PRINCIPLES

Tables, graphs, charts, maps, and diagrams should give the viewer a rapid, objective, and coherent grasp of the data. Whether the table or graphic serves to help the investigator understand the data or explain the data in a report or to an audience, their organization should quickly reveal the principal patterns and the exceptions to those patterns. When using tables or graphics to communicate, first decide on the main point and then choose the method of display.

Tables, graphs, charts, maps, and diagrams all have the following three elements in common:

- A title that includes the "what, where, and when" that completely identify the data they introduce.
- Footnotes that explain abbreviations, data sources, units of measurement, and other necessary details or data that was lost in the data summarization.
- Text that points out the main patterns of the data. This text may appear with the table or graphic or in the body of the report.

## TABLES

Tables are the best way to show numerical values. Tables are preferable for many small data sets. They also work well when data presentation requires many localized comparisons.[22] A well-structured table that is organized to focus on comparisons may prove superior to a graph or chart. In addition to the previously mentioned elements common to all data displays, tables will have column and row headings. These headings should include an identification of the data and any units of measurement that apply to all the data in the column or row. Abbreviations may be needed to conserve space in column headings, and these will need to be explained in the footnotes.

Careful attention to data arrangement in your tables will go far toward enhancing your readers' understanding. Although little empirical evidence exists concerning the ideal structure of a table for data presentation, statisticians in several fields espouse the following guidelines, proposed by Ehrenberg.[32, 33]

- Round data to two significant or effective figures. Rarely is more precision needed for epidemiologic data, and more than two significant figures interferes with comparison and comprehension. *Effective figures* refers to numbers that contain additional, leading non-zero digits that do not vary (e.g. 123, 145, 168, 177) within a column or row.
- Provide marginal averages, rates, totals, or other summary statistics.
- Use columns for the more important data comparisons. Numbers are more easily compared down a column than across a row.
- Organize data by magnitude in columns and if possible also in rows. It helps also to organize data columns and rows by the magnitude of the marginal summary statistics. When the row or column headings have an intrinsic numerical order (e.g. age groups), the row or column headings should govern the order.
- Utilize the table layout to guide the eye. This involves paying attention to alignment of numbers (aligned on the decimal), placing numbers close together for comparisons, and avoiding grids and other unnecessary ornamentation.

To show the effect of applying these guidelines, two tables of the same made-up data are presented (Tables 9–5A and 9–5B). The first ignores these guidelines, and the second shows the same data after rearrangement according to the guidelines. Note that these guidelines apply to presentation of data for identification, comparison, and communication of patterns. Tables that are designed purely to look up a statistic (reference tables) should be organized to allow the user to quickly find the desired statistic.

**Table 9-5 A.** Incidence Rates (per 10,000 per year) for Disease X by Ethnicity and Sex

| ETHNICITY | MALES | | | FEMALES | | | BOTH SEXES | | |
|---|---|---|---|---|---|---|---|---|---|
| | CASES | POP.[a] | RATE | CASES | POP.[a] | RATE | CASES | POP.[a] | RATE |
| White, non-Hispanic | 51 | 34,233 | 14.9 | 36 | 35,621 | 10.1 | 87 | 69,854 | 12.5 |
| Black, non-Hispanic | 23 | 12,561 | 18.3 | 13 | 14,888 | 8.7 | 31 | 27,449 | 11.3 |
| Hispanic | 12 | 5,843 | 20.5 | 7 | 5,072 | 13.8 | 19 | 10,915 | 17.8 |
| Asian/Pacific Islander | 4 | 2,311 | 17.3 | 3 | 2,076 | 14.5 | 7 | 4,387 | 14.9 |
| American Indian/Alaskan Native | 13 | 4,874 | 26.7 | 8 | 4,412 | 18.1 | 21 | 9,286 | 22.4 |
| Other | 2 | 907 | 22.1 | 0 | 823 | 0.0 | 2 | 1,730 | 10.3 |
| All | 105 | 60,729 | 17.3 | 67 | 62,892 | 10.7 | 167 | 123,621 | 13.5 |

a. Population estimate from 2000 census.

**Table 9-5 B.** Incidence Rates (per 10,000 per year)[a] for Disease X by Ethnicity and Sex, City A, 2005

| ETHNICITY | MALES | | FEMALES | | BOTH SEXES | | RATE | | |
|---|---|---|---|---|---|---|---|---|---|
| | CASES | POP.[b] | CASES | POP.[b] | CASES | POP.[b] | M | F | BOTH |
| American Indian/Alaskan Native | 13 | 4,900 | 8 | 4,400 | 21 | 9,300 | 27 | 18 | 22 |
| Hispanic | 12 | 5,800 | 7 | 5,100 | 19 | 11,000 | 21 | 14 | 18 |
| Asian/Pacific Islander | 4 | 2,300 | 3 | 2,100 | 7 | 4,400 | 17 | 14 | 15 |
| White, non-Hispanic | 51 | 34,000 | 36 | 36,000 | 87 | 70,000 | 15 | 10 | 13 |
| Black, non-Hispanic | 23 | 13,000 | 8 | 15,000 | 31 | 28,000 | 18 | 5 | 11 |
| Other | 2 | 910 | 0 | 820 | 2 | 1,700 | 22 | 0 | 10 |
| All | 105[c] | 61,000 | 62 | 63,000 | 167[c] | 124,000 | 17 | 10 | 13 |

a. All numbers rounded to 2 significant digits unless otherwise indicated.
b. Population estimate from 2000 census.
c. Not rounded.

## GRAPHS

The simplest graphs are most effective. No more lines or symbols should be used in a single graph than the eye can easily follow or than the viewer can easily understand. To compare several strata, use several miniaturized and identically scaled graphs arranged on the page to facilitate comparison. Avoid unnecessary decoration. Above all, emphasize the data without distortion. The best graphs synthesize large amounts of data yet preserve the necessary detail in the data. For more comprehensive coverage of graphic techniques, the reader is referred to Cleveland and a series of books by Tufte.[23, 34–36]

Follow these guidelines:

- When more than one variable is shown on the graph, each should be clearly differentiated by legends or keys.
- Frequencies are usually represented on the vertical scale and method of classification on the horizontal scale.
- Adhere to basic mathematical principles in plotting data and scaling axes.
- On an arithmetic scale, equal numerical units must be represented by equal distances on the scale.
- When comparing two graphs (e.g. Figs. 9–13 and 9–15) use appropriate scales. Usually these are identical, but if this destroys resolution, different scales may be used.
- Scale divisions should be clearly indicated, as well as the units into which the scale is divided.
- Use visually prominent symbols to plot and emphasize data.
- Keep tick marks, keys, legends, markers, and other annotations out of the data space. Instead put them just outside the data region.
- Overlapping plotting symbols should be distinguishable.
- Superimposed data sets must be visually discriminated. This problem occurs when two or more data sets are plotted in the same data space.
- Minimize frames, gridlines, tick marks (6–10 per axis are sufficient) to avoid interference with the data.
- Scale the graph to fill the data space and improve resolution. If this means that you must exclude the zero level, exclude it.
- Use graphic designs that reveal the data from the broad overview to the fine detail.
- Proofread your graphs.

## Graphing Time and other Numerically Scaled Variables

The basic options for displaying and assessing epidemiologic rates include arithmetic and semi-logarithmic graphs. Time or other numerically scaled variables (e.g., age) are best shown on the x axis either on a continuous scale or divided into intervals. Case counts, rates, or ratios are best shown on the y axis.

## Arithmetic scale line graph

In an arithmetic scale line graph, an equal distance on the y axis represents an equal quantity anywhere on a given x axis. The shape of the line will depend upon the scaling of the axes, and judgment should be used to avoid distorting the data or obscuring important features of the line. The scale should be defined in such a way as to make it easy to understand. When possible, a break in the scale should *not* be used with a scale line graph. If large differences in rates must be shown, then consider a semilogarithmic graph (Fig 9–20) or use a box inset into the graph to show a portion of the line at a different scale.

## Semilogarithmic scale line graph

Data on graphs may be transformed to different scales for better understanding and increased clarity. The most common and versatile rescaling of graphs in epidemiology is the semi-logarithmic scale line graph. In the semi-logarithmic line graph, one coordinate or axis (usually the y axis) is transformed to logarithms of units, whereas the other axis is scaled in arithmetic units. Consider this approach for examining the relative changes rather than the absolute change (i.e., actual amount of change). It is particularly helpful when comparing two or more variables whose rates differ by several orders of magnitude (Fig 9–20). The advantages of semi-logarithmic graphing are that:

- A straight line indicates a constant rate of change,
- The slope of the line indicates the rate of change,
- Two or more lines following parallel paths show identical rates of change, and
- A wide range of values (three to four orders of magnitude) can be displayed effectively on a single graph.

## Scatter plots

Scatter plots are versatile instruments for exploring and for communication data. Indeed, both spot maps (Fig 9–16) and line graphs (without the lines) are forms of the scatter plot. They are used to show the relationship between two numerically scaled variables. Each spot represents the joint magnitude of the two variables. One of the variables is scaled according to the x axis and the other according to the y axis. The averages and variances of each of the two variables may also be shown on the plot and on the respective axes. Scatter plots are often used in epidemiology to show the relationship between rates and some explanatory variable thought to be related to that rate. As a convention the explanatory variable is plotted against the *x* axis and the rate against the y axis.

When the pattern of the spots forms a compact, linear pattern, one can suspect a strong relationship between the two variables. In the example (Figures 9–22), there is a distinctive pattern of rapidly increasing cholera death rates as the altitude approaches the level of the river Thames. Note that this does not indicate that altitude causes cholera but suggests that some geographic feature (e.g., poor drainage of sewage) may contribute to cholera incidence.

*Graphing counts*   A histogram presents the frequency distribution of individual measurements. A measurement—normally a continuous variable, such as time, age, height, weight, or blood pressure—is partitioned into intervals along the *x* axis. Counts of individuals or cases are then shown as vertical columns scaled against the y axis. The area under the curve represents the *frequency distribution*. Thus, adjacent columns are not separated by space, and scale breaks should not be used. Do not use unequal intervals. However, if unequal intervals are unavoidable (e.g., for a frequency distribution by age), the height of each column should be adjusted to maintain the ratio of area to frequency. The most common use of histograms in field epidemiology is the *epidemic curve* (Figs. 9–4 to 9–13). In general, only lines representing the height of each column are drawn. With only a few cases, a common practice is to divide each column to show individual cases.

Comparing the frequency distributions of two or more subgroups will often be necessary. For example, you may want to compare epidemic curves by districts of a city. To allow the eye to rapidly compare graphs of individual strata, use multiple histograms—one for each stratum—with the same scaling. These may be reduced

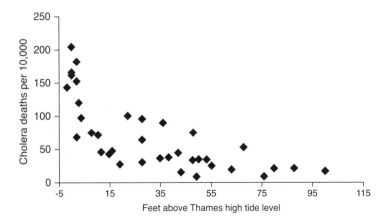

**Figure 9–22.**   Cholera deaths per 10,000 inhabitants and altitude above the average high tide level by district, London, 1849 [*Source:* Registrar-General, 1852.[37]]

in size of inclusion in reports without losing sight of the data pattern or comparison (Fig. 9–13) Avoid stacking subgroups or strata upon one another on the same baseline as this can hopelessly distort the individual patterns and their interpretation. Also consider using *frequency polygons* for comparing strata. Frequency polygons are constructed from histograms. A line is drawn between the midpoints of the tops of each column. Several frequency polygons may then be plotted on the same axes as long as the individual lines do not become entangled and difficult to interpret.

*Seasonal curves*   For a single year, either a simple histogram of case counts or a line graph of monthly rates may be constructed. Since the idea of the seasonal curve is to observe the relative difference from month to month, comparisons of seasonal curves in different places may be adjusted to depict relative rather than absolute differences. The epidemiologist may make semi-logarithmic plots. This method has the advantage of conserving the comparison of rates but tends to suppress the visual perception of peaks and valleys in the distribution. A second method converts the data to percentage of total (see Fig. 9–14). This will put all localities on the same relative axis and accentuate the visual perception of seasonal peaks. However, localities with more extended seasonal increases or more than one peak will appear as if they had less intense incidence. Consider including a redundant beginning point and end point (see Fig. 9–14). This allows the viewer to see the trend between the last and first intervals of the cycle.

*Maps*   Maps should have a scale that reflects the actual distance. This scale may be shown as a scale bar, scaling of the $x$ and $y$ axes (longitude and latitude), and a numerical key showing the ratio of distance on the map to actual distance. For example 1:100,000 indicates that 1 cm on the map represents 1 km (100,000 cm) in actual distance. These distance relationships are critical in interpreting the spread or distribution of diseases and should always be shown on epidemiologic maps. Maps also need an indicator of orientation. Usually this is shown by a simple arrow pointing north. Finally, maps need to have an indicator of location on the earth. This is normally shown with longitude and latitude grid or tick marks which may also serve as a scale.

Most maps will also have a key or legend to allow the viewer to understand the meaning of shading, spots, or other symbols that indicate disease and possible exposures and other environmental factors. You should take care in coloring maps, particularly area maps. To show rates and other quantitative information about the same disease, use different intensities of the same color. Shading maps with varying shades of gray between white and pure black gives the best discrimination (Fig 9–18). To show nominative or qualitative data, use different colors. Two colors may be used to show divergence of rates or ratios from an average or reference level toward high and low extremes.

## CHARTS

Charts are instruments for presenting statistical information symbolically using only one coordinate.

## Bar Charts

Bar charts allow rapid visualization and comprehension of differences in rates or counts among nominative categories. Alternatively, a table may show the same data with similar effectiveness. Avoid using bar charts for showing different categories of a numerically scaled variable. These are better presented as line graphs.

All categories in a bar chart have a uniform column width. The columns are separated by spaces. The bars may be arranged horizontally or vertically. Arrangement in either an ascending or descending order helps interpretation. Scale breaks should never be used in bar charts. However, the columns may be shaded, hatched, or colored to index the variable shown by each bar. Bars should be labeled at their base.

### Simple bar chart

Counts, rates, percentages, ratios, or any other numerical derivative of several categories of a nominative variable may be compared using this basic format (Fig. 9–23).[37] Each column rises from a baseline. The length of the column is gauged against the other columns and the y axis or, if a horizontal chart, the x axis. The numerical scale may be arithmetic or logarithmic, ratio-scaled or by any other derivative of the basic data. The tabular equivalent of this chart is a two-variable table.

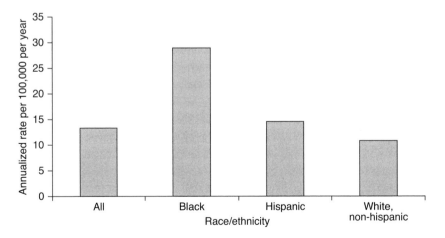

**Figure 9-23.** Annualized rates per 100,000 population for firearm-related injuries by race/ethnicity—United States, 1993–1998. [*Source:* CDC, 2001.[38]]

### Two-category bar charts

Several designs allow simultaneous comparisons of a numerical variable among different categories and subcategories of a nominative value variable. For example, a major category, ETHNIC GROUP, could be divided into a secondary nominative variable such as EDUCATION ATTAINED. A legend is needed to index the subcategories. These charts correspond to three-variable tables.

### Grouped (clustered) bar chart

A grouped bar chart can also be thought of as an aggregation of miniaturized, simple bar charts, each one representing a different primary category (Fig. 9–24).[37] Bars within each primary category are usually adjoining, whereas bar groupings are separated. Grouped bar charts may be shown as a series of charts along a single baseline or as miniaturized multiples arranged in columns and rows. Since all bars are on the same baseline, differences in bar length are easily visualized. Grouped bar charts do not clearly show the differences in the totals among the major categories. Moreover, the display becomes confusing with more than a few subcategories.

### Stacked bar chart, 100% bar chart, and pie charts.

Stacked bar chart, 100% bar charts, and pie charts should be avoided. Empirical evidence has shown that they do not communicate data or data patterns as quickly or accurately as simple bar charts, dot charts, line graphs or tables.[22, 34]

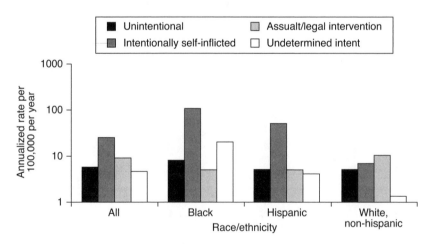

**Figure 9–24.** Annualized rates per 100,000 population for firearm-related injuries by race/ethnicity and intent of injury—United States, 1993–1998. [*Source:* CDC, 2001.[38]]

## A FINAL SUGGESTION FOR THE DESIGN AND USE OF TABLES, GRAPHS, AND CHARTS

Effective communication entails not only the ability to transfer facts to the viewer so that understanding is reached, but to do so in a believable and persuasive way. So, remember who your audience is. Are they professional epidemiologists, other scientists, policy makers, administrators, news media, or the general public? Your data presentations and language should fit their level of understanding and intellect. However, no matter who the audience is, your challenge is to inform and simplify while showing as undistorted a picture of the data as possible.

## REFERENCES

1. Centers for Disease Control and Prevention (1999). Intussusception among recipients of rotavirus vaccine—United States, 1998–1999. *Morb Mortal Wkly Rep* 48, 577–81.
2. Centers for Disease Control and Prevention. (1992). *Principles of Epidemiology. A Self-Study Course*, 2nd ed., Atlanta.
3. Centers for Disease Control and Prevention (1997). Injuries and deaths associated with use of snowmobiles—Maine, 1991–1996. *Morb Mortal Wkly Rep* 46,1–4.
4. Centers for Disease Control and Prevention (1992). Summary of notifiable diseases, United States. *Morb Mortal Wkly Rep* 41, 38.
5. Abulrahi, H.A., Bohlega, E.A., Fontaine, R.E., et al. (1997). *Plasmodium falciparum* malaria transmitted in hospital through heparin locks. *Lancet* 349, 23–5.
6. Centers for Disease Control and Prevention (1994). Outbreak of measles among Christian Science students—Missouri and Illinois, 1994. *Morb Mortal Wkly Rep* 43, 463–5.
7. Ministry of Health (1999). Field Epidemiology Training Program, Jordan. Unpublished data.
8. Tauxe, R.V., Tormey, M.P., Mascola, L., et al. (1987). Salmonellosis outbreak in trans-atlantic flights; Foodborne illness on aircraft: 1947–1984. *Am J Epidemiol* 125, 150–7.
9. Mausner, J.S., Bahn, A.K. (1974). *Epidemiology: An Introductory Text*, W.B. Saunders, Philadelphia.
10. Anderson, R.M., May, R.M. (1992). *Infectious Diseases of Humans: Dynamics and Control*, Oxford University Press, Oxford.
11. Fontaine, R.E., Cohen, M.L., Martin, W.T., et al. (1980). Epidemic salmonellosis from cheddar cheese: surveillance and prevention. *Am J Epidemiol* 111, 247–53.
12. Centers for Disease Control and Prevention (1999). Rubella outbreak—Westchester County, New York, 1997–1998. *Morb Mortal Wkly Rep* 48, 560–3.
13. Ko, A.I., Mitermayer, G.R., Ribero Dourado, C.M., et al. (1999). Urban epidemic of severe leptospirosis in Brazil. *Lancet* 354, 820–5.
14. Centers for Disease Control and Prevention (1999). Update: West Nile virus encepha-litis—New York, 1999. *Morb Mortal Wkly Rep* 48, 944–55.
15. Ministry of Health (1996). Field Epidemiology Training Program, Saudi Arabia. Unpublished data.
16. Al-Qarawi, S.M., El Bushra, H.E., Fontaine, R.E., et al. (1995). Typhoid fever from water desalinized using reverse osmosis. *Epidemiol Infect* 114, 41–50.

17. Centers for Disease Control and Prevention (1992). Summary of notifiable diseases, United States. *Morb Mortal Wkly Rep* 41, 64.
18. Fontaine, R.E., van Severin, M., Houng, A. (1984). The stratification of malaria in El Salvador using available malaria surveillance data. Abstract 184, XIth International Congress for Tropical Medicine and Malaria, Calgary, Canada.16–22 September 1984.
19. Heukelbach, J., de Oliveira, F.A., Kerr-Pontes, L.R., et al. (2001). Risk factors associated with an outbreak of dengue fever in a *favela* in Fortaleza, northeast Brazil. *Trop Med Int Health*. 8, 635–42.
20. Kenyon, T.A., Valway, S.E., Ihle, W.W., et al. (1996). Transmission of multidrug-resistant *Mycobacterium tuberculosis* during a long airplane flight. *N Engl J Med* 334, 933–8.
21. Centers for Disease Control and Prevention (1999). Unpublished data.
22. Tufte, E.R. (1987). *The Visual Display of Quantitative Information*, Graphics Press, Cheshire, Conn.
23. Robinson, A.H., Sale, R.D., Morrison, J.L., et al. (1985). *Elements of Cartography*, 5th ed., John Wiley & Sons, New York.
24. Cliff, A.D., Haggett, P. (1988). *Atlas of Disease Distributions: Analytic Approaches to Epidemiological Data*, Blackwell Publishers, Cambridge, Mass.
25. Xie, S., Zeng, G., Lei, J., Li, Q., et al. (2003). A highly efficient transmission of SARS among extended family and hospital staff in Beijing, China, April 2003. 2nd Southeast Asian and Western Pacific Bi-regional TEPHINET Scientific Conference, November 24–28, 2003, Borocay, Philippines.
26. Goodman, R.A., Smith, J.D., Sikes, R.K., et al. (1985) An epidemiologic study of fatalities associated with farm tractor injuries. *Public Health Rep* 100, 329–33.
27. National Center for Health Statistics (2001). http://www.cdc.gov/nchs/data/mx190039.pdf. April 2001.
28. National Center for Health Statistics (2001). http://www.cdc.gov/nchs/data/mx195059.pdf. April 2001.
29. National Center for Health Statistics (2001). http://www.cdc.gov/nchs/data/nvsr/nvsr48/nvsr48_11.pdf. April 2001.
30. Fleiss, J.C. (1981). *Statistical Methods for Rates and Proportions*, John Wiley & Sons, New York.
31. Mokdad, A.H., Serdula, M.K., Dietz, W.H., et al. (1999). The spread of the obesity epidemic in the United States, 1991–1998. *JAMA* 282, 1519–22.
32. Ehrenberg, A.C. (1981). The problem of numeracy. *Am Statistician* 35, 67–71.
33. Bailar, J.C. III, Mosteller, F. (1988). Guidelines for statistical reporting in articles for medical journals. Amplifications and explanations. *Ann Intern Med* 108(2), 266–73.
34. Cleveland, W.S. (1985). *The Elements of Graphing Data*, Wadsworth Advanced Books and Software, Monterey, Calif
35. Tufte, E.R. (1990). *Envisioning Information*, Graphics Press, Cheshire, Conn.
36. Tufte, E.R. (1997). *Visual Explanations*, Graphics Press, Cheshire, Conn.
37. Registrar-General (1852). Report on the mortality of cholera in England 1848–1849. Her Majesty's Stationery Office.
38. Centers for Disease Control and Prevention (2001). Surveillance for fatal and nonfatal firearm-related injuries—United States, 1993–1998. *Morb Mortal Wkly Rep* CDC Surveillance Summaries 50, 27–8.

# 10

# ANALYZING AND INTERPRETING DATA

Richard C. Dicker

The purpose of many field investigations is to identify causes, risk factors, sources, vehicles, routes of transmission, or other factors that put some members of the population at greater risk than others of having an adverse health event. In some field investigations, identifying a "culprit" is sufficient; if the culprit can be eliminated, the problem is solved. In other field settings, the goal is to quantify the relationship between exposure (or any population characteristic) and a health outcome. Quantifying this relationship may lead not only to appropriate interventions but also to advances in knowledge about disease causation. Both types of field investigation require appropriate but not necessarily sophisticated analytical methods. This chapter describes the strategy for planning an analysis, methods for conducting the analysis, and guidelines for interpreting the results.

## PREANALYSIS PLANNING

### What to Analyze

The first step of a successful analysis is to lay out an analytic strategy in advance. A thoughtfully planned and carefully executed analysis is just as critical for a field investigation as it is for a protocol-based study. Planning is necessary to assure that the appropriate hypotheses will be considered and that the relevant data will be appropriately collected, recorded, managed, analyzed, and interpreted to evaluate those hypotheses. Therefore, the time to decide on what (and how) to analyze the data is before you design your questionnaire, *not* after you have collected the data. As illustrated in Figure 10–1, the hypotheses that you wish to evaluate drive the analysis. (These hypotheses are usually developed by considering the common causes and modes of transmission of the condition under investigation; talking with patients and with local medical and public health staff; observing the dominant

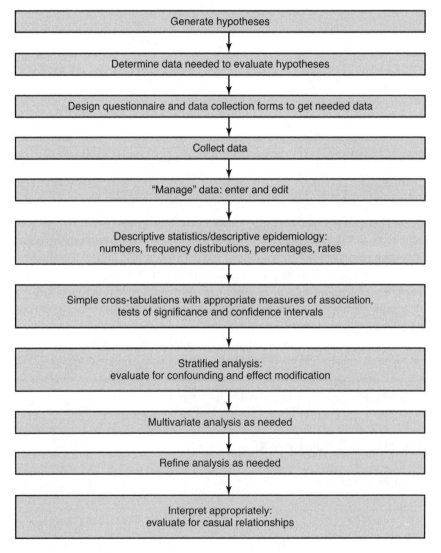

**Figure 10–1.** Steps in an analysis.

patterns in the descriptive epidemiologic data; and scrutinizing the outliers in these data.) Depending on the health condition being investigated, the hypotheses should address the source of the agent, the mode (and vehicle or vector) of transmission, and the exposures that caused disease. They should obviously be testable, since the role of the analysis will be to evaluate them.

Once you have determined the hypotheses to be evaluated, you must decide which data to collect in order to test the hypotheses. (You will also need to determine the best study design to use, as described in Chapter 8.) There is a saying in clinical medicine that "if you don't take a temperature, you can't find a fever."[1] Similarly, in field epidemiology, if you neglect to ask about a potentially important risk factor in the questionnaire, you cannot evaluate its role in the outbreak. Since the hypotheses to be tested dictate the data you need to collect, the time to plan the analysis is before you design the questionnaire.

Questionnaires and other data collection instruments are not limited to risk factors, however. They should also include identifying information, clinical information, and descriptive factors. Identifying information (or ID codes linked to identifying information stored elsewhere) allows you to recontact the respondent to ask additional questions or provide follow-up information. Sufficient clinical information should be collected to determine whether a patient truly meets the case definition. Clinical data on spectrum and severity of illness, hospitalization, and sequelae may also be useful. Descriptive factors related to time, place, and person should be collected to adequately characterize the population, assess comparability between groups (cases and controls in a case control study; exposed and unexposed groups in a cohort study), and help you generate hypotheses about causal relationships.

## Data Editing

Usually, data for an analytic study are collected on paper questionnaires. These data are then entered into a computer. Increasingly, data are entered directly into a computer or an online questionnaire database. In either situation, good data management practices will facilitate the analysis. These practices include, at the very least,

- Ensuring that you have the right number of records, with no duplicates
- Performing quality-control checks on each data field

Check that the number of records in the computerized database matches the number of questionnaires. Then check for duplicate records. It is not uncommon for questionnaires to be skipped or entered twice, particularly if they are not all entered at one sitting.

Two types of quality-control checks should be performed before beginning the analysis: range checks and logic (or consistency) checks. A *range check* identifies values for each variable that are "out of range" (i.e., not allowed, or at least highly suspicious). If, for the variable "gender," "male" is coded as 1 and "female" as 2, the range check should flag all records with any value other than 1 or 2. If 3's, F's, or blanks are found, review the original questionnaire, recontact the respondent, or recode those values to "known missing." For the variable "weight (in pounds)," an allowable range for adults might be 90 to 300. It is quite possible that some respondents will weigh more or less than this range, but it is also possible that values outside that range represent coding errors. Again, you must decide whether to attempt to verify the information or leave it as entered. The effort needed to confirm and complete the information should be compared with the effect of lost data in the analysis—for a small study, you can ill-afford missing data for the key variables but can tolerate it for less important variables. Under no circumstances should you change a value just because "it doesn't seem right."

A logic check compares responses to two different questions and flags those that are inconsistent. For example, a record in which "any symptoms?" is coded as "no" and "vomiting" is coded as "yes" should be flagged. Dates can also be compared—date of onset of illness should usually precede date of hospitalization (except in outbreaks of nosocomial infection, when date of hospitalization *precedes* date of onset), and date of onset should precede date of report. Again you must decide how to handle inconsistencies.

Two additional principles should guide data management. First, document everything, particularly your decisions. Take a blank copy of the questionnaire and write the name of each variable next to the corresponding question on the questionnaire. If, for the variable "gender," you decide to recode F's as 2's and recode 3's and blanks as 9's for "known missing," write those decisions down as well, so that you and others will know how to recode unacceptable values for gender in the future.

Note that you cannot create logic checks in advance for every possible contingency. Many inconsistencies in a database come to light during the analysis. Treat these inconsistencies the same way—decide how best to resolve the inconsistency (short of making up better data!) and then document your decision.

The second principle is, "Never let an error age." Deal with the problem as soon as you find it. Under the pressures of a field investigation, it is all too common to forget about a data error, analyze the data as they are, and then be embarrassed during a presentation when calculations or values in a table do not seem to make sense.

## Developing the Analysis Strategy

After the data have been edited, they are ready to be analyzed. But before you sit down to analyze the data, first develop an *analysis strategy* (Table 10–1).

**Table 10-1.**   Sequence of an Epidemiologic Analysis Strategy

1. Establish how the data were collected and plan to analyze accordingly.

2. Identify and list the most important variables in light of what you know about the subject matter, biologically plausible hypotheses, and the manner in which the study will be (or was) conducted:
Exposures of interest
Outcomes of interest
Potential confounders
Variables for subgroup analysis

3. Plan to perform frequency distributions and descriptive statistics on the variables identified in step 2.

4. Create tables of clinical features and descriptive epidemiology (table shells should be created in advance).

5. To assess exposure-disease associations, create two-way tables based on study design, prior knowledge, and hypotheses (table shells should be created in advance).

6. Create additional two-way tables based on interesting findings in the data.

7. Create three-way tables, refinements (e.g., dose-response; sensitivity analysis) and subgroup analysis based on design, prior knowledge, hypotheses, or interesting findings in the data.

The analysis strategy is comparable to the outline you would develop before sitting down to write a term paper. It lays out the key components of the analysis in a logical sequence and provides a guide to follow during the actual analysis. An analytic strategy that is well planned in advance will expedite the analysis once the data are collected.

The first step in developing the analysis strategy is to recognize how the data were collected. For example, if you have data from a cohort study, think in terms of exposure groups and plan to calculate rates. If you have data from a case control study, think in terms of cases and controls. If the cases and controls were matched, plan to do a matched analysis. If you have survey data, review the sampling scheme—you may need to account for the survey's design effect in your analysis.

The next step is to decide which variables are most important. Include the exposures and outcomes of interest, other known risk factors, study design factors such as variables you matched on, any other variables you think may have an impact on the analysis, and variables you are simply interested in. With a short questionnaire, perhaps all variables will be deemed important. Plan to review the frequency of responses and descriptive statistics for each variable. This is the best way to become familiar with the data. What are the minimum, maximum, and average values for each variable? Are there any variables that have many missing responses? If you hope to do a stratified or subgroup analysis by, say, race, are there enough responses in each race category?

The next step in the analysis strategy is to sketch out table shells. A *table shell* (sometimes called a "dummy table") is a table such as a frequency distribution or two-way table that is titled and fully labeled but contains no data. The numbers will be filled in as the analysis progresses.

You should sketch out the series of table shells as a guide for the analysis. The table shells should proceed in a logical order from simple (e.g., descriptive epidemiology) to complex (e.g., analytic epidemiology). The table shells should also indicate which measures (e.g., odds ratio and 95% confidence interval) and statistics (e.g., chi-square and *P*-value) you will calculate for each table. Measures and statistics are described later in this chapter.

One way to think about the types and sequence of table shells is to consider what tables you would want to show in a report. One common sequence is as follows:

Table 1:  Clinical features (e.g., signs and symptoms, percent lab-confirmed, percent hospitalized, percent died, etc.)
Table 2:  Descriptive epidemiology
          Time: usually graphed as line graph (for secular trends) or epidemic curve
          Place: county of residence or occurrence, spot or shaded map
          Person: "Who is in the study?" (age, race, gender, etc.)

For analytic studies,

Table 3:  Primary tables of association (i.e., risk factors by outcome status)
Table 4:  Stratification of Table 3 to separate effects and to assess confounding and effect modification
Table 5:  Refinements of Table 3 (e.g., dose–response, latency, use of more sensitive or more specific case definition, etc.)
Table 6:  Specific subgroup analyses

The following table shells (10–A, 10–B, and 10–C) were designed for a case control study of a cluster of mysterious deaths in Panama in 2006.[2] The clinical information about the cases had already been gathered, so the case control study focused on the cause, or vehicle. At this point in the investigation, speculation about the cause or vehicle centered around consumption of prescribed, over-the-counter, and traditional medications. Table 10–C is an example of what each medication table would look like.

**Table Shell 10–A.**   Descriptive Characteristics of the Study Participants

| | | CASES | | CONTROLS | |
| | | (N=42) | | (N=140) | |
| DEMOGRAPHIC | CHARACTERISTIC | NUMBER | PERCENT | NUMBER | PERCENT |
|---|---|---|---|---|---|
| Age | 18–24 yr | — | (%) | — | (%) |
| | 25–34 yr | — | (%) | — | (%) |
| | 35–44 yr | — | (%) | — | (%) |
| | 45–54 yr | — | (%) | — | (%) |
| | 55–64 yr | — | (%) | — | (%) |
| | 65–74 yr | — | (%) | — | (%) |
| | 75 yr and older | — | (%) | — | (%) |
| Gender | Female | — | (%) | — | (%) |
| | Male | — | (%) | — | (%) |
| Region | Cocle | — | (%) | — | (%) |
| | Colon | — | (%) | — | (%) |
| | Herrera | — | (%) | — | (%) |
| | Los Santos | — | (%) | — | (%) |
| | Metropolitana | — | (%) | — | (%) |
| | Panama Este | — | (%) | — | (%) |
| | Panama Oeste | — | (%) | — | (%) |
| | San Miguelito | — | (%) | — | (%) |
| | Veraguas | — | (%) | — | (%) |

Since descriptive epidemiology has been covered in Chapter 9, the remainder of this chapter addresses the analytic techniques most commonly used in field investigations.

Figure 10–2 depicts output from Epi Info's Analysis module (see Chapter 7). It shows the output from the TABLES command for data from a typical field investigation. Note the four elements of the output: (1) a two-by-two table, (2) parameters or measures of association, (3) confidence intervals for each point

**Table Shell 10–B.**  Association Between Preexisting Medical Conditions and Case-Control Status

| | CASES (N=42) | | CONTROLS (N=140) | | ODDS RATIO* (95% CONFIDENCE INTERVAL) |
|---|---|---|---|---|---|
| | NO. | PCT. | NO. | PCT. | |
| Diabetes | — | (%) | — | (%) | __ (__ - __) |
| Hypertension | — | (%) | — | (%) | __ (__ - __) |
| Cardiovascular Disease | — | (%) | — | (%) | __ (__ - __) |
| Other | — | (%) | — | (%) | __ (__ - __) |
| Any ACE inhibitor† | — | (%) | — | (%) | __ (__ - __) |

\* Statistically significant findings are in boldface type
† ACE inhibitors include enalapril, ramipril, and lisinopril

**Table Shell 10–C.**  Association Between Prescribed Liquid Cough Syrup and Case-Control Status

| | CASES (N=42) | | CONTROLS (N=140) | | CRUDE OR* (95% CI) | ADJUSTED OR*† (95% CI) |
|---|---|---|---|---|---|---|
| | NO. | PCT. | NO. | PCT. | | |
| LIQUID COUGH SYRUP | | | | | | |
| Yes | — | (%) | — | (%) | __ (__ - __) | __ (__ - __) |
| No | — | (%) | — | (%) | | |

\* Statistically significant findings are in boldface type
† Odds ratio adjusted for ...
[*Source:* Barr et al., 2008]

estimate, and (4) statistical tests, also known as "tests of statistical significance." Each of these elements is discussed below.

## The Two-by-Two Table

Every epidemiologic study can be summarized in a two-by-two table.

—H. Ory

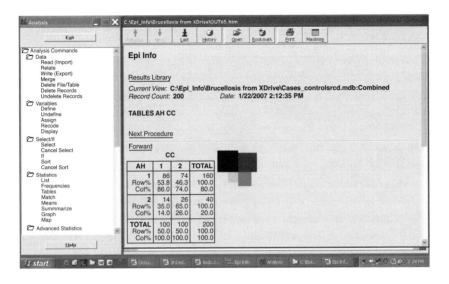

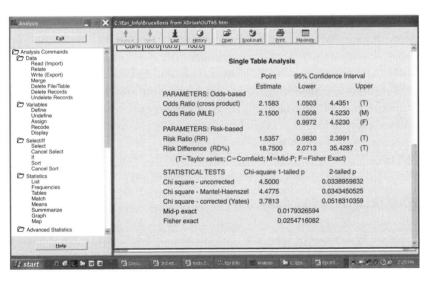

**Figure 10–2.** Typical Epi Info output from the analysis module, using the tables command. [*Source:* Dean et al., 1994]

In many epidemiologic studies, exposure and the health event being studied can be characterized as binary variables (e.g., "yes" or "no"). The relationship between exposure and disease can then be cross-tabulated in a *two-by-two table*, so named because both the exposure and disease have just two categories (Table 10–2). Disease status (e.g., ill vs. well) is usually represented along the top, and exposure

**Table 10–2.** Layout and Standard Notation of a Two-by-Two Table

|  |  | ILL | WELL | TOTAL | ATTACK RATE |
|---|---|---|---|---|---|
| Exposed? | Yes | a | b | $H_1$ | $a/H_1$ |
|  | No | c | d | $H_0$ | $c/H_0$ |
|  | Total | $V_1$ | $V_0$ | T | $V_1/T$ |

status along the side. (Epi Info follows this convention, but a few epidemiologic textbooks do not.) The intersection of a row and a column in which a count is recorded is known as a *cell*. The letters a, b, c, and d within the four cells of the two-by-two table refer to the number of persons with the disease status indicated in the column heading and the exposure status indicated to the left. For example, c is the number of unexposed ill/case subjects in the study. The *horizontal* row totals are labeled $H_1$ and $H_0$ (or $H_2$), and the *vertical* column totals are labeled $V_1$ and $V_0$ (or $V_2$). The total number of subjects included in the two-by-two table is written in the lower right corner and is represented by the letters T or N. If the data are from a cohort study, attack rates (the proportion of a group of people who develop disease during a specified time interval) are sometimes provided to the right of the row totals. Risk ratios (or odds ratios) and confidence intervals and/or P-values are often provided to the right of, or below, the table.

Data from an outbreak investigation in Virginia are presented in Table 10–3.[4] The table provides a cross-tabulation of beef (exposure) by presence or absence of *Salmonella* gastroenteritis (outcome). Attack rates (65.4% for those who answered that they ate beef; 11.4% for those who denied eating beef) are given to the right of the table.

## MEASURES OF ASSOCIATION

A *measure of association* quantifies the strength or magnitude of the statistical association between the exposure and the health problem of interest. Measures of

**Table 10–3.** Beef Consumption and *Salmonella* Gastroenteritis, Virginia, December 2003

|  |  | ILL | WELL | TOTAL | ATTACK RATE |
|---|---|---|---|---|---|
| Ate beef? | Yes | 53 | 28 | 81 | 65.4% |
|  | No | 4 | 31 | 35 | 11.4% |
|  | Total | 57 | 59 | 116 | 49.1% |

[*Source:* Jani et al., 2004.]

association are sometimes called *measures of effect* because—if the exposure is causally related to the disease—the measures quantify the effect of having the exposure on the incidence of disease. In cohort studies, the measure of association most commonly used is the risk ratio. In case control studies, the odds ratio is the most commonly used measure of association. In cross-sectional studies, either a prevalence ratio or a prevalence odds ratio may be calculated.

## Risk Ratio (Relative Risk)

The *risk ratio* (RR) is the risk in the exposed group divided by the risk in the unexposed group:

$$\text{Risk ratio (RR)} = \text{risk}_{exposed} / \text{risk}_{unexposed} = (a/h_1) / (c/h_0)$$

The risk ratio reflects the excess risk in the exposed group compared with the unexposed (background, expected) group. The excess is expressed as a ratio. In acute outbreak settings, risk is represented by the attack rate. The data presented in Table 10–3 show that the risk ratio of illness, given beef consumption, was $0.654/0.114 = 5.7$. That is, persons who ate beef were 5.7 times as likely to become ill as those who did not eat beef. Note that the risk ratio will be greater than 1.0 when the risk is greater in the exposed group than in the unexposed group. The risk ratio will be less than 1.0 when the risk in the exposed group is less than the risk in the unexposed group, as happens when the exposure is vaccination, prophylactic antibiotics, or another factor that protects against occurrence of disease.

## Odds Ratio (Cross-Product Ratio, Relative Odds)

In most case control studies, because the true size of the exposed and unexposed groups are not known, you do not have a denominator with which to calculate an attack rate or risk. However, using case-control data, the risk ratio can often be approximated by an *odds ratio* (OR). The odds ratio is calculated as

$$\text{Odds ratio (OR)} = ad/bc$$

In an outbreak of group A *Streptococcus* (GAS) surgical wound infections in a community hospital, 10 cases had occurred during a 17-month period. [5] Investigators used a table of random numbers to select controls from the 2600 surgical procedures performed during the epidemic period. Since many clusters of GAS surgical wound infections can be traced to a GAS carrier among operating room personnel, investigators studied all hospital staff associated with each patient.

**Table 10–4.** Surgical Wound Infection and Exposure to Nurse A, Hospital M, Michigan, 1980

|              |       | CASE | CONTROL | TOTAL |
|--------------|-------|------|---------|-------|
| Exposed to   | Yes   | 8    | 5       | 13    |
| Nurse A?     | No    | 2    | 49      | 51    |
|              | Total | 10   | 54      | 64    |

[*Source:* Berkelman et al. 1982.]

They drew a two-by-two table for exposure to each staff member and calculated odds ratios. The two-by-two table for exposure to Nurse A is shown in Table 10–4. The odds ratio is calculated as $8 \times 49/2 \times 5 = 39.2$. Strictly speaking, this means that the *odds* of being exposed to Nurse A were 39 times higher among cases than among controls. It is also reasonable to say that the odds of developing a GAS surgical wound infection were 39 times higher among those exposed to Nurse A than among those not exposed. For a rare disease (say, less than 5%), the odds ratio approximates the risk ratio. So in this setting, with only 10 cases out of 2600 procedures, the odds ratio could be interpreted as indicating that the *risk* of developing a GAS surgical wound infection was 39 times higher among those exposed to Nurse A than among those not exposed.

The odds ratio is a very useful measure of association in epidemiology for a variety of reasons. As noted above, when the disease is rare, a case control study can yield an odds ratio that closely approximates the risk ratio from a cohort study. From a theoretical statistical perspective (beyond the scope of this book), the odds ratio also has some desirable statistical properties and is easily derived from multivariate modeling techniques.

## Prevalence Ratio and Prevalence Odds Ratio

Cross-sectional studies or surveys generally measure the prevalence (existing cases) of a health status (such as vaccination status) or condition (such as hypertension) in a population rather than the incidence (new cases). For a disease, prevalence is a function of both incidence (risk) and duration of illness, so measures of association based on prevalent cases reflect both the exposure's effect on incidence and its effect on duration or survival.

The prevalence measures of association analogous to the risk ratio and the odds ratio are the *prevalence ratio* and the *prevalence odds ratio*, respectively.

In the two-by-two table (Table 10–5), the prevalence ratio is 4.0 (0.20/0.05). That is, exposed subjects are four times as likely as unexposed subjects to have

**Table 10–5.**   Data from a Hypothetical Cross-Sectional Survey

|          |       | YES | NO  | TOTAL | PREVALENCE |
|----------|-------|-----|-----|-------|------------|
| Exposed? | Yes   | 20  | 80  | 100   | 20.0%      |
|          | No    | 20  | 380 | 400   | 5.0%       |
|          | Total | 40  | 460 | 500   | 8.0%       |

the condition. In the example above, the prevalence odds ratio = (20) (380)/(80) (20) = 4.75. The *odds* of having disease are 4.75 times higher for the exposed than the unexposed group. Note that the overall prevalence is 0.08, or 8.0%. The lower the prevalence, the closer the values of the prevalence ratio and the prevalence odds ratio will be.

## MEASURES OF PUBLIC HEALTH IMPACT

A measure of public health impact places the exposure–disease association in a public health perspective. It reflects the apparent contribution of an exposure to the frequency of disease in a particular population. For example, for an exposure associated with an increased risk of disease (e.g., smoking and lung cancer), the *attributable risk percent* represents the expected reduction in disease load if the exposure could be removed (or never existed). The *population attributable risk percent* represents the proportion of disease in a population attributable to an exposure. For an exposure associated with a decreased risk of disease (e.g., vaccination), a prevented fraction could be calculated that represents the actual reduction in disease load attributable to the current level of exposure in the population.

## Attributable Risk Percent (Attributable Fraction [or Proportion] among the Exposed, Etiologic Fraction)

The *attributable risk percent* is the proportion of cases in the exposed group presumably attributable to the exposure. This measure assumes that the level of risk in the unexposed group (assumed to be the baseline or background risk of disease) also applies to the exposed group, so that only the *excess* risk should be attributed to the exposure. The attributable risk percent can be calculated with either of the following formulas (which are algebraically equivalent):

$$\text{Attributable risk percent} = (\text{risk}_{\text{exposed}} - \text{risk}_{\text{unexposed}}) / \text{risk}_{\text{exposed}}$$
$$= (RR - 1) / RR$$

The attributable risk percent can be reported as a fraction or can be multiplied by 100 and reported as a percent. Using the beef consumption data in Table 10–3, the attributable risk percent is $(0.654 - 0.114) / 0.654 = 82.6\%$. Therefore, most of the gastroenteritis that occurred among persons who ate beef could be attributed to their beef consumption. In theory, the other 17.4% might be attributed to other causes, such as the baseline occurrence of gastroenteritis in that population. In practice, even some of these other cases are probably attributable to beef as a result of cross-contamination or imperfect data collection.

In a case control study, if the odds ratio is thought to be a reasonable approximation of the risk ratio, you can calculate the attributable risk percent as

$$\text{Attributable risk percent} = (OR - 1) / OR$$

## Population Attributable Risk Percent (Population Attributable Fraction)

The *population attributable risk percent* is the proportion of cases in the entire population (both exposed and unexposed groups) presumably attributable to the exposure. Algebraically equivalent formulas include:

$$\text{Population attributable risk percent} = (\text{risk}_{\text{overall}} - \text{risk}_{\text{unexposed}}) / \text{risk}_{\text{overall}}$$
$$= P(RR - 1) / [P(RR - 1) + 1]$$

where P = proportion of population exposed = $H_1/T$.

Applying the first formula to the beef consumption data, the population attributable risk percent is $(0.466 - 0.114) / 0.466 = 75.6\%$. In situations in which most of the cases are exposed, the attributable risk percent and population attributable risk percent will be close. For diseases with multiple causes (e.g., many chronic diseases) and uncommon exposures, the population attributable risk percent may be considerably less than the attributable risk percent.

The population attributable risk percent can be estimated from a population-based case control study by using the OR to approximate the RR and by using the proportion of controls exposed to approximate P; that is, $P = b/V_0$, assuming that the controls are representative of the entire population.

## Prevented Fraction in the Exposed Group (Vaccine Efficacy)

If the risk ratio is less than 1.0, you can calculate the prevented fraction, which is the proportion of potential new cases that would have occurred in the absence of the exposure. In other words, the prevented fraction is the proportion of potential cases prevented by some beneficial exposure, such as vaccination. The prevented fraction in the exposed group is calculated as

$$\text{Prevented fraction among the exposed} = (\text{risk}_{\text{unexposed}} - \text{risk}_{\text{exposed}}) / \text{risk}_{\text{unexposed}}$$
$$= 1 - RR$$

Table 10–6 presents data from a varicella (chickenpox) outbreak in an elementary school in Nebraska in 2004.[6] As shown in Table 10–6, the risk of varicella was 13.0% among vaccinated children and 66.7% among unvaccinated children. The resulting vaccine efficacy is 80.5%, indicating that vaccination prevented about 80% of the cases that would have otherwise occurred among vaccinated children had they not been vaccinated.

Note that the terms *attributable* and *prevented* convey much more than statistical association. They imply a cause-and-effect relationship between the exposure and disease. Therefore, these measures should be presented, not routinely, but only after thoughtful inference of causality.

## TESTS OF STATISTICAL SIGNIFICANCE

Tests of statistical significance are used to determine how likely it is that the observed results could have occurred by chance alone, if exposure was not actually related to disease. This section describes the key features of the tests used most commonly with two-by-two tables. For discussion of theory, derivations, and other topics beyond the scope of this book, you should consult a statistics or biostatistics textbook.

In statistical testing, you assume that the study population is a sample from some large "source population." Then assume that, in the source population,

**Table 10–6.** Vaccination Status and Occurrence of Varicella, Elementary School Outbreak, Nebraska, 2004

| | VARICELLA | NO VARICELLA | TOTAL | RISK OF VARICELLA |
|---|---|---|---|---|
| Vaccinated | 15 | 100 | 115 | 13.0% |
| Unvaccinated | 18 | 9 | 27 | 66.7% |
| Total | 33 | 109 | 142 | 23.2% |

Risk ratio = 13.0 / 66.7 = 0.195

Vaccine efficacy = (66.7 − 13.0) / 66.7 = 80.5%

[*Source:* CDC, 2006.]

incidence of disease is the same for exposed and unexposed groups. In other words, assume that, in the source population, exposure is not related to disease. This assumption is known as the *null hypothesis*. (The *alternative hypothesis*, which will be adopted if the null hypothesis proves to be implausible, is that exposure *is* associated with disease.) Next, compute a measure of association, such as a risk ratio or odds ratio. Then, calculate the test of statistical significance such as a chi-square (described below). This test tells you the probability of finding an association as strong as (or stronger than) the one you have observed if the null hypothesis were really true. This probability is called the *P-value*. A very small *P*-value means that you would be very unlikely to observe such an association if the null hypothesis were true. In other words, a small *P*-value indicates that the null hypothesis is implausible, given the data at hand. If this *P*-value is smaller than some predetermined cutoff (usually 0.05 or 5%), you discard ("reject") the null hypothesis in favor of the alternative hypothesis. The association is then said to be "statistically significant."

In reaching a decision about the null hypothesis, be alert to two types of error. In a *type I error* (also called *alpha error*), the null hypothesis is rejected when in fact it is true. In a *type II error* (also called *beta error*), the null hypothesis is not rejected when in fact it is false.

Both the null hypothesis and the alternative hypothesis should be specified in advance. When little is known about the association being tested, you should specify a null hypothesis that the exposure is not related to disease (e.g., RR = 1 or OR = 1). The corresponding alternative hypothesis states that exposure and disease are associated (e.g., RR ≠ 1 or OR ≠ 1). Note that this alternative hypothesis includes the possibilities that exposure may either increase or decrease the risk of disease.

When you know more about the association between a given exposure and disease, you may specify a narrower (*directional*) hypothesis. For example, if it is well established that an exposure increases the risk of developing a particular health problem (e.g., smoking and lung cancer), you can specify a null hypothesis that the exposure does not increase risk of that condition (e.g., RR ≤ 1 or OR ≤ 1) and an alternative hypothesis that exposure does increase the risk (e.g., RR > 1 or OR > 1). Similarly, if you were studying a well-established protective relationship [measles-mumps-rubella (MMR) vaccine and measles], you could specify a null hypothesis that RR ≥ 1 and an alternative hypothesis that RR < 1.

A nondirectional hypothesis is tested by a *two-tailed* test. A directional hypothesis is tested with a *one-tailed* test. In general, the cutoff for a one-tailed test is twice the cutoff of a two-tailed test (i.e., 0.10 rather than 0.05). Since raising the cutoff for rejecting the null hypothesis increases the likelihood of making a type I error, epidemiologists in field situations generally use a two-tailed test.

Two different tests, each with some variations, are used for testing data in a two-by-two table. These two tests, described below, are the Fisher exact test and the chi-square test. These tests are not specific to any particular measure of association. The same test can be used regardless of whether you are interested in risk ratio, odds ratio, or attributable risk percent.

## Fisher Exact Test and Mid-P

The *Fisher exact test* is considered the "gold standard" for a two-by-two table and is the test of choice when the numbers in a two-by-two table are small. Assume that the null hypothesis is true in the source population and that the values in the four cells of the two-by-two table could change but the row and column totals are fixed. The Fisher exact test involves computing the probability (*P*-value) of observing an association in a sample equal to or greater than the one observed. The mid-P is a variation of the Fisher Exact *P*-value in which half rather than all of the observed probability is used, so it is always smaller.

As a rule of thumb, the Fisher exact or mid-*P* test is the test of choice when the *expected* value in any cell of the two-by-two table is less than 5. The expected value is calculated by multiplying the row total by the column total and dividing by the table total.

## Chi-Square Test

When you have at least 30 subjects in a study and the expected value in each cell of the two-by-two table is at least 5, the *chi-square test* provides a reasonable approximation to the Fisher exact test. Plugging the appropriate numbers into the chi-square formula, you get a value for the chi-square. Each chi-square value corresponds to a particular *P*-value. Nowadays, analytic software packages routinely provide both chi-square values and *P*-values.

At least three different formulas of the chi-square for a two-by-two table are in common use; Epi Info presents all three.

$$\text{Pearson uncorrected } \chi^2 = \frac{T(ad-bc)^2}{(V_1)(V_0)(H_1)(H_0)}$$

$$\text{Mantel-Haenszel uncorrected } \chi^2 = \frac{(T-1)(ad-bc)^2}{(V_1)(V_0)(H_1)(H_0)}$$

$$\text{Yates corrected } \chi^2 = \frac{T(|ad-bc|-(T/2))^2}{(V_1)(V_0)(H_1)(H_0)}$$

For a given set of data in a two-by-two table, the *Pearson chi-square formula* gives the largest chi-square value and hence the smallest *P*-value. This *P*-value is often somewhat smaller than the "gold standard" *P*-value calculated by the Fisher exact method. So the Pearson chi-square is more apt to lead to a type I error (concluding that there is an association when there is not). The *Yates corrected chi-square* gives the largest *P*-value of the three formulas, sometimes even larger than the corresponding Fisher exact *P*-value. The Yates correction is preferred by epidemiologists who want to minimize their likelihood of making a type I error, but it increases the likelihood of making a type II error (failing to find a statistically significant association when an association truly exists). The *Mantel-Haenszel formula*, popular in stratified analysis, yields a *P*-value that is slightly larger than that from the Pearson chi-square but often smaller than the *P*-value from the Yates corrected chi-square and Fisher exact *P*-value. Fortunately, for most analyses the three chi-square formulas provide similar enough *P*-values to make the same decision regarding the null hypothesis based on all three. When the different chi-square formulas point to different decisions, as in Figure 10–2, epidemiologic judgment is required.

## Which Test to Use?

The Fisher exact test is the commonly accepted standard when the expected value in any cell is less than 5. Remember that the expected value for any cell can be determined by multiplying the row total by the column total and dividing by the table total.

If all expected values in the two-by-two table are 5 or greater, then you can choose among the chi-square tests. Each of the three formulas shown above has its advocates among epidemiologists, and Epi Info provides all three. Some field epidemiologists prefer the Yates-corrected formula because they are least likely to make type I error (but most likely to make a type II error). Others acknowledge that the Yates correction often overcompensates, so they prefer the uncorrected formula. Epidemiologists who frequently perform stratified analyses are accustomed to using the Mantel-Haenszel formula, so they tend to use this formula even for simple two-by-two tables.

## Measure of Association versus Test of Significance

The measures of association, such as risk ratio and odds ratio, reflect the strength of the relationship between an exposure and a disease. These measures are generally independent of the size of the study and may be thought of as the "best guess" of the true degree of association in the source population. However, the measure gives no indication of its reliability (i.e., how much faith one should put in it).

In contrast, a test of significance provides an indication of how likely it is that the observed association is due to chance. Although the chi-square test statistic is influenced both by the magnitude of the association and the study size, it does not distinguish the contribution of each one. Thus the measure of association and the test of significance (or a confidence interval, see below) provide complementary information.

## Interpreting Statistical Test Results

"Not significant" does not necessarily mean "no association." The measure of association (risk ratio, odds ratio) indicates the direction and strength of the association. The statistical test indicates how likely it is that the observed association may have occurred by chance alone. Nonsignificance may reflect no association in the source population but may also reflect a study size too small to detect a true association in the source population.

Statistical significance does not by itself indicate a cause–effect relationship. An observed association may indeed represent a causal relationship, but it may also be due to chance, selection bias, information bias, confounding, and other sources of error in the design, execution, and analysis of the study. Statistical testing relates only to the role of chance in explaining an observed association, and statistical significance indicates only that chance is an unlikely (though not impossible) explanation of the association. You must rely on your epidemiologic judgment in considering these factors as well as the consistency of the findings with those from other studies, the temporal relationship between exposure and disease, biological plausibility, and other criteria for inferring causation. These issues are discussed at greater length in the last section of this chapter.

Finally, "statistical significance" does not necessarily mean "public health significance." With a large study, a weak association with little public health (or clinical) relevance many nonetheless be "statistically significant." More commonly, relationships of public health and/or clinical importance fail to be "statistically significant" because the studies are too small.

## CONFIDENCE INTERVALS FOR MEASURES OF ASSOCIATION

We have just described the use of a statistical test to determine how likely it is that the difference between an observed association and the null state is consistent with chance variation. Another index of the statistical variability of the association is the *confidence interval*. Statisticians define a 95% confidence interval as the interval that, given repeated sampling of the source population, will include or "cover" the true association value 95% of the time. The epidemiologic concept of a 95% confidence interval is the range of values consistent (statistically compatible) with the data in the study.[7]

The chi-square test and the confidence interval are closely related. The chi-square test uses the observed data to determine the probability (*P*-value) under the null hypothesis, and you "reject" the null hypothesis if the probability is less than some preselected value, called *alpha*, such as 5%. The confidence interval uses a preselected probability value, alpha, to determine the limits of the interval, and you can reject the null hypothesis if the interval does not include the null association value. Both indicate the precision of the observed association; both are influenced by the magnitude of the association and the size of the study group. While both measure precision, neither addresses validity (lack of bias).

You must select a probability level (alpha) to determine limiting values of the confidence interval. As with the chi-square test, epidemiologists traditionally choose an alpha level of 0.05 or 0.01. The "confidence" is then 100 x (1 − alpha)% (e.g., 95% or 99%).

Unlike the calculation of a chi-square, the calculation of a confidence interval is a function of the particular measure of association. That is, each association measure has its own formula for calculating confidence intervals. In fact, each measure has several formulas, including exact ones and a variety of approximations.

## Interpreting the Confidence Interval

As noted above, a confidence interval can be regarded as the range of values consistent with the data in a study. Suppose that you conducted a study in your area in which the risk ratio for smoking and disease X was 4.0, and the 95% confidence interval was 3.0 to 5.3. Your single best guess of the association in the general population is 4.0, but your data are consistent with values anywhere from 3.0 to 5.3. Note that your data are *not* consistent with a risk ratio of 1.0; that is, your data are *not* consistent with the null hypothesis. Thus, the values that are included in the confidence interval and values that are excluded both provide important information.

The width of a confidence interval (i.e., the values included) reflects the precision with which a study can pinpoint an association such as a risk ratio. A wide confidence interval reflects a large amount of variability or imprecision. A narrow confidence interval reflects little variability and high precision. Usually, the larger the number of subjects or observations in a study, the greater the precision and the narrower the confidence interval.

As stated earlier, the measure of association provides the "best guess" of your estimate of the true association. If you were in a casino, that "best guess" would be the number to bet on. The confidence interval provides a measure of the confidence you should have in that "best guess"; that is, it tells you how much to bet! A wide confidence interval indicates a fair amount of imprecision in the best guess, so you should not bet too much on that one number. A narrow confidence interval indicates a more precise estimate, so you might want to bet more on that number.

Since a confidence interval reflects the range of values consistent with the data in a study, you can use the confidence interval to determine whether the data are consistent with the null hypothesis. Since the null hypothesis specifies that the risk ratio (or odds ratio) equals 1.0, a confidence interval that includes 1.0 is consistent with the null hypothesis. This is equivalent to deciding that the null hypothesis cannot be rejected. On the other hand, a confidence interval that does not include 1.0 indicates that the null hypothesis should be rejected, since it is inconsistent with the study results. Thus the confidence interval can be used as a surrogate test of statistical significance.

## SUMMARY EXPOSURE TABLES

If the goal of the field investigation is to identify one or more vehicles or risk factors for disease, it may be helpful to summarize the exposures of interest in a single table, such as Table 10–7. For a food-borne outbreak, the table typically includes each food item served, numbers of ill and well persons by food consumption history, food-specific attack rates (if a cohort study was done), risk ratio (or odds ratio), chi-square and/or $P$-value, and, sometimes, a confidence interval. To identify a culprit, you should look for a food item with two features:

1. An elevated risk ratio, odds ratio, or chi-square (small $P$-value), reflecting a substantial difference in attack rates among those exposed to the item and those not exposed.
2. Most of the ill persons had been exposed, so that the exposure could "explain" or account for most if not all of the cases.

In Table 10–7, beef had the highest risk ratio (and smallest $P$-value) and could account for 53 of the 57 cases.

## STRATIFIED ANALYSIS

Although it has been said that any epidemiologic study can be summarized in a two-by-two table, many such studies require more sophisticated analyses than

**Table 10-7.** Attack Rates By Items Served at Company A's Holiday Banquet, Virginia, December 2003

| FOOD ITEMS SERVED | NUMBER OF PERSONS WHO ATE SPECIFIED FOOD | | | | NUMBER OF PERSONS DID NOT EAT SPECIFIED FOOD | | | | RISK RATIO |
|---|---|---|---|---|---|---|---|---|---|
| | ILL | NOT ILL | TOTAL | ATTACK RATE | ILL | NOT ILL | TOTAL | ATTACK RATE | |
| Beef | 53 | 28 | 81 | 65% | 4 | 31 | 35 | 11% | 5.7 |
| Ravioli | 43 | 35 | 78 | 55% | 14 | 24 | 38 | 37% | 1.5 |
| Cajun sauce* | 19 | 11 | 30 | 63% | 37 | 48 | 85 | 44% | 1.5 |
| Pesto cream* | 37 | 29 | 66 | 56% | 19 | 30 | 49 | 39% | 1.4 |
| California rolls* | 21 | 14 | 35 | 60% | 34 | 44 | 78 | 44% | 1.4 |
| Mushrooms* | 32 | 26 | 58 | 55% | 24 | 31 | 55 | 44% | 1.3 |
| Broccoli* | 34 | 30 | 64 | 53% | 22 | 29 | 51 | 43% | 1.2 |
| Carrots* | 34 | 30 | 64 | 53% | 23 | 28 | 51 | 43% | 1.2 |
| Potatoes* | 39 | 41 | 80 | 49% | 17 | 17 | 34 | 50% | 1.0 |

*Excludes 1 or more persons with indefinite history of consumption of that food.
[*Source:* Jani et al., 2004.]

those described so far in this chapter. For example, two different exposures may appear to be associated with a disease. How do you analyze both at the same time? Even when you are only interested in the association of one particular exposure and one particular outcome, a third factor may complicate the association. The two principal types of complications are *confounding* and *effect modification*. Stratified analysis, which involves examining the exposure–disease association within different categories of a third factor, is one method for dealing with these complications.

Stratified analysis is an effective method for looking at the effects of two different exposures on the disease. Consider a hypothetical outbreak of hepatitis A among junior high school students. The investigators, not knowing the vehicle, administered a food consumption questionnaire to 50 students with hepatitis A and to 50 well controls. Two exposures had elevated odds ratios and statistically significant *P*-values: milk and donuts (Table 10–8). Donuts were often consumed with milk, so many people were exposed to both or neither. How do you tease apart the effect of each item?

Stratification is one way to tease apart the effects of the two foods. First, decide which food will be the exposure of interest and which will be the stratification variable. Since donuts has the larger odds ratio, you might choose donuts as the primary exposure and milk as the stratification variable. The results are shown in Table 10–9. The odds ratio for donuts is 6.0, whether milk was consumed or not. Now, what if you had decided to look at the milk–illness association, stratified by donuts? Those results are shown in Table 10–10. Clearly, from Table 10–9, consumption of donuts remains strongly associated with disease, regardless of milk consumption. On the other hand, from Table 10–10, milk consumption is not independently associated with disease, with an odds ratio of 1.0 among those who

**Table 10–8.** Hepatitis A and Consumption of Milk and Donuts

| DRANK MILK? | CASES | CONTROLS | TOTAL | |
|---|---|---|---|---|
| Yes | 37 | 21 | 58 | Odds ratio = 3.9 |
| No | 13 | 29 | 42 | Yates-corrected $\chi^2 = 9.24$ |
| Total | 50 | 50 | 100 | *P*-value = 0.0002 |

| ATE DONUTS? | CASES | CONTROLS | TOTAL | |
|---|---|---|---|---|
| Yes | 40 | 20 | 60 | Odds ratio = 6.0 |
| No | 10 | 30 | 40 | Yates-corrected $\chi^2 = 15.04$ |
| Total | 50 | 50 | 100 | *P*-value = 0.0001 |

**Table 10–9.** Hepatitis A and Donut Consumption, Stratified by Milk

| | DRANK MILK | | | DID NOT DRINK MILK | |
| --- | --- | --- | --- | --- | --- |
| ATE DONUTS? | CASES | CONTROLS | ATE DONUTS? | CASES | CONTROLS |
| Yes | 36 | 18 | Yes | 4 | 2 |
| No | 1 | 3 | No | 9 | 27 |
| | Odds Ratio = 6.0 | | | Odds Ratio = 6.0 | |

did and did not eat donuts. Milk only *appeared* to be associated with illness because so many milk drinkers also ate donuts.

An alternative method for analyzing two exposures is with a two-by-four table, as shown in Table 10–11. In that table, Exposure 1 is labeled "Exp 1"; Exposure 2 is labeled "Exp 2." To calculate the risk ratio for each row, divide the attack rate ("risk") for that row by the attack rate for the group not exposed to either exposure (bottom row in Table 10–11). To calculate the odds ratio for each row, use that row's values for a and b in the usual formula, ad/bc.

With this presentation, it is easy to see the effect of Exposure 1 alone (row 3) compared with the unexposed group (row 4), Exposure 2 alone (row 2) compared with the unexposed group (row 4), and Exposure 1 and 2 together (row 1) compared with the unexposed group (row 4). Thus the separate and joint effects can be assessed.

From Table 10–12, you can see that donuts alone had an odds ratio of 6.0, whereas milk alone had an odds ratio of 1.0. Together, donuts and milk had an odds ratio of 6.0, the same as donuts alone. In other words, donuts, but not milk, were associated with illness. The two-by-four table summarizes the stratified tables in one and eliminates the need to designate one food as the primary exposure and the other as the stratification variable.

**Table 10–10.** Hepatitis A and Milk Consumption, Stratified by Donuts

| | ATE DONUTS | | | DID NOT EAT DONUTS | |
| --- | --- | --- | --- | --- | --- |
| DRANK MILK? | CASES | CONTROLS | DRANK MILK? | CASES | CONTROLS |
| Yes | 36 | 18 | Yes | 1 | 3 |
| No | 4 | 2 | No | 9 | 27 |
| | Odds Ratio = 1.0 | | | Odds Ratio = 1.0 | |

**Table 10–11.**  Data Layout for Two-by-Four Table, Analyzing Two Exposures at Once

| EXP I | EXP 2 | ILL OR CASE | WELL OR CONTROL | TOTAL | RISK | RISK RATIO | ODDS RATIO |
|-------|-------|-------------|-----------------|-------|------|------------|------------|
| Yes | Yes | $a_{YY}$ | $b_{YY}$ | $H_{YY}$ | $a_{YY}/H_{YY}$ | $Risk_{YY}/Risk_{NN}$ | $a_{YY}d/b_{YY}c$ |
| No | Yes | $a_{NY}$ | $b_{NY}$ | $H_{NY}$ | $a_{NY}/H_{NY}$ | $Risk_{NY}/Risk_{NN}$ | $a_{NY}d/b_{NY}c$ |
| Yes | No | $a_{YN}$ | $b_{YN}$ | $H_{YN}$ | $a_{YN}/H_{YN}$ | $Risk_{YN}/Risk_{NN}$ | $a_{YN}d/b_{YN}c$ |
| No | No | c | d | $H_{NN}$ | $c/H_{NN}$ | 1.0 (Reference) | 1.0 (Reference) |
| Total | | $V_1$ | $V_0$ | T | $V_1/T$ | | |

## Confounding

Stratification also helps in the identification and handling of confounding. *Confounding is the distortion of an exposure–disease association by the effect of some third factor (a "confounder").* A third factor may be a confounder and distort the exposure–disease association if it is:

- Associated with the outcome independent of the exposure—that is, even in the nonexposed group. (In other words, it must be an independent "risk factor.")
- Associated with the exposure but not a consequence of it.

To separate out the effect of the exposure from the effect of the confounder, stratify by the confounder.

Consider the mortality rates in Alaska versus Arizona. In 1988, the crude mortality rate in Arizona was 7.9 deaths per 1000 population, over twice as high

**Table 10–12.**  Hepatitis A and Consumption of Milk and Donuts, in Two-by-Four Table Layout

| DONUT | MILK | CASE | CONTROL | ODDS RATIO |
|-------|------|------|---------|------------|
| Yes | Yes | 36 | 18 | 6.0 |
| No | Yes | 1 | 3 | 1.0 |
| Yes | No | 4 | 2 | 6.0 |
| No | No | 9 | 27 | 1.0 (Reference) |
| | Total | 50 | 50 | |

as the crude mortality rate in Alaska (3.9 deaths per 1000 population). Is living in Arizona more hazardous to one's health? The answer is no. In fact, for most age groups, the mortality rate in Arizona was about equal to or slightly lower than the mortality rate in Alaska. The population of Arizona was older than the population of Alaska, and death rates rise with age. Age is a confounder that wholly accounts for Arizona's apparently elevated death rate—the age-adjusted mortality rates for Arizona and Alaska are 7.5/1000 and 8.4/1000, respectively. Note that age satisfies the two criteria described above: increasing age is associated with increased mortality, regardless of where one lives; and age is associated with state of residence (Arizona's population is older than Alaska's).

Return to the sequence in which an analysis should be conducted (see Fig. 10–1). After you have assessed the basic exposure–disease relationships using two-by-two tables, you should stratify the data by "third variables"—variables that are cofactors, potential confounders, or effect modifiers (described below). If your simple two-by-two table analysis has identified two or more possible risk factors, each should be stratified by the other or others. In addition, you should develop a list of other variables to be assessed. The list should include the known risk factors for the disease (one of the two criteria for a confounder) and matching variables. Then stratify or separate the data by categories of relevant third variables. For each stratum, compute a stratum-specific measure of association. Age is so often a real confounder that it is reasonable to consider it a potential confounder in almost any data set. Using age as an example, you could separate the data by 10-year age groups (strata), create a separate two-by-two table of exposure and outcome for each stratum, and calculate a measure of association for each stratum.

The result of this type of analysis is that, within each stratum, "you compare like with like." If the stratification variable is gender, then in one stratum the exposure–disease relationship can be assessed for women and in the other the same relationship can be assessed for men. Gender can no longer be a confounder in these strata, since women are compared with women and men are compared with men.

To look for confounding, first look at the smallest and largest values of the stratum-specific measures of association and compare them with the crude value. If the crude value does not fall within the range between the smallest and largest stratum-specific values, confounding is surely present.

Often, confounding is not quite that obvious. So the next step is to calculate a summary "adjusted" measure of association as a weighted average of the stratum-specific values. The most common method of controlling for confounding is by stratifying the data and then computing measures that represent weighted averages of the stratum-specific data. One popular technique was developed by Mantel and Haenszel. (This and other methods are described in Reference 7.)

After calculating a summary value, compare the summary value to the crude value to see if the two are "appreciably different." Unfortunately, there are no hard-and-fast rules or statistical tests to determine what constitutes "appreciably different." In practice, we assume that the summary adjusted value is more accurate. The question then becomes, "Does the crude value adequately approximate the adjusted value, or would the crude value be misleading to a reader?" If the crude and adjusted values are close, you can use the crude because it is not misleading and it is easier to explain. If the two values are appreciably different (10%? 20%?), use the adjusted value.

After deciding whether the crude or adjusted or stratum-specific measures of association are appropriate, you can then perform hypothesis testing and calculate confidence intervals for the chosen measures.

## Effect Modification

The third use of stratification is in assessing effect modification. *Effect modification* means, simply, that the degree of association between an exposure and an outcome differs in different subgroups of the population. For example, a measles vaccine (exposure) may be highly effective (strong association) in preventing disease (outcome) if given after a child is 12 months of age (stratification variable = age at vaccination, stratum 1 = ≥12 months), but less effective (weaker association) if given before 12 months (age stratum 2 = <12 months). As a second example, tetracycline (exposure) may cause (strong association) tooth mottling (outcome) among children (stratifier = age, stratum 1 = children), but tetracycline does not cause tooth mottling among adults. In both examples, the association or effect is a function of, or is modified by, some third variable. Effect modification is enlightening because it raises questions for further research. Why does the effect vary? In what way is one group different from the other? Studying these and related questions can lead to insights into pathophysiology, natural history of disease, and genetic or acquired host characteristics that influence risk.

Basically, evaluation for effect modification involves determining whether the stratum-specific measures of association differ from one another. Identification of effect modification is really a two-part process involving these questions:

1. Is the range of associations wide enough to be of public health or scientific importance? (A credo of field epidemiology is that "a difference, to be a difference, has to make a difference.")
2. Is the range of associations likely to represent normal sampling variation? Evaluation can be done either qualitatively ("eyeballing the results") or quantitatively (done with multivariate analysis such as logistic regression or with statistical tests of heterogeneity).

Another difference is important to note: confounding is extremely common because it is just an artifact of the data. True effect modification, on the other hand, usually represents a biological phenomenon and hence is much less common.

## ADDITIONAL ANALYSES

Two additional areas are worth mentioning, although technical discussions are beyond the scope of this book. These two areas are the assessment of dose–response relationships and modeling.

### Dose Response

In epidemiology, *dose–response* means increased risk of disease with increasing (or, for a protective exposure, decreasing) amount of exposure. Amount of exposure may reflect intensity of exposure (e.g., milligrams of 1-tryptophan or number of cigarettes per day) or duration of exposure (e.g., number of months or years of exposure) or both.

If an association between an exposure and a health problem has been established, epidemiologists often take the next step to look for a dose–response effect. Indeed, the presence of a dose–response effect is one of the well-recognized criteria for inferring causation. Statistical techniques are available for assessing such relationships, even when confounders must be taken into account.

The first step, as always, is organizing your data. One convenient format is a 2-by-H table, where H represents the categories or doses of exposure.

As shown in Table 10–13, an odds ratio (or a risk ratio for a cohort study) can be calculated for each dose relative to the lowest dose or the unexposed group. You can calculate confidence intervals for each dose as well.

Merely eyeballing the data in this format can give you a sense of whether a dose–response relationship is present. If the odds ratios increase or decrease monotonically, a statistically significant dose–response relationship may be present.

### Modeling

There comes a time in the life of many epidemiologists when neither simple nor stratified analysis can do justice to the data. At such times, epidemiologists may turn to modeling. *Modeling* is a technique of fitting the data to particular statistical equations. One group of models are regression models, where the outcome is a function of exposure variables, confounders, and interaction terms (effect modifiers).

**Table 10–13.** Data Layout and Notation for Dose-Response Table

| DOSE | ILL OR CASE | WELL OR CONTROL | TOTAL | RISK | RISK RATIO | ODDS RATIO |
|------|------|------|------|------|------|------|
| Dose 5 | $a_5$ | $b_5$ | $H_5$ | $a_5 / H_5$ | $Risk_5 / Risk_0$ | $a_5 d / b_5 c$ |
| Dose 4 | $a_4$ | $b_4$ | $H_4$ | $a_4 / H_4$ | $Risk_4 / Risk_0$ | $a_4 d / b_4 c$ |
| Dose 3 | $a_3$ | $b_3$ | $H_3$ | $a_3 / H_3$ | $Risk_3 / Risk_0$ | $a_3 d / b_3 c$ |
| Dose 2 | $a_2$ | $b_2$ | $H_2$ | $a_2 / H_2$ | $Risk_2 / Risk_0$ | $a_2 d / b_2 c$ |
| Dose 1 | $a_1$ | $b_1$ | $H_1$ | $a_1 / H_1$ | $Risk_1 / Risk_0$ | $a_1 d / b_1 c$ |
| Dose 0 | $c$ | $d$ | $H_0$ | $c / H_0$ | 1.0 (Reference) | 1.0 (Reference) |
| Total | $V_1$ | $V_0$ | | | | |

The types of data usually dictate the type of regression model that is most appropriate. For example, logistic regression is the model most epidemiologists choose for binary outcome variables (ill/well, case/control, alive/dead, etc.).

In logistic regression, the binary outcome (dependent) variable is modeled as a function of a series of independent variables. The independent variables should include the exposure or exposures of primary interest and may include confounders and more complex interaction terms. Software packages provide beta coefficients for each independent term. If the model includes only the outcome variable and the primary exposure variable coded as (0,1), then $e^{\beta}$ should equal the odds ratio you could calculate from the two-by-two table. If other terms are included in the model, then $e^{\beta}$ equals the odds ratio adjusted for all the other terms. Logistic regression can also be used to assess dose–response relationships, effect modification, and more complex relationships. A variant of logistic regression called *conditional logistic regression* is particularly appropriate for pair-matched data.

Other types of models used in epidemiology include *Cox proportional hazards models* for life-table analysis, *binomial regression* for risk ratio analysis, and *Poisson regression* for analysis of rare-event data.

Keep in mind that *sophisticated analytic techniques cannot atone for sloppy data*. Analytic techniques such as those described in this chapter are only as good as the data to which they are applied. Analytic techniques, whether they be simple, stratified, or multivariate, use the information at hand. They do not ask or assess whether the proper comparison group was selected, whether the response rate was adequate, whether exposure and disease were properly defined, or whether the data coding and entry were free of errors. Analytic techniques are merely tools; as the analyst, you are responsible for knowing the quality of the data and interpreting the results appropriately.

## MATCHING IN CASE CONTROL STUDIES

Early in this chapter we noted that different study designs require different analytic methods. *Matching* is one design that requires methods different from those described so far. Because matching is so common in field studies, this section addresses this important topic.

Matching generally refers to a case control study design in which controls are intentionally selected to be similar to case-subjects on one or more specified characteristics (other than the exposure or exposures of interest). The goal of matching, like that of stratified analysis, is to "compare like with like." The characteristics most appropriately specified for matching are those that are potential confounders of the exposure–disease associations of interest. By matching cases and controls on factors such as age, gender, or geographic area, the distribution of those factors among cases and controls will be identical. In other words, the matching variable will not be associated with case-control status in the study. As a result, if the analysis is properly done, the matching variable will not confound the association of primary interest.

Two types of matching schemes are commonly used in epidemiology. One type is *pair matching*, where each control is selected according to its similarity to a *particular* case. This method is most appropriate when each case is unique in terms of the matching factor; for example, 50 cases widely scattered geographically. Each case could be matched to a friend or neighborhood control. A particular control is suitably matched to a particular case, but not to any other case in the study. The matching by design into these unique pairs must be maintained in the analysis.

The term *pair matching* is sometimes generalized to include not only matched pairs (case and one control), but matched triplets (case and two controls), quadruplets, and so on. The term also refers to studies in which the number of matched controls per case varies, as long as the controls are matched to a specific case.

The other type of matching is *category matching*, also called *frequency matching*. Category matching is a form of stratified sampling of controls, wherein controls are selected in proportion to the number of cases in each category of a matching variable. For example, in a study of 70 male and 30 female case-subjects, if 100 controls were also desired, you would select 70 male controls at random from the pool of all non-ill males and 30 female controls from the female pool. The pairs are not unique; any male control is a suitable match to any male case-subject. Data collected by category matching in the study design must be analyzed using stratified analysis.

Matching has several advantages. Matching on factors such as neighborhood, friendship, or siblingship may control for confounding by numerous social factors that would be otherwise impossible to measure and control. Matching may be cost- and time-efficient, facilitating enrollment of controls. For example, matched friend controls may be identified while interviewing each case-subject, and these friends are more likely to cooperate than controls randomly selected from the general population. And finally, matching on a confounder increases the statistical efficiency of an analysis and thus provides narrower confidence intervals.

Matching has disadvantages, too. The primary disadvantage is that matching on a factor prevents you from examining its association with disease. If the age and gender distribution of case-subjects and controls are identical because you matched on those two factors, you cannot use your data to evaluate age and gender as risk factors themselves. Matching may be both cost- and time-inefficient, if considerable work must be performed to identify appropriately matched controls. The more variables to be matched on, the more difficult it will be to find suitably matched controls. In addition, matching on a factor that is not a confounder or having to discard cases because suitable controls could not be found decreases statistical efficiency and results in wider confidence intervals. Finally, matching complicates the analysis, particularly if other confounders are present.

In summary, matching is desirable and beneficial when you know beforehand that (1) you do not wish to examine the relationship between the matching factor and disease; (2) the factor is related to risk of disease so it is a potential confounder; and (3) matching is convenient or at least worth the potential extra costs to you. When in doubt, do not match, or match only on a strong risk factor that is likely to be distributed differently between exposed and unexposed groups and that is not a risk factor you are interested in assessing.

## Matched Pairs

The basic data layout for a matched-pair analysis appears at first glance to resemble the simple unmatched two-by-two tables presented earlier in this chapter, but in reality the two are quite different. In the matched-pair two-by-two table, each cell represents the number of matched pairs who meet the row and column criteria. In the unmatched two-by-two table, each cell represents the number of individuals who meet the criteria.

In Table 10–14, E+ denotes "exposed" and E– denotes "unexposed." Cell f thus represents the number of pairs made up of an exposed case and an unexposed control. Cells e and h are called *concordant pairs* because the case and control are both exposed or unexposed. Cells f and g are called *discordant pairs*.

In a matched-pair analysis, only the discordant pairs are informative. The odds ratio is computed as

$$\text{Odds ratio} = f / g$$

**Table 10–14.**  Data Layout and Notation for Matched-Pair Two-by-Two Table

|        |           | CONTROLS ||  TOTAL |
|        |           | EXPOSED | UNEXPOSED | TOTAL |
|--------|-----------|---------|-----------|-------|
| CASES  | Exposed   | e       | f         | e + f |
|        | Unexposed | g       | h         | g + h |
|        | Total     | e + g   | f + h     | e + f + g + h pairs |

The test of significance for a matched pair analysis is the *McNemar chi-square test*. Both uncorrected and corrected formulas are commonly used.

$$\text{Uncorrected McNemar test} = (f - g)^2 / (f + g)$$

$$\text{Corrected McNemar test} = (|f - g| - 1)^2 / (f + g)$$

Table 10–15 presents the data from a pair-matched case control study conducted in 1980 to assess the association between tampon use and toxic shock syndrome.[8]

## Larger Matched Sets and Variable Matching

In some studies, two, three, four, or a variable number of cases are matched to controls. A general formula for calculating the odds ratio with *any* number of controls per case is

$$OR = \frac{\text{Number of unexposed controls matched with exposed cases}}{\text{Number of exposed controls matched with unexposed cases}}$$

An alternative way of analyzing matched sets is to consider each set as a separate stratum, and analyze the data using Mantel-Haenszel techniques to summarize the strata.[9] Such data are best analyzed with appropriate computer software, such as Epi Info.

## Does a Matched Design Require a Matched Analysis?

Does a matched design require a matched analysis? Usually, yes. In a pair-matched study, if the pairs are unique (siblings, friends, etc.), then pair-matched analysis is needed. If the pairs were based on a non-unique characteristic such as gender

**Table 10–15.** Continual Tampon Use During Index Menstrual Period in Case-Control Pairs, Toxic Shock Syndrome Study, 1980

|  |  | CONTROLS | | TOTAL |
|---|---|---|---|---|
|  |  | EXPOSED | UNEXPOSED |  |
| CASES | Exposed | 33 | 9 | 42 |
|  | Unexposed | 1 | 1 | 2 |
|  | Total | 34 | 10 | 44 pairs |

Odds Ratio = 9 / 1 = 9.0
McNemar uncorrected chi-square = $(9 - 1)^2 / (9 + 1) = 6.40 \ (P = 0.01)$
McNemar corrected chi-square = $(|9 - 1| - 1)^2 / (9 + 1) = 4.90 \ (P = 0.03)$

[*Source:* Shands et al., 1980.]

or race, stratified analysis is preferred. In a frequency matched study, stratified analysis is necessary.

In practice, some epidemiologists perform the appropriate matched analysis, then "break the match" and perform an unmatched analysis on the same data. If the results are similar, they may opt to present the data in unmatched fashion. In most instances, the unmatched odds ratio will be closer to 1.0 than the matched odds ratio ("bias toward the null"). Less frequently, the "broken" or unmatched odds ratio will be further from the null. These differences, which are related to confounding, may be trivial or substantial. The chi-square test result from unmatched data may be particularly misleading, usually being larger than the McNemar test result from the matched data. The decision to use a matched analysis or unmatched analysis is analogous to the decision to present crude or adjusted results. You must use your epidemiologic judgment in deciding whether the unmatched results are misleading to your audience or, worse, to yourself!

## INTERPRETING FIELD DATA

> Skepticism is the chastity of the intellect …. Don't give it away to the first attractive hypothesis that comes along.
> —M. B. Gregg, after George Santayana

Does an elevated risk ratio or odds ratio or a *P* value less than 0.05 automatically mean that the exposure is a true cause of disease? Certainly not. Although the association may indeed be causal, flaws in study design, execution, and analysis can result in apparent associations that are actually artifacts. Chance, selection bias, information bias, confounding, and investigator error should all be evaluated as possible explanations for an observed association.

One possible explanation for an observed association is chance. Under the null hypothesis, you assume that your study population is a sample from some source population and that incidence of disease is not associated with exposure in the source population. The role of chance is assessed by using tests of statistical significance. (As noted above, confidence intervals can be used as well.) A very small *P*-value indicates that the null hypothesis is an *unlikely* explanation of the result you found. Keep in mind that chance can never be ruled out entirely. Even if the *P*-value is small, say 0.01, yours may be the one sample in a hundred in which the null hypothesis is true and chance *is* the explanation! Note that tests of significance evaluate only the role of chance. They do not say anything about the roles of selection bias, information bias, confounding, or investigator error, discussed below.

Another explanation for the observed explanation is selection bias. *Selection bias* is a systematic error in the designation of the study groups or in the enrollment of study participants that results in a mistaken estimate of an exposure's effect on the risk of disease. In more simplistic terms, selection bias may be thought of as a problem arising from who gets into the study. Selection bias may arise either in the design or in the execution of the study. Selection bias may arise from the faulty design of a case control study if, for example, too loose a case definition is used (so some persons in the case group do not actually have the disease being studied), asymptomatic cases go undetected among the controls, or an inappropriate control group is used. In the execution phase, selection bias may result if eligible subjects with certain exposure and disease characteristics choose not to participate or cannot be located. For example, if ill persons with the exposure of interest know the hypothesis of the study and are more willing to participate than other ill persons, then cell a in the two-by-two table will be artificially inflated compared to cell c, and the odds ratio will also be inflated. So to evaluate the possible role of selection bias, you must look at how cases and controls were specified and how they were enrolled.

Another possible explanation of an observed association is information bias. *Information bias* is a systematic error in the collection of exposure or outcome data about the study participants that results in a mistaken estimate of an exposure's effect on the risk of disease. Again, in more simplistic terms, information bias is a problem with the information you collect from the people in the study. Information bias may arise in a number of ways, including poor wording or understanding of a question on a questionnaire, poor recall (can you remember exactly what you had for lunch a week ago Tuesday?), or inconsistent interviewing technique. Information bias can also arise if a subject knowingly provides false information, either to hide the truth or, as is common in some cultures, in an attempt to please the interviewer.

As discussed earlier in this chapter, confounding can also distort an association. To evaluate the role of confounding, ensure that a list of potential confounders has been drawn up, that they have been evaluated for confounding, and that they have been controlled for as necessary.

Finally, investigator error has been known to be the explanation for some apparent associations. A misplaced semicolon in a computer program, an erroneous transcription of a value, or use of the wrong formula can all yield artifactual associations! Check your work, or have someone else try to replicate it.

So, before considering whether an association may be causal, consider whether the association may be explained by chance, selection bias, information bias, confounding, or investigator error. Now suppose that an elevated risk ratio or odds ratio has a small $P$-value and narrow confidence interval, so chance is an unlikely explanation. Specification of cases and controls is reasonable and participation was good, so selection bias is an unlikely explanation. Information was collected using a standard questionnaire by an experienced and well-trained interviewer. Confounding by other risk factors was assessed and found not to be present or to have been controlled for. Data entry and calculations were verified. But before you conclude that the association is causal, you should consider the strength of the association, its biological plausibility, consistency with results from other studies, temporal sequence, and dose–response relationship, if any.

## Strength of the Association

In general, the stronger the association, the more likely one is to believe it is real. Thus we are generally more willing to believe that a risk ratio of 9.0 may be causal than a risk ratio of 1.5. This is not to say that a risk ratio of 1.5 cannot reflect a causal relationship; it can. It is just that a subtle selection bias, information bias, or confounding could easily account for a risk ratio of 1.5. The bias would have to be quite dramatic to account for a risk ratio of 9.0!

## Biological Plausibility

Does the association make sense? Is it consistent with what is known of the pathophysiology, the known vehicles, the natural history of disease, animal models, or other relevant biological factors? For an implicated food vehicle in an infectious disease outbreak, can the agent be identified in the food, or will the agent survive (or even thrive) in the food? While some outbreaks are caused by new or previously unrecognized vehicles or risk factors, most are caused by those that we already know.

## Consistency with Other Studies

Are the results consistent with those from other studies? A finding is more plausible if it can be replicated by different investigators, using different methods in different populations.

## Exposure Precedes Disease

This criterion seems obvious, but in a retrospective study it may be difficult to document that exposure precedes disease. Suppose, for example, that persons with a particular type of leukemia are more likely than controls to have antibodies to a particular virus. It might be tempting to conclude that the virus causes the leukemia, but from the serologic evidence at hand you could not be certain that exposure to the virus preceded the onset of leukemic changes.

## Dose–Response Effect

Evidence of a dose–response effect adds weight to the evidence for causation. A dose–response effect is not a *necessary* feature for a relationship to be causal; some causal relationships may exhibit a threshold effect, for example. In addition, a dose–response effect does not rule out the possibility of confounding. Nevertheless, it is usually thought to add credibility to the association.

In many field investigations, a likely culprit may not meet all the criteria listed above. Perhaps the response rate was less than ideal, or the etiologic agent could not be isolated from the implicated food, or the dose–response analysis was inconclusive. Nevertheless, if the public's health is at risk, failure to meet every criterion should not be used as an excuse for inaction. As stated by George Comstock, "The art of epidemiologic reasoning is to draw sensible conclusions from imperfect data."[10] After all, field epidemiology is a tool for public health action to promote and protect the public's health based on science (sound epidemiologic methods), causal reasoning, and a healthy dose of practical common sense.

> All scientific work is incomplete—whether it be observational or experimental. All scientific work is liable to be upset or modified by advancing knowledge. That does not confer upon us a freedom to ignore the knowledge we already have, or to postpone the action it appears to demand at a given time.
>
> —Sir Austin Bradford Hill[11]

# REFERENCES

1. Shem, S. (1978). *The House of God*, Richard Marek Publishers, New York.
2. Barr, D.B., Barr, J.R., Weerasekera, G., et al. (2008). Identification and quantification of diethylene glycol in pharmaceuticals implicated in poisoning epidemics: an historical laboratory perspective. *J Anal Toxicol* 32, 106–115.
3. Dean, A.G., Arner, T.G., Sunki, G.G., et al. (2002). Epi Info™, a database and statistics program for public health professionals. Centers for Disease Control and Prevention, Atlanta.
4. Jani, A.A., Barrett, E., Murphy, J., et al. (2004). A steamship full of trouble: an out-break of Salmonella typhimurium DT104 gastroenteritis at a holiday banquet—Virginia, 2003. Presented at the 53th Annual Epidemic Intelligence Service Conference, 2003 April 19–23, Atlanta.
5. Berkelman, R.L., Martin, D., Graham, D.R., et al. (1982). Streptococcal wound infections caused by a vaginal carrier. *JAMA* 247, 2680–2.
6. CDC (2006). Varicella outbreak among vaccinated children—Nebraska, 2004. *Morb Mortal Wkly Rep* 55 749–52.
7. Rothman, K.J., Greenland, S. (1988). *Modern Epidemiology*, 2$^{nd}$ ed., Williams & Wilkins, Philadelphia.
8. Shands, K.N., Schmid, G.P., Dan, B.B., et al. (1980). Toxic-shock syndrome in menstruating women: Association with tampon use and *Staphylococcus aureus* and clinical features in 52 cases. *N Engl J Med* 303, 1436–42.
9. Mantel, N., Haenszel, W. (1959). Statistical aspects of the analysis of data from retrospective studies of disease. *J Natl Cancer Inst* 22, 719–48.
10. Comstock, G.W. (1990). Vaccine evaluation by case-control or prospective studies. *Am J Epidemiol*, 131, 205–7.
11. Hill, A.B. (1965). The environment and disease: association or causation? *Proc R Soc Med* 58, 295–300.

# 11

# DEVELOPING INTERVENTIONS

Richard A. Goodman
Robert E. Fontaine
James L. Hadler
Duc J. Vugia

All scientific work is incomplete—whether it be observational or experimental.
All scientific work is liable to be upset or modified by advancing knowledge.
That does not confer upon us a freedom to ignore the knowledge we already
have, or to postpone the action that it appears to demand at a given time.
—Sir Austin Bradford Hill[1]

Epidemiologic field investigations are often done in response to disease outbreaks
and other acute public health problems. Disease outbreaks usually create an urgent
need to identify the source and/or cause of the problem as a basis for initiating
control measures or other interventions. Alternatively, the identification of environmental or occupational hazards frequently demands evaluation of exposed
persons and an assessment of the risks of disease. Regardless of the nature of such
problems, there will be an immediate need to investigate, to recommend control
and preventive measures, and to both educate and persuade the affected community to accept public health recommendations.

When circumstances require an immediate response, public health officials
must take and/or recommend specific public health actions often without evidence
supporting incontrovertible epidemiologic "proof," such as the determination of
a causal relation. Under such circumstances, the key issue for the field epidemiologist and decision makers is the answer to the following question: To what extent
must an acute health problem be epidemiologically defined and understood before
action should be initiated?

This chapter discusses decision-making regarding the implementation of interventions during the course of epidemiologic field investigations. Specifically, this chapter first outlines principles that public health officials should take into account when considering interventions. Next, the chapter examines key determinants often involved in making such decisions about interventions, including the severity of the problem being investigated and the extent to which causation has been established. It then presents a spectrum of intervention options from which public health officials can select as a function of multiple factors involving the field investigation, and briefly discusses selected issues and evolving approaches in interventions. The chapter concludes with a summary listing of actions relating to interventions that should be considered at each stage of the field investigation. In this chapter, the term *intervention* is used to represent control and/or prevention measures public health officials select and implement at one or more points in time following the initiation of a field investigation.

## GUIDING PRINCIPLES FOR INTERVENTIONS

Public health officials who have responsibility and legal authority for making decisions about interventions should take into account certain key principles when considering putting an intervention into place, selecting the appropriate intervention, facilitating implementation of the intervention, and assessing the effectiveness of the intervention. These principles are summarized in the following box.

---

Guiding principles for interventions used during epidemiologic field investigations of acute public health problems.

- As soon as an acute public health problem is detected, there is a public health responsibility and societal expectation for public health officials to intervene as soon as possible to minimize preventable morbidity and mortality.
- Public health interventions should be scientifically driven, based on established facts and data, on current investigation findings, and on knowledge from previous investigations and studies. While there may be salient sociopolitical forces (e.g., public fear or political outcry) that create pressures for rapid public health interventions, the sociopolitical context should be acknowledged but not become the driving force for interventions.
- For a given problem, the type(s) and number of interventions to be implemented will vary depending upon the nature of the acute problem, including its cause, mode of spread, and other factors.
- The type(s) and number of interventions used may evolve as a function of incremental gains in information developed during the investigation.
- Most public health interventions demand—and even may be potentiated by—open, two-way communication between involved government agencies and the public.

---

# DETERMINANTS FOR EMPLOYING INTERVENTIONS

As noted above, field epidemiologists must consider several important determinants in the course of making a decision about whether there is a scientifically rational basis for employing an intervention and when selecting one or more specific interventions optimally matched to the public health problem. These determinants, many of which are both interrelated and not mutually exclusive, encompass a constellation of factors such as specific knowledge of causative agent(s), and of reservoirs and/or mode(s) of acquisition or spread; and recognition of other causal determinants as reflected, in part, by assessing the investigation's ability to address the criteria of causation (see below). This section examines three highly interrelated key determinants: severity of the problem, levels of certainty about key epidemiologic factors, and criteria for causation. In addition, it considers the sociopolitical context and its possible role in determining interventions.

## Severity of the Problem

The severity of a specific problem is a key determinant of the urgency and course of a field investigation, and indeed of any early intervention. The greater the severity of the problem, the sooner a public health intervention is expected. Severity is indicated by factors such as the degree and nature of complications, mortality, duration of illness, need for treatment and hospitalization, and economic impact. For example, virtually all cases of botulism in the United States trigger extensive epidemiologic investigations because of the vital need to prevent deaths by quickly identifying the source food and other exposed or ill individuals, and by administering antitoxin as indicated. Similarly, medical errors such as clusters of health-care-acquired infection—especially those in postsurgical or immune-compromised patients—are often investigated because of the potential for serious complications and greatly prolonged hospitalization, the possibility of iatrogenic illness as an unnecessary medical event, and the need to quickly resolve questions about the safety of continuing to admit patients to the hospital.[2]

## Levels of Certainty about Agents, Sources, and Modes of Spread

In addition to the severity of a problem, a spectrum of other factors influences the aggressiveness, extent, and scientific rigor of an epidemiologic field investigation. In the prototypical investigation, control measures are formulated only after a series of other steps have been carried out (see Chapter 5). In practice, however, control measures may be appropriate or warranted at any step in the sequence. For most outbreaks of acute disease, the scope of an investigation is dictated by the levels of certainty about (*1*) the etiology of the problem (e.g., the specific pathogen or toxic agent), and (*2*) the source and/or mode of spread (e.g., water-borne or airborne).[3] When the problem initially is identified, the levels of certainty regarding the etiology, source, and mode of spread may range from known to unknown (Figure 11–1). These basic dichotomies are illustrated in the figure by four examples that represent the extremes. In many situations, control measures follow policy or practice guidelines; in others, interventions are appropriate only after exhaustive epidemiologic investigation. Preliminary control measures often can be started based on limited initial information, and then can be modified as investigations proceed.

For example, the occurrence of a suspected norovirus outbreak associated with a restaurant or food preparation establishment may warrant a spectrum of interventions such as the prompt exclusion of food service employees if symptomatic with vomiting or diarrhea, temporarily closing the restaurant, replacing all food items, sanitizing all surfaces and equipment, monitoring food-handling practices until more specific information is available from the epidemiologic investigation, education on norovirus containment for food handlers, and training and education on the food code for restaurant owners.[4] In an instance such as this,

**Source/transmission mode**

|  | | Known | Unknown |
|---|---|---|---|
| **Etiology** | **Known** | Investigation +<br>Control +++<br>Example: Suspected Norovirus in restaurants and other food establishments[4] | Investigation +++<br>Control +<br>Example: *Salmonella* in marijuana[5] |
| | **Unknown** | Investigation +++<br>Control +++<br>Example: Eosinophilia myalgia syndrome[6,7] | Investigation +++<br>Control +<br>Example: Legionnaires' disease[8] |

**Figure 11–1.** Relative emphasis of investigative and control efforts (intervention options) in disease outbreaks as influenced by levels of certainty about etiology and source/mode of transmission. *Investigation* means extent of the investigation; *control* means the basis for rapid implementation of control/intervention measures at the time the problem is initially identified. Pluses show the level of response indicated (+ = low; +++ = high). [*Source:* Goodman et al., 1990.[3]]

the response will be based on knowledge of possible continuing sources of norovirus or some other enteric pathogen exposure in the restaurant and removal of those sources. Moreover, while this sort of prompt and appropriate response addresses the possibility of continued transmission based on known agent-specific facts and experience, the epidemiologist sometimes may need to extend the investigation, depending upon the circumstances and needs (e.g., when a traceback might be indicated to identify a continuing primary source for a restaurant-associated outbreak, such as shellfish that were contaminated before being harvested).

More commonly, there is some degree of uncertainty about the etiology or about sources and the mode of spread (Figure 11–1). In most outbreaks of gastrointestinal disease, the control measures selected will depend on knowing whether transmission is from person-to-person, food-borne, or waterborne, and, if either of the two latter modes, on identifying the source. For example, an outbreak of *Salmonella muenchen* in several states in 1981 required an extensive epidemiologic field investigation, including an analytic (case control) study, before the mode of spread was found to be personal use of or household exposure to marijuana.[5] The converse situation—involving a presumed source, but unknown etiology—is illustrated by the nationwide outbreak of eosinophilia myalgia syndrome in the United States in 1989.[6, 7] In that outbreak, L-tryptophan, a dietary supplement, was initially implicated as the source of the exposure, and contaminants in specific brands were eventually implicated through laboratory analysis. In the interim, epidemiologists were able to make recommendations for preventing further exposures and cases. Finally, as illustrated by the Legionnaires' disease outbreak in 1976, an extensive field investigation can fail to identify the cause, the source, and mode of spread in time to control the acute problem, but still enable advances in knowledge that ultimately lead to preventive measures.[8]

## Causation and the Field Investigation

In his seminal article on criteria for assessing causal associations in epidemiology, Austin Bradford Hill concluded with a call to base action on weighing the strength of the epidemiologic evidence against the severity of the consequences of delaying action and of taking premature action.[1] These same issues commonly confront epidemiologists during field investigations. The criteria specified by Hill (including temporality, strength of association, biologic gradient, consistency, plausibility, coherence, experiment, and analogy) provide a useful framework for assessing the strength of epidemiologic evidence developed during a field investigation. Assessing causality at each step in an investigation is important, not only to assess the strength of evidence developed up to that point, but also to help identify what evidence is missing or requires further attention, and to plan additional approaches, such as data gathering and analysis essential to support decisions regarding interventions.

Some criteria (such as strength of association, dose–response, and temporality) may increase confidence in initiating actions. Moreover, at any step in the investigation, evidence to satisfy a specific criterion may not be readily available. Nonetheless, field investigators should try to collect available data to examine causality by using as many criteria as may be feasible. While a single criterion may not be convincing in a given context or fully accepted based on the interpreter's viewpoint, a combination of well-assessed criteria pointing to a common exposure can strengthen confidence and facilitate support for directed interventions.

Epidemiology, and particularly field epidemiology are relatively young scientific disciplines in the medical world, acquiring academic, and then public, acceptance only gradually over the past four to five decades. Among some sectors—including, for example, the legal profession, private enterprise, and even regulatory agencies—acceptance of epidemiologic conclusions has come at a slower rate, in part because of the nature of causation in epidemiology: epidemiologic evidence establishes associations, not hard, irrefutable proof. At the same time, epidemiologic evidence often is the first basis for implicating a causative agent and/or mode of spread before the results of more in-depth and lengthier scientific investigations become available to support decision-making about interventions. Moreover, and lamentably, epidemiologic evidence that compels epidemiologists to take prompt action may not readily convince others whose cooperation is necessary to initiate action. For example, several years elapsed after field studies had clearly implicated antecedent aspirin use as a risk factor for Reye syndrome[9] before industry and the Food and Drug Administration accepted the association and issued warnings to that effect. The story of toxic shock syndrome (see Chapter 20) further illustrates the reluctance of some to accept epidemiologic evidence in the face of an acute public health problem on the scale of a nationwide epidemic. These examples underscore the practical challenges in balancing the need to assess causality through the process of scientific inquiry with the potentially conflicting need to intervene quickly to protect the public's health.

In any outbreak, multiple groups of persons may be exposed, affected, or involved in some respect. Because of differences in knowledge, beliefs, and perceived impact of the outbreak, each group may draw different conclusions regarding causality from the same information. For example, in a suspected restaurant-associated food-borne outbreak, restaurant patrons, the public, owners and management, media, attorneys, and public health officials are each likely to have a different threshold for judging the degree of association between eating food from the restaurant and illness. In this situation, the public health field epidemiologist's concerns might focus especially on the criteria of strength of association and dose–response effect between exposure to a certain food item and illness, while a restaurant patron's primary concern may simply be plausibility. On the other hand, attorneys—who either are representing plaintiff-patrons, who putatively acquired their cases of illness as a result of restaurant exposure, or are defending a restaurant epidemiologically associated with a food-borne epidemic— will approach such a problem by using a legal framework for causation that varies from epidemiologic causation.[10] In civil cases, the plaintiff's attorney, in particular, must meet a preponderance of evidence standard of proof, which means that the fact finders (e.g., the jury) must believe that the plaintiff's version of events is more probable than not in order for the plaintiff to prevail[11]; this standard also has been analogized to a probability of 0.51.[12]

## Sociopolitical Context

Often, field investigations take place in the public limelight, whether intended to or not. When a problem is perceived as severe (e.g., a death has occurred) and possibly ongoing, there may be a public demand for information and action. In addition, when there is intense interest from politicians, including executive-branch leaders such as governors and mayors, they may wish to be visible and demonstrate their interest in protecting the public. For example, a death from meningitis in a school child may lead to pressure to close the school. A death from Legionnaire's disease in a hospital patient may lead to pressure to consider closing the hospital.

As part of the deliberation of when and how to intervene, it is essential to have effective and continuous communication with all concerned entities. They need to be aware of the possibilities, the ongoing risks, if any, and how to best address them given the level of information available. An essential component of intervention is effective communication with political leaders and with the public. Such communication will assist in enabling the use of the scientific factors to be the determinants for selecting the intervention(s) to protect the public against disease and should help minimize the potential for unnecessary, costly and misleading interventions.

## INTERVENTION OPTIONS

Interventions for preventing and controlling public health problems—including infectious disease outbreaks and non-infectious diseases, injuries, and disabilities— can be approached through a variety of classification schemes. Examples of these approaches include: (1) interventions targeting specific aspects of the relationship between the host, environment, and disease- or injury-causing agent; (2) primary, secondary, and tertiary prevention options; and (3) Haddon's injury prevention model, which keys on intervention strategies at the pre-event, event, and post-event phases.[13–16] In addition to the specific nature of the etiologic agent, these and other models may take into account other factors, such as the agent's reservoir or source, the mode of spread or transmission, host-related risk factors, environmental and other mediating factors, *a priori* evidence of the effectiveness of the intervention, operational and logistical feasibility, and the legal authority necessary to support implementation of the measure. Public health interventions that are used to control infectious disease outbreaks include, for example, post-exposure prophylaxis with antibiotics, antiviral agents, or vaccines; cohorting and/or isolating infected persons; and recommendations for hand-washing or other modifications in personal behavior and hygiene practices.

In this chapter, the model used to systematically identify and characterize the spectrum of intervention options for outbreaks and other acute health threats focuses on two basic biological and environmental dimensions: (*1*) interventions that can be directed at the source(s) of most infectious and other disease-causing agents; and (*2*) interventions that can be directed at persons who are susceptible to such agents. These two categories and specific intervention options are listed in Table 11–1. The first category of interventions—those directed at the source—most obviously includes measures that would eliminate the disease-causing agent's presence as a risk to susceptible populations, such as seizure and destruction of contaminated foods, or barring an infected person from preparing or serving food until s/he is no longer infectious as a result of treatment or natural resolution. An additional point about this two-category approach is that both sets encompass some of the same options and, in that regard, are not completely mutually exclusive. For example, during a sexually transmitted disease outbreak, the behavior-modifying measure of condom use probably would be recommended to infected persons to interrupt transmission to susceptible contacts, as well as to known or presumed susceptibles to decrease their risk of exposure. During the SARS epidemic in 2003, public health officials in Toronto employed a combination of intervention measures directed at persons who met the SARS case definition and at their close contacts (i.e., isolation and quarantine, respectively), as well as temporarily restricting movement of all essential hospital staff (work quarantine) and barring all nonessential hospital staff members and visitors from entering hospitals in the province.[17]

Selections from measures listed in Table 11–1 and other alternatives may be considered at any stage of a field investigation. During early stages, interventions based on established guidelines for disease control may be applied. For example, as indicated earlier in this chapter, excluding symptomatic employees and removing all possible existing sources of an enteric pathogen like norovirus from a food preparation facility can be done regardless of the actual source of the outbreak.[4] If, at a subsequent time, the nature of the risk of infection is more sharply defined,

**Table 11-1**.   Selected public health intervention options for outbreaks and other acute health threats, by interventions that can be directed at the source(s) of most infectious and other disease-causing agents, and by interventions that can be directed at persons who are susceptible to such agents.

Intervention efforts directed at source

- Treat infected persons/animals
- Isolate infected persons (includes cohorting)
- Quarantine exposed persons
- Quarantine contaminated sites/sources
- Implement cordon sanitaire, close public places, and prevent gatherings (to freeze/limit movement and minimize likelihood of mixing groups by exposure/infection status)
- Seize and/or destroy contaminated food, property, animals, or other sources
- Clean and disinfect contaminated surfaces and other environmental repositories
- Modify environment through vector control
- Modify environment by restricting/controlling contaminants
- Modify behavior to reduce risks to self and/or others
- Deter through civil suits or criminal prosecution

Interventions efforts directed at susceptibles

- Administer post-exposure prophylaxis
- Immunize/vaccinate in advance
- Exclude unvaccinated persons from cohorts of vaccinated persons
- Employ barrier techniques
- Implement cordon sanitaire, close public places, and prevent gatherings (to freeze/limit movement and minimize likelihood of mixing groups by exposure/infection status)
- Modify behavior to reduce risks to self and/or others
- Use shelter-in-place (reverse quarantine)
- Employ contact tracing, partner notification, and treatment
- Issue press releases, health alerts, and other information regarding risk reduction

then additional, tailored corrective measures can be directed at the source and/or mode of spread. In this and similar situations—such as the well-known, intentionally caused outbreak of *Salmonella typhimurium* occurring in Oregon in 1984[18]— it also may be important for the investigation to continue because of the possibility of identifying novel or unusual causes of the problem demanding equally atypical interventions.

## ISSUES AND EVOLVING APPROACHES IN INTERVENTIONS

While this chapter has developed a science-based foundation for the identification, selection, and implementation of public health interventions, field investigators also must contend with a spectrum of new and evolving issues that challenge decision-making about interventions. This section briefly addresses three such issues, including: first, the dilemma public health officials face in selecting and implementing interventions, or planning for the use of interventions, when science-based information may be limited about the appropriateness and/or effectiveness of such interventions; second, the paramount importance of increasing the affected community's understanding of the nature of the public health problem and the rationale for the recommended intervention(s); and third, the sometimes complex nature of making a decision about when to terminate an intervention or, alternatively, how to institutionalize or to sustain the intervention over a longer period of time.

For some infectious diseases and other public health problems, recent efforts to plan for the selection and use of different interventions have, paradoxically, encountered controversy and or other challenges because of limitations in the availability of science-based information regarding key aspects of the interventions. For example, the deliberations about what measures might be appropriate for responding to a problem of the magnitude of an influenza A(H5N1) pandemic have suggested the need to consider whether there is enough science-based evidence to support widespread use of some relatively draconian social-distancing measures to restrict the movement of and exposures for large groups of people.

An important trend in selecting and implementing interventions is the increasing role of community involvement. For example, over the past decade, public health agencies have had to innovatively modify their responses to problems such as outbreaks of multidrug-resistant tuberculosis, clusters of cases of human immunodeficiency virus infection, and resurgent sexually transmitted diseases.[19, 20] For some of these problems, traditional methods for investigation and contact evaluation have been supplanted by newer "social network" approaches—interventions that require increased involvement of community representatives. In such settings, community support is essential to the success of the investigation and longer-term prevention and control measures; conversely, failure to obtain community trust and support actually can disable or constrain the impact of an investigation. This may be especially true when problems disproportionately affect groups who are marginalized and who otherwise may be initially reluctant to work with public health officials. The need to obtain community trust also implicates the important role of health and risk communications, as well as the importance of explaining to the community both the rationale for and potential limitations of an intervention (e.g., why the intervention may not work or may not be 100% effective). The increasing role of community involvement in and support for public health interventions applies, not only to infectious diseases, but also to the prevention and control of environmental hazards, injuries, and other noninfectious disease problems.

The final challenge encompasses the needs to assess the effectiveness of interventions and make decisions about whether and when to terminate (or sustain) intervention measures. At the earliest possible moment following implementation of public health interventions to address an acute problem, data being generated by the epidemiologic investigation should be used to assess the appropriateness and effectiveness of the intervention. Such information as developed by the investigation also guides decision-making regarding modification or termination of already-implemented interventions, or, as the investigation and situation evolve, the selection and use of additional or new measures. A decision to leave an intervention in place long-term or permanently might be made in situations where the public health risk cannot be eliminated and remains an ongoing threat, as is the case for many childhood and adult infectious diseases preventable through vaccination, as well as the ban on the use of lead-based paint.

## SUMMARY

Epidemiologic field investigations usually are initiated in response to epidemics or the occurrence of other acute disease, injury, or environmental health problems. Under such circumstances, the primary objective of the field investigation will be to employ the scientific principles of epidemiology to determine a rational and appropriate response for ending or controlling the problem. Key factors that influence decisions about the timing and choice of public health interventions include a carefully crafted balance of the severity of the problem, the levels of scientific certainty of the findings, the extent to which causal criteria have been established, the intervention's operational and logistical feasibility, and, increasingly, the public and political perceptions of what is the best course of action, and legal considerations.

This chapter has examined essential factors epidemiologists and other public health officials must consider when making decisions about the selection and implementation of public health interventions during epidemiologic field investigations. Taking these factors into account, the following actions should be reconsidered at each progressive stage of the field investigation:

- Define the scope of the public health problem with available information by assessing: severity of the illness; nature of the suspected etiologic agent; number of possible susceptibles and extent of exposure; and potential reasons for the outbreak's occurrence.
- Determine whether possible reasons for the outbreak could be ongoing and, for all potentially ongoing reasons and exposures for which intervention(s) might be offered, consider what empirical interventions could be used to reduce or eliminate any ongoing risk of exposure and/or illness.

- For each potential intervention, consider the costs and benefits of implementing the intervention at that stage of the investigation in the absence of additional information.
- Implement all reasonable empirical interventions.
- Communicate the rationale for implementing (or not implementing) interventions at any moment in time to those within the community who have been exposed and/or affected, as well as others who may need to know.
- Continuously assess the effectiveness of and modify the interventions as new information from the investigation becomes available.

Adherence to these and other steps during epidemiologic field investigations can be integral to helping to attain and optimize a scientifically rational basis for selecting and implementing public health interventions to control or terminate the problem.

## NOTE

Portions of this chapter as incorporated within the first and second editions of this book were adapted with permission of the editors of R.A. Goodman et al., (1990), The epidemiologic field investigation.[3]

ACKNOWLEDGMENT   We acknowledge James W. Buehler and Jeffrey P. Koplan, whose work on Chapter 9, "Developing Interventions," in the first and second editions of this text contributed in part to this chapter.

## REFERENCES

1. Hill, A.B. (1965). The environment and disease: association or causation? *Proc R Soc Med* 58, 295–300.
2. Gaynes, R., Richards, C., Edwards, J., et al. (2001). Feeding back surveillance data to prevent hospital-acquired infections. *Emerg Infect Dis* 7, 295–8.
3. Goodman, R.A., Buehler, J.W., Koplan, J.P. (1990). The epidemiologic field investigation: science and judgment in public health practice. *Am J Epidemiol* 132, 91–6.
4. CDC (2006). Multisite outbreak of norovirus associated with a franchise restaurant—Kent County, Michigan, May 2005. *Morb Mortal Wkly Rep* 55, 395–7.
5. Taylor, D.N., Wachsmuth, K., Yung-Hui, S., et al. (1982). Salmonellosis associated with marijuana: a multistate outbreak traced by plasmic fingerprinting. *N Engl J Med* 306, 1249–53.
6. CDC (1989). Eosinophilia-myalgia syndrome—New Mexico. MMWR 38, 765–7.
7. CDC (1989). Eosinophilia-myalgia syndrome and L-tryptophan-containing products—New Mexico, Minnesota, Oregon, and New York. *Morb Mortal Wkly Rep* 38, 785–8.

8. Fraser, D.W., Tsai, T.R., Orenstein, W., et al. (1977). Legionnaires' disease: description of an epidemic of pneumonia. *N Engl J Med* 297, 1189–97.

9. Hurwitz, E.S., Schonberger, L.B. (1997). Editorial Note—1997. *Morb Mortal Wkly Rep* 46, 750–5.

10. Goodman, R.A., Loue, S., Shaw, F.E. (2006). Law in epidemiology. In: R. Bownson, D. Petiti (eds.), *Applied Epidemiology*, 2nd ed., New York, Oxford University Press. pp. 289–326.

11. Freer, R.D., Perdue, W.C., eds. (1997). *Civil Procedure: Cases, Materials, and Questions*, 2nd ed., Anderson Publishing Co., Cincinnati.

12. Lazzarini, Z., Goodman, R.A., Dammers, K. (2007). Criminal law and public health practice. In: R.A. Goodman, R.E. Hoffman, et al. (eds.), *Law in Public Health Practice*, 2nd ed., New York, Oxford University Press. pp. 136–67.

13. Wenzel, R.P. (1998). Overview: Control of communicable diseases. In: R.B. Wallace, B.N. Doebbeling, J.M. Last (eds.), *Maxcy-Rosenau-Last Public Health and Preventive Medicine*, 14th ed., Appleton & Lange, Stamford, Conn. pp. 69–71.

14. Kim-Farley, R.J. (2002). Global strategies for control of communicable diseases. In: R. Detels, J. McEwen, R. Beaglehole, et al. (eds.), *Oxford Textbook of Public Health*, 4th ed., Oxford University Press, New York. pp. 1839–59.

15. Olsen, J. (2002). Disease prevention and control of non-communicable diseases. In: R. Detels, J. McEwen, R. Beaglehole, et al. (eds.), *Oxford Textbook of Public Health*, 4th ed., Oxford University Press, New York.

16. Peek-Asa, C., Dean, B., Kraus, J.F. (2002). Injury Control: The public health approach. In: R. Detels, J. McEwen, R. Beaglehole, et al. (eds.), *Oxford Textbook of Public Health*, 4th ed., Oxford University Press, New York, pp. 1533–47.

17. Svoboda, T., Henry, B., Shulman, L., et al. (2004). Public health measures to control the spread of the Severe Acute Respiratory Syndrome during the outbreak in Toronto. *N Engl J Med* 350, 2352–61.

18. Torok, T.J., Tauxe, R.V., Wise, R.P., et al. (1997). A large community outbreak of salmonellosis caused by intentional contamination of restaurant salad bars. *JAMA* 278, 396–8.

19. CDC (2001). Outbreak of syphilis among men who have sex with men—Southern California, 2000. *Morb Mortal Wkly Rep* 50, 117–20.

20. CDC (2000). HIV-related tuberculosis in a transgender network—Baltimore, Maryland, and New York City area, 1998–2000. *Morb Mortal Wkly Rep* 49, 317–20.

# 12

## COMMUNICATING EPIDEMIOLOGIC FINDINGS

Michael B. Gregg

Among the skills of a field epidemiologist is knowing how to communicate effectively. This chapter deals with some of the elements of both written and oral communication skills.

The single most important lesson to take home on this subject is that the data you collect are no more useful to fellow scientists and the public than your ability to communicate these findings convincingly.[1] Meaningful transfer of facts and their implications shapes medical and public health practice and drives the need to acquire new data. Therefore, communication is a prime function of the field epidemiologist.

A key word here is "convincingly." Supreme Court Justice Oliver Wendell Holmes once said "a page of history is worth a volume of logic." What he meant was that if you want to move people to act, real-life illustrations, present-day success stories, and past experiences are much more persuasive than spelling out a series of logical analyses, which tend to be cold, academic, and detached from reality.

Another quotation from a famous American epidemiologist may also bring to light some of the more fundamental aspects of communicating epidemiologic findings. In defining epidemiology, Wade Hampton Frost, considered by many the "father" of American epidemiology, wrote, "Epidemiology is something more than the total of its established facts. It includes the orderly arrangement of facts into chains of inference that extend more or less beyond the bounds of direct observation."

This tells us at least two things: first, that good epidemiology includes putting information into sensible order and, second, that the whole may be greater than the sum of the parts. Thus, once you assemble all the components, you may be able to draw more inferences from the aggregate than would appear to be possible when each fact is interpreted separately.

## WRITING AN EPIDEMIOLOGIC PAPER

### Basic Structure

Although varying somewhat from journal to journal, most formats of scientific papers include an introduction, a materials and methods section, and sections for results, discussion (or comment), and conclusions. Some articles have a summary, and most have an abstract of the article at the very beginning. Sometimes, particularly in epidemiologic papers, there is a background section. Over the past few years some medical journals changed their abstract to include subheadings such as: objective, design, setting, participants, interventions, main outcome measures, results, and conclusions. Because these divisions can be helpful to you in the overall organization of your epidemiologic paper,[2] let us look at each of the major sections briefly to get some ideas of their function.

### Introduction

The introduction of virtually all scientific papers gives a very brief historical perspective. Epidemiologic papers are no exception. You should usually give some indication of why the investigation was done (i.e., because of an outbreak of illness or an apparent need to explain or explore why certain health events happened). You should also indicate the overall purpose of the paper and give some indication of the specific area to be covered. If the topic is cancer or an outbreak of salmonella infection, say what particular facet will be emphasized. Look at published papers in the target journal to get the acceptable format.

The introduction is not a literature review. You should pick out only the pertinent material and try to guide the reader's thinking into your own thought processes—where you are going and what will be covered.

### Materials and methods

Tell the readers what tools and methods you used, what was the design of the study, what rules and definitions were used, how they were applied, and what operations you actually did.

In an epidemiologic paper, a case definition is an absolute necessity because, if the readers do not know your definition, they do not know exactly what you are counting. Describe the case-finding techniques—contacting physicians, visiting all relevant clinics, doing a survey, analyzing an existing database, or various other methods of case finding. Outline the laboratory methods (but probably not in great detail in an epidemiologic paper). Describe surveys or other sampling techniques you used, statistical tests applied, and any allied areas such as animal, vector, and environmental studies.

Also, a statement concerning background or setting may fit appropriately here. Describe the area under investigation, the size of the community, or the hospital. Give the reader a denominator: "The community hospital served a population of 24,000 people"; "There were 200 discharges per month"; or "The community has a maximum population of 15,000 people, most of whom are migrant workers who come in during the peak harvesting season." Some detail about geographic, climatic, or physical features of where the investigation took place may be necessary. What was there when the investigation started, and who was there? Key people may need to be identified (usually by title rather than by name). Such a section can also appear as part of the introduction or even be included in the results. After the first drafts of the paper are prepared, you will almost certainly have a better feeling of where a background statement best belongs.

## Results

For a field investigation, the results section very often, but not always, starts with how the problem or epidemic was recognized and a very short description of the pertinent time, place, and person findings. Such a short paragraph prepares the reader and gives a feeling of time moving and a sense of the whole picture—important components of good communication.

Now comes the first major area of the results: *descriptive epidemiology*. Start with the clinical and laboratory aspects first. Usually, there will be a range of signs and symptoms from mild to very serious and even death. So describe the clinical findings in some detail. They will give the more clinically oriented reader an idea of the spectrum of disease and will often help justify the case definition. State what laboratory tests were done and their results. Avoid the tendency to defend the methods or to interpret the results at this point; that follows later in the discussion.

Next, in whatever detail is necessary, orient the reader to the time, the place, and the person of the investigation. This may involve considerable discussion about the timing and distribution of cases. It is the logical place to show an epidemic curve, if appropriate. Describe the figure and analyze it for the reader. Then describe the findings according to where the persons became ill or where they were placed at risk. Present the pertinent characteristics of the cases (age, gender, race, occupation, etc.) This section is still descriptive, but it should be as detailed as needed to help build the best possible foundation for developing a hypothesis and subsequent analysis. Include, if possible, pertinent negative findings. Such data are often as important as "positive" data and can materially help you lead the readers' minds in the direction you want them to go. You are not doing any real analysis yet, but you are setting the scene to do so.

Next comes the *transition of thought* between descriptive and analytic epidemiology. This often can be a difficult task, particularly for the beginner. Essentially, you are now taking the readers by the hand and leading them through an objective interpretation of the clinical, laboratory, and epidemiologic descriptive data. You should guide them down plausible avenues of inference that can be considered and discarded or considered and established as the most reasonable and defensible explanation for what was found. Present the pertinent information in an orderly way, blending the findings and existing knowledge in a persuasive path of logic. A possible order of considerations might be the following:

- What health problem (disease) do the clinical and laboratory data confirm or support?
- What do the facts of time, place, and person suggest? And, almost simultaneously:
- How well does the existing knowledge of this disease's pathogenesis and epidemiology fit with the investigative findings? Can these facts help one understand or suggest what happened?
- What possible exposures occurred, and how can one postulate a chain of events happening that would explain the health problem?
- What hypotheses come to mind?

Here is an example, in somewhat truncated form:

*Descriptive facts:* In August 1980, a community hospital in Michigan recognized seven cases of streptococcal wound infection in postoperative patients spanning the previous four months. Since this number represented more cases than usual, an investigation was begun.[3] A total of 10 cases of streptococcal infection, all of the same serotype, was ultimately found over the previous four months, all of whom were inpatients on several surgical wards. *Transition:* The temporal and geographic clustering of cases, the fact that all infections developed within one to two days after surgery, and the fact that all infections were of the same serotype strongly suggested a common exposure—presumably in the operating rooms. Since most streptococcal infections in the hospital setting are transmitted by humans, the field team hypothesized that contact with or exposure to a member of the hospital staff posed the unique risk to the infected patients.

This example shows how the descriptive data plus a knowledge of the epidemiology of the infectious agent were combined to lead the reader to the same logical hypothesis as the investigators.

Now comes *analytic epidemiology;* that is, comparisons of cases and controls or those exposed and not exposed (see Chapter 8). If there were no apparent associations between exposure and illness, you would probably not be writing the paper. If there were associations, what are the probabilities of their occurring? Here you will logically select risks and/or exposures that you compared and present them to the reader. Consider starting with the comparisons that showed no statistically significant differences, then lead on to those where differences were noted and focus on them.

To continue with the above example: The field team then compared infected patients to comparable noninfected postsurgical patients with respect to contact with 38 surgeons, anesthesiologists, and nursing staff. Rates of exposure to various hospital staff were not statistically different between cases and controls, except for one nurse. The nurse was then found to be a carrier of the epidemic strain of streptococcus. When she was removed from the surgical wards, no more cases of streptococcal infection occurred.

Sometimes the first analyses reveal nothing, requiring another level of analysis and/or collection of new data. This is particularly characteristic of nosocomial infections where numbers of cases are often small, such as in the outbreak above. In any event take your reader, logically, step by step through your analyses.

If control and/or prevention measures were taken, this is the place to include them in the paper.

## Discussion

A good discussion highlights the significant findings without reviewing everything all over again. The most salient points can be restated for emphasis. You can now express your own judgment as to what the results mean and show how your findings relate to the current state of knowledge. You should weigh the possible inferences of all of your data as you go along, and then you should give your judgment in terms of a conclusion.

The discussion section is also a good place to integrate your findings with what is known about the subject. Moreover, consider how your investigation might serve as a stimulus for further research in the area of concern.

Be sure to review critically the definitions, the measurements, and the analytic tools that you used; for example, case definitions, survey instruments, levels of sensitivity and specificity, and statistical tests. How good were they? Were they the most appropriate instruments for the study? Weigh them fairly for the readers so they know how you view them. What were the weaknesses or difficulties you had in collecting important information? Did lack of relevant data have significant impact with regard to confounding or effect modification? Be a critic of your methods, yet defend them objectively and honestly. You will be much more believable if you do so. Exactly where in the discussion you include these remarks will depend a great deal upon their importance in verifying your findings. In fact, you may want to discuss the pros and cons of your methods as you interpret the findings. That is quite acceptable. However, in general, evaluations of methods will fall after the major points of the discussion.

## Conclusions

Summarize the results and inferences of the work in one short paragraph. You may also want to include in a sentence or two what further work or research is needed to clarify or expand the findings of your study.

## Order of Writing

Let us next talk about the sequence you might consider in starting to write an article. You have done the investigation, and you know the component parts; how do you write the article? The temptation is to start at the beginning—namely, the introduction—and go to the end. Consider avoiding this temptation and describe the facts first. It is a much more comfortable process. Some fledgling authors spend a great deal of time and effort spinning their wheels trying to write an introduction, not knowing how much of the literature to review, not yet knowing what their major points are going to be, not knowing how they want to orient the reader. So forget about the introduction, sit down and write about what you did and what you found—that is, what you know as nobody else knows.

Consider writing the body of the study—the background, the material and methods, and the results—first. The discussion and the introduction will still be there waiting and may appear in a better perspective if you first write about what you did and what you found out. Also, you will have exercised your descriptive and analytic mind so that by the time the discussion, the introduction, and the conclusion are ready to be written, you will see the major and minor findings quite clearly. In truth, you may not really be aware of some of the key issues, the new facts, and their ramifications and interplay until the facts are laid out in logical order in the descriptive and analytic narrative. Putting things on paper gives a perspective on what you know compared to what you thought you knew almost better than anything else you can do.

Lastly, after the first or second draft has been written, wait ten days to two weeks before looking at your paper again. You will then often see your writing more objectively and critically. The evidence, the inferences, the logic, the "flow" of your paper may appear in a very different light and may need more changes.

## Guidelines

Here are several guidelines that may help in presenting the results and in the discussion. Remember you are trying to convince and to persuade people to believe you.

1. Develop your findings logically. Write from the general to the specific; do not start with the minutiae and then try to encompass the whole world afterward. In the results section, try to grasp and explain the full extent of the findings at the beginning. Then focus on the individual elements one by one. In the discussion, start with the big picture to provide an overall context or consideration, and then fix attention upon the more specific aspects of your study. If the subject is influenza in the United States or about cancer of a particular type, write several sentences about influenza or cancer in general that orient the reader, so that all the subsequent facts and findings will fit into a more understandable context. In other words, concentrate on the unfolding of facts and transition in thought.

2. Consider "friendly persuasion" in the discussion. Do not hit your reader over the head with the hardest material to understand or even the best evidence at the beginning. Start with simple, understandable, and accepted statements. Present the weakest supporting evidence at the beginning, then slowly build to the strongest and most plausible explanation at the end. Let your sentences grow in complexity, all the while recognizing other possible explanations as you slowly present your case. Leave the really controversial aspects to the end of the discussion—you do not want to divert the readers' attention away from the conclusions you want them to accept.

3. Develop your thesis with an overall pathogenesis in mind. That is, when you elaborate on the factors that putatively contributed to the disease or health problem, consider the attributes of the inciting agent, the development of symptoms and signs, and the full-blown clinical presentations. How do they square with, support, and advance your presentation of the epidemiologic findings?

4. Make your style as simple as possible. Use short words (which are usually Anglo-Saxon in derivation), short sentences, and straightforward constructions. Use the active voice when possible. It is easier to understand and more forceful. Select words that denote rather than connote: you are an epidemiologist, not a poet.

5. Use plenty of transition devices. Transitions are extremely important in any kind of writing. They prepare or cue the reader for further elaboration, a change in thinking, an exception, or an unusual observation. Additionally, transitions can create a time frame that helps move the action in a desired direction. Ideally, your exposition will have transitions in thought, but if it does not, at least transitional words will help. Subheadings also cue the reader to what is to come, including the size and complexity of the subject's component parts.

## Problems

Here are a few problem areas to avoid:

1. Being wrong. One of the easiest ways to "turn readers off" is to be wrong. If you state the wrong percentage or the wrong bibliographical reference or your numbers do not add up correctly, the reader may discount everything else you say. You have then lost the battle of communicating, of convincing.
2. "Talking down" to the reader. Declarative, unmodified statements, such as "all malaria is caused by mosquitoes," often invite error and make most readers angry. The use of long and highly technical words may seemingly command power and persuade, but seldom do these expressions, per se, convince scientifically experienced and critical audiences. More often, such words confuse rather than clarify, and their frequent use suggests a kind of professional insecurity.
3. Mixing opinion with fact. One may frequently see a statement or even a phrase stating a conclusion before all the evidence is presented. This most often happens when the author states the incubation period before the exposure has been established. Those inferences and opinions belong in the discussion after all the facts have been presented.

## PRESENTING A SCIENTIFIC PAPER

### Advance Preparation

#### The audience

Before preparing a scientific paper, you should know something about your audience. For the lay public, students, or scientists, you will necessarily select a special format of presentation, a vocabulary, appropriate audiovisuals, and perhaps even a demeanor or style of presentation. This means that you need to think carefully of how to communicate best—how to serve the needs and desires of that audience.

#### The facilities

How large is the auditorium? How is it lighted? How many does it seat? How many people will be there? Who controls the lights and the projector? What kind of microphone will be used? Is there a lectern, a chalkboard, a flipchart? Do you have choices for any of those facilities? How far will you be from the first row of the audience, and how good are the acoustics? Sometimes the acoustics with a microphone are so bad that you are best understood by raising your voice unaided by the electronic amplifier. Try to get answers to these questions as soon as possible. At scientific meetings, at least try to attend several sessions in the same room a few hours in advance.

## Slides, transparencies, or presentation software

The first rule of thumb is: do not use more than one kind of projection method for your talk. To do so is confusing, wastes time, and can easily lead to errors by you or the projectionist.

Slides and computer projections usually require a dark room. They are generally quicker to change. One can show the "real thing," that is, pictures of patients, places, and things. But slides are sometimes hard to make quickly and at the last minute. Equipment failures are not uncommon and can be absolutely devastating at an important scientific meeting or formal presentation. Parenthetically, it would be very smart to be sure, before you give your talk, that there are extra bulbs available for immediate replacement. With both slides and computer projections you frequently lose significant eye contact with your audience.

Transparencies are very easy to make at the last minute. They tend to promote good eye contact with the audience, particularly if you point at the transparency (not the screen) as you speak. However, they are often awkward to use because they collect static electricity, make noise, and there often is no logical place to put them when you are through. Moreover, unless you look at and check each transparency, one by one, as you show them, you can easily not center them correctly on the screen. For some, using transparencies gives the impression of teaching rather than lecturing or giving a scientific presentation. On the other hand, one can use transparencies for that delicate mixture of teaching and presenting material, because you can write on a transparency as you progress through your talk, underline, or circle, and emphasize certain points.

In some situations handouts can be very useful. They are particularly good for teaching and leaving your audience with the most important points you want to make, giving, in truth, a "take-home" lesson. They are ideal to use when, at the end of a field investigation, you are summarizing your findings to the local health officers. They are clearly very useful when you are concerned about electrical supply or the real possibility of equipment failure. Unfortunately, handouts have to be reproduced, they are noisy, the audience attention is not on you, but on the paper, and you lose control over them. Last, they really are not that frequently used at major scientific meetings.

The use of slides, presentation software, transparencies, or handouts is a personal choice. Knowing the setting and the formality of your talk, the nature of your audience, and the ultimate purpose of your presentation will be the best guides for deciding what audiovisual devices to use.[4]

## To read or not to read

Another serious consideration is whether to read or not to read your presentation. Ideally, you will probably communicate best if you do not have to read your paper or talk. However, it usually requires years of practice, innate ability to extemporize, and a great deal of self-confidence to communicate scientific material effectively without reading it.

Again, the circumstances surrounding your talk will often dictate whether reading is essential, important, or inconsequential. Formal, major scientific presentations or guest lectureships will more likely than not necessitate reading a substantial part of your paper. This is particularly true if you are new at the game and not experienced in presenting scientific material. It is also true if there is a major time constraint (and there usually is). At most scientific meetings, one is given 10, maybe 15 minutes at most for presentations, and it is absolutely critical not to exceed your allotted time. This can best be accomplished by writing out the presentation and rehearsing it so that you are within 10 to 20 seconds of your allotted time. And, indeed, practice your talk—perhaps to a few of your colleagues or even your spouse. Get their reaction and input; it is well worth the time.

The size of the audience sometimes can help you decide whether to read or extemporize. Small audiences of 30 persons usually permit an informal atmosphere where your presentation can be done ad lib. When the audience is 50 or more, again depending upon a variety of circumstances, you may still be able to ad lib your presentation and refer frequently to notes to jog your memory. Scientific presentations to 75 persons or more probably dictate a formal, airtight presentation that is best read, unless you are a real professional. It is the rare professional who can present a paper ad lib at a scientific meeting in exactly 10 minutes in first-rate, smooth, and clear fashion. The vast majority of presenters read their papers; and with enthusiasm, knowledge of the subject, good projection of words, and modest eye contact, they can communicate extremely well to the audience.

The rule of thumb: when in doubt, read it out loud. If you rehearse and are enthusiastic, articulate, knowledgeable, and coherent, you should have little difficulty in informing and convincing by communication.

## The Actual Presentation

Be aware that you, almost as much as the substance of your talk, are under the close scrutiny of your audience. So try to eliminate any possible barriers that might arise between yourself and the audience such as: unfamiliar or odd clothing, unusual or inappropriate body language, or visible distractions. Suitable language and recognition of cultural norms go a long way to good communication as well. And do not endanger your credibility as an epidemiologist by self-deprecation or apologies.

When called upon to make your talk, walk briskly to the lectern. There is nothing more disappointing than seeing a lecturer or presenter saunter casually up to the stage. It gives the impression of not caring, of not being prepared. Get comfortable before you start talking. Make sure the microphone is exactly where you want it. Get your visuals, your notes, your glass of water, your position behind the lectern exactly the way you want them before you start. Frequently you may need to acknowledge the person who introduced you with thanks or perhaps a joke. More often, at a true scientific meeting, there will be no introduction, but it is usually good manners to acknowledge the moderator. Listen to a few talks before your own so you will know what manners are expected and appropriate.

Position yourself close to the images on the screen so you do not have to walk halfway across the stage to point out something or find it yourself. Usually this is no problem. Minimize walking around on the stage unless you are really in a teaching mode or you are going to create a dialogue with your audience. Make eye contact with your audience as frequently as possible, not contact with the microphone, the screen, or the papers you are reading from. Look about the audience, not at one place or one person. This brings them in to you as you are talking. If there is a pointer, or electric arrow, keep it as still as possible and turn it off when you are not actively pointing out something. Speak slowly and clearly. The adrenalin circulating through you will almost always make your words come out faster. Speak distinctly, and try to project the words to the back of the auditorium.

It usually takes about two minutes to read one page of double-spaced text reasonably slowly and clearly. This means, if you have a 10-minute talk, your paper should be no longer than 4½ to 5½ pages at the very most. Regarding projections, recall that it takes varying lengths of time to get the projectionist's attention, turn the lights off and on, and show the material. Many presenters read their paper at the same time they show slides. However, quite often speakers ad lib when the slides appear. This then adds time to the presentation—about 5–15 seconds per slide, because it takes the audience at least that time to digest the material.

Do not hesitate to bring in props, or the real things that you used or found in your investigation. A can of tainted food or pesticide, or a piece of equipment that was associated with disease is very convincing, can be very useful, and "lightens" your presentation.[5]

### Content

A 10-minute presentation should include most of the key components of a scientific article. There often will be acknowledgments at the beginning and then a brief introduction with a statement of background and purpose. Your materials and methods must emphasize the most important parts of your investigation or analysis. You cannot go into detail here—simply state the barest essentials so your audience will know exactly what you did. Avoid referring to methods that you do not have time to explain (i.e., there should be no "black box").

State the most important results, recalling that you cannot tell the audience everything you found. This part will be the longest of your presentation. This is where you may use tables, figures, and charts, which, if well used, will generally increase comprehension and minimize explanation. Discussion comes next, when, as in a written paper, you highlight what was most important, how it fits in with what is presently known, and your interpretation of the findings. Then state your conclusion: a very brief summary and what it all means, including control and prevention, if appropriate.

When you are finished, say "Thank you." Do not simply stop talking at the end of your presentation. The audience does not know what to expect. Also, it is simple courtesy to thank them for listening to you.

### How to alienate your audience

There are some relatively simple rules that, if broken, can seriously impair your ability to communicate with your audience and at the same time make you lose credibility and/or stature.

1. Probably the greatest offense is taking more time than you are allotted. This is selfish, it is unfair, and, if there is a discussion period set aside for your paper, you are using time that is not yours. The discussion is time for the audience to react to your presentation. Exceeding your time will infuriate most moderators, and if this constraint is grossly abused, you stand to suffer the major embarrassment of being asked to stop talking and sit down. Furthermore, taking more time than allowed implies you were not well prepared and did not know what were the important points to make. All of which boils down to the simple fact that you must not and cannot expect to present everything you did or found. You must be selective. Perhaps the discussion will touch on some areas that you could not present during your allotted time.

2. The next major problem concerns visual aids. You are responsible for the quality and order of your projections. If they are out of order or upside down or illegible, they will materially detract from your ability as a communicator and even your credibility as an investigator. For some strange reason, some people simply do not care about their visual aids. They seem to be above it all. Do not be one of them. If at all possible, bring your own slide carousel or laptop to the auditorium. Put your slides in the carousel yourself. Check them or the computer order at least two times before you make your presentation. Nothing can ruin a first-rate presentation faster than out-of-order, upside down, or backwards visual aids.

3. Do not use projections that are illegible or have too much data on them. Avoid this simply by projecting the material in a room roughly the size of the room where the meeting is. If you cannot read them easily at the back of the room, you have no business wasting everyone's time showing them.

4. Do not talk down to the audience. This is hard to define easily, but avoid pompous attitudes, long words, or an air of superiority. Along the same line, remember that the moderator is your supervisor; do not disregard his or her requests. If you do not follow the moderator's instructions, this can cause great embarrassment and loss of credibility.
5. Do not become angry or upset in front of your audience. This is especially a hazard during the discussion period. Compliment the questioner on his or her question; stay composed; say you don't know if you don't know; respect the opinions of others, even if they are outrageous; and remain calm and pleasant, even if you are furious underneath.

## SUMMARY

Whether you are writing or speaking, your primary purpose is to transfer facts and ideas so your audience will understand and believe you. Keep your words simple, your logic clear and understandable, and your tone one of friendly persuasion. And, always remember Gregg's Law #12: "Never tell your audience everything you know."

## REFERENCES

1. King, L.S. (1991). *Why Not Say It Clearly: A Guide to Expository Writing*, 2nd ed., Little, Brown, Boston.
2. Huth, E.J. (1987). *Medical Style and Format: An International Manual for Authors, Editors, and Publishers*, ISI Press, Philadelphia.
3. Berkelman, R.L., Martin, D., Graham, D.R., et al. (1982). Streptococcal wound infections caused by a vaginal carrier. *JAMA* 248, 2680–2.
4. Mandel, S. (1987). *Effective Presentation Skills: A Practical Guide for Better Speaking*, Crisp Publications, Los Altos, Calif.
5. Heinich, R., Molenda, M., Russell, J.D. (eds.) (1993). *Instructional Media and the New Technologies of Instruction*, 4th ed., MacMillan Publishing Co., New York. pp. 54–57.

## SUGGESTED READING

1. *American Medical Association Manual of Style*, 8th ed. (1989). Williams & Wilkins, Baltimore.
2. Fowler, H.R. (1980). *The Little, Brown Handbook*, Little, Brown, Boston.

# 13

# DEALING WITH THE PUBLIC AND THE MEDIA

Bruce B. Dan

Early in a field investigation, the variety of problems facing an epidemiologist can be daunting—sketchy information, wary local officials, long hours, and a looming crisis. Certainly the last thing the field team wants to add to their tasks is confronting the news media. But once the media learn of an investigation in the community, they will naturally insist on knowing what's happening in their own backyard. And while those charged with working up the problem are reticent to speculate on causes early in an investigation, it is precisely then that the public wants simple, direct, black-and-white answers. Every epidemic investigation has its own unique facets, and every local situation will have its own peculiarities, but this chapter attempts to provide helpful guidelines in dealing with an investigation under the spotlight of the news media.

## BACKGROUND

Until recently, virtually the only way the public learned about medical information was by talking to their personal physicians. Now anyone can become educated about health and disease by reading newspaper articles, health magazines, and diet and nutrition books, or by watching television news, celebrity fitness

DVDs, and late-night infomercials, or by typing a few words into Google, or downloading the latest health tip as a podcast.[1] In fact, the average time that a household spends viewing television is estimated to be more than eight hours each day, almost an hour more than when surveyed a decade earlier.[2]

There are now in excess of 1700 commercial and public television stations in the United States, and their broadcasts reach 99% of the households with television sets. Add to that, cable and satellite TV systems, satellite radio, and AM and FM radio stations sending signals to 99% of households with radios, and the 1500 major newspapers with a combined circulation of almost 60 million, and you can see we are awash in information. Moreover, the Internet now provides access to an almost unlimited amount of medically related material. Of the 113 million adult Internet users in the U.S., 80% have searched for information on health topics, with increasing interest in subjects such as diet, fitness, drugs, and experimental treatments.[3]

Medical information may emanate from a variety of sources: for example, medical journals, scientific meetings, federal and state health bulletins, or hospital press releases. But no matter whence it comes, medical news ends up in the public arena having been first filtered through and disseminated by the mass media. The public naturally wants to hear from medical experts during times of uncertainty. Indeed, their health may well depend upon the immediate advice of medical authorities during a serious disease outbreak, or they may just need to have their fears calmed during the almost annual occurrence of head lice in elementary schools.

Surveys have shown that the high volume of media coverage that medical reports invariably generate has not always brought clarity to health issues.[4] A large portion of the problem can be laid at the feet of health professionals themselves who often do not interact well with the media. Understanding how the media provide information to their audiences, and knowing how to deliver a message, can determine whether or not the public takes effective action. The reality is that if health care providers want to improve public health, they must be as comfortable and skilled at appearing in the media as they are in taking a history, listening to the chest, or filling out a prescription. Health information is of little use unless it can be communicated effectively and clearly to those who will benefit from it most—the public.

The public health community confronted the reality of these issues on an enormous scale during the events surrounding the bioterrorism attacks with anthrax in September, 2001. While health officials must always be adept at communicating health information, they must be unerring when the situation has the potential of a national epidemic. Often, as in the case of the anthrax threat (with only 22 cases discovered), the actual number of persons becoming ill may be small, but the consequences—cultural, financial, and political—may be immense.

The missteps of public health officials during the early phases of the anthrax investigation were not the result of diagnostic errors, badly constructed case definitions, or imprecise laboratory techniques. The problems occurred because responsible health officials did not possess the necessary communication skills and strategies to deal with an epidemic of that order. The CDC has admitted that the lessons learned from this outbreak changed the way the institution now operates.[5]

## News

While everyone knows what news is when we see it or hear it, it's not so easy to define. When you read about new medical breakthroughs or new discoveries, you know that's news. But what exactly makes an event newsworthy? It helps to know how reporters define "news." News happens when something strays from the ordinary—news, in its essence, is the unusual, or to put it into our biostatistical parlance, two standard deviations from the mean. Reporters and their media outlets are interested in change, change that has significance, change that appears threatening, anything that disrupts the status quo—new diseases, new victims. That's news!

As the person being interviewed, you actually have no way of controlling what reporters write—no more than they control how you conduct surveillance or choose a case definition. More problematic, you will not know what other interviews or elements are going into the story. What you *can* do is to ensure that the most favorable aspects, reflecting on you and your organization, are put into the mix. It takes communications skills and strategy, but once they are mastered you may even enjoy being part of the process.

Journalists and broadcasters divide news into two categories: *soft* news and *hard* news. Soft news (also called a *feature*) is the story behind the story. Features are not *the* events so much as the *background* behind them. Features can include a report on the issues of a particular story or trend, such as a television documentary on food-borne illnesses in America, a radio series on low-birth-weight infants, or an article on health-care budget cuts.

Hard news concerns the events that precipitate coverage by the media—they *are* the story. Many news outlets refer to hard news as "breaking" news. It's the plane crash, the bomb explosion, the epidemic.

## Deadlines

Each of the traditional media (print, radio, and television) suffers from a particular form of pressure—the deadline. Unlike most other enterprises, journalism runs under a continuous and unrelenting schedule. News reporters must get their stories in print or on the air under exacting constraints. For them, news a day late is no longer news. This pervasive pressure explains many of the quirks of the news business. When reporters seem curt or abrupt, it often merely reflects the conditions under which they must work.

Monthly magazines generally have long lead times, and reporters often have weeks to work on a story. And even newspaper reporters can work on a story for an entire day for the next day's edition. Even at deadline, a rapidly transcribed quote may be all that is necessary for the next morning's edition.

Radio news needs to conform to a much more precise broadcast schedule. Hourly news programs are the rule, but 10-minute updates are common during the early morning and late afternoon drive times. The emergence of "all news" radio stations means that they need to keep up on a minute-by-minute basis. However, even breaking medical news can be written rapidly and read over the air if need be. A quick phone call can provide a radio station with the information and voice it needs to make the story real.

Television correspondents work under the tightest deadlines. The reason that television news is the most rigidly constrained is because it is a visual medium. Obviously, it takes time to edit and put video images together in a logical and orderly sequence—and for TV, if there are no pictures, then there is no story. For most afternoon and evening news broadcasts on commercial stations, interviews must be set up early in the day in order to schedule camera crews and reporters. With the proliferation of cable channels and 24-hour news programs, television news has become a hungry and competitive business looking for the latest breaking stories.

With the emergence of 24-hour news programming and the Internet, reporters and their editors are under even greater pressure to provide information to the public as quickly as possible. This really means that when reporters call about a story, they generally need it then (not tomorrow or next week), and they may need to talk to you at that moment, not later that day. While it is important that you respond when the news media call, it is also critical that you be prepared when they speak to you. We will discuss later the proper balance and timing of interviews.

## The News Business

It's also of vital importance to understand the interplay between reporter and news source. Each has an agenda.[4] The media are part of a journalistic exercise in the principles of the First Amendment, and they are also part of the free enterprise system; that is, they are businesses. It is critical to understand that they are not in the business of public health. While it may seem that news organizations are doing a public service by communicating important health information, they do it only to sell more newspapers or charge higher rates for commercial time. The priorities for public health organizations and news organizations are different. Public health officials need the media to disseminate important information; the media need medical stories to sell news. But in the end, good relationships between these two diverse groups benefit the public at large.

## THE INTERVIEW

All journalists share a common tool in their work: the interview. The interview is the most frequent interaction between you and a journalist, and it is also the most flexible format. A print or radio reporter may interview you on the telephone. A television reporter may ask you to participate in a videotaped interview arranged at a convenient place and time. Reporters will want to give their source of news some sort of attribution, not only to identify the source but to give an air of credibility: "Dr. John Smith, epidemic specialist in diarrheal diseases." Develop a title that the audience you are speaking to will easily understand. Few lay people are familiar with terms such as "nephrologist," "neonatologist," or "hematologist-oncologist." And labeling yourself as a "medical epidemiologist" is certainly treading on unfamiliar ground.

In conducting an interview, journalists may visit you at your office or may even intercept you unexpectedly in the field (the dreaded "ambush" interview). Most reporters and news organizations use a combination of formats, depending on the nature of their story. News reporters, like health officials, vary in their characteristics and their backgrounds. Not surprisingly, the story reported by the science writer for a local newspaper may differ from that of the health correspondent for a major network, but all reporters are looking for the answers to the same six questions: Who/ What/ Where/ When/ How/Why. It is your job to have the answers to those questions ready and to present them in a clear and concise manner.

But before consenting to any interview, those same six questions should be asked of the interviewer. Who is going to do the interview and from what organization? What is the subject matter to be discussed and what questions will be asked? Where will it be done (in the comfort of your office or in some strange TV studio)? When will the interview take place and when will it appear (tonight's evening news or in next month's health magazine)? How will the interview be conducted (videotaped or live, one-on-one with the reporter or in a group)? And, perhaps, most important, *why* is it being done?

Unless you have all of those questions answered, the interview should not be granted. There is a tendency to feel honored, important, and in the spotlight when asked to be quoted in *Time* magazine or appear on *Nightline*, but be wary of the temptation. An overeager and ill-prepared health official usually does more damage than good.

Additionally, it is imperative that you check with local, state, or national public information personnel about any prospective interviews. Each level may have its own rules of engagement with the press. Regardless, the media relations experts can give you sound advice on carrying out an interview, and it is imperative to keep them abreast of press inquiries. That knowledge will allow them to coordinate interviews, keep track of media attention, and prevent miscommunication with the press.

## Interview Objective

By far, the most important thing to remember is that a news interview is solely an opportunity to deliver your message to an important audience. Despite its appearance, a news interview is not a venue to answer the reporter's questions or to make him or her happy. You are there to communicate an idea that you believe is critically important. An interview is not an intellectual exercise or a debate. It is certainly not an argument or a friendly chat.

Often reporters come to an interview with a mental story already written. The challenge to you is to make certain they have the *right* story. Too many people who are interviewed try to tell a reporter everything they know about a subject, and their basic point gets lost in the clutter. Your primary duty is to make a comment that captures the reporter's attention and gets your point across. That task is accomplished by constructing a single critical message and learning how to deliver it.

That unique message has been referred to as the Single Overriding Communication Objective (SOCO), pronounced *SOCK-oh*. It is by definition the single, most important message you can deliver about your topic. In fact, it is fair to say that your goal is to turn each and every question during an interview into an opportunity to relay your SOCO.

Here are some rules of thumb:

- Construct a single cogent idea and write it down (your SOCO)
- Find a means for getting your SOCO across in the interview
- Get your SOCO across early (the interview may end abruptly)
- Get your SOCO in as many times as possible
- Learn to relate your SOCO in a language the audience will understand

Exercising this art of good communication requires a great deal of preparation. Avoid the temptation to "wing it." Remember that no professional goes to a performance without a script.

## Language

In attempting to get a single message delivered, you will be most successful if the words you use are understandable to the greatest number of people. Avoid medical jargon. It works well in a clinical setting but not with the lay public. Learn to say it simply. For instance:

- Instead of "communicate," try "say"
- Instead of "disseminate," try "send"
- Instead of "metastasize," try "spread"

Use single-syllable words instead of polysyllabic ones. Use Anglo-Saxon words with easily pronounced guttural consonants; leave Latin and Greek to the textbooks. Stay away from potentially confusing words and phrases like "atypical," "subclinical," "negative test results," or "positive cultures." Avoid esoteric terminology such as "relative risk," "odds ratio," "controls," "sensitivity," and "specificity." Try to find alternatives to prefixes such as "pre-," "post-," and "pseudo-."

## Interview Techniques

### Bridging

You can prevent reporters from straying from your message or turning the interview into an interrogation by anticipating the tough questions and using the technique called *bridging*. Bridging is simply transitioning—forming a bridge between one point and another. In other words, moving from where the reporter is going to where you want the interview to go. Rather than ignoring or evading the question you simply recognize it briefly and then move or *bridge* to your SOCO. Rather than having to develop answers to dozens of potential questions, you merely need a few transitional phrases to bridge to your SOCO. These are some very simple bridges to use:

- *Don't know* to *do know*—"I don't know the answer to that, but I *can* say . . ."
- *Time*—"That was true in the past, but now we know that . . ."
- *Importance*—"That's a factor, but what's more important is . . ."

- *Affirmation*—"Yes, but in addition to that . . ."
- *Contradiction*—"No not really, let me explain . . ."
- *Contrast*—"That's the number-one cause in women, but for men . . ."
- *Focusing*—"In general that's true, but let's take a closer look at . . ."

You can construct innumerable ways to get back to the main point: "You alluded to something else I should mention . . ."; "Let me put that into perspective . . ."; "What that means is. . . ." Find comfortable phrases that fit easily into your own style of conversation. But the important point is to take the subject back to your message. Do not attempt to answer a question about which you are not knowledgeable. You can easily lose your credibility, but more important, you may misinform your audience.

## Flagging

You can punctuate your message and make it more memorable to the reporter and the audience by calling attention to your SOCO using the technique called *flagging*. It is simply using a phrase to *flag* your comment as the major component of the conversation. Flagging statements include:

- The most important thing I could say about frostbite is . . .
- If a woman who is sexually active asked me . . .
- The bottom line for people living near nuclear plants is . . .
- The single fact a food handler needs to remember is . . .
- The take-home message for people with tuberculosis is . . .

## Handling Difficult Interviews

In dealing with a potentially troublesome or even hostile interview, just make certain that your responses bridge to your messages. Because professionals in many occupations have a natural tendency to defend their positions when questioned, clever reporters will use this to lead you from curious questions to what often seems like a heated debate. Your opportunity to deliver your message gets lost in the intellectual fisticuffs. However, you are not required to justify your thoughts or actions, and you are not on the witness stand. Simply use the interviewer's statements to bridge to your SOCO. Do not repeat negative phrases. Pause and give thoughtful, positive responses. Take control, have conviction, and do not wait for permission to tell your side of the story.

Interviews may be on-the-record, off-the-record, or something in between, called "background." If you cannot give an interview that is "on-the-record" (meaning that everything you say or do can be used and attributed to you), then you probably should not be talking to the press. Never agree to an off-the-record interview. You have no guarantee that it will remain so. Do not say anything to a reporter that you would be uncomfortable seeing in the next morning's headlines.

## Planning for an Interview

Interviews should not be hit-or-miss affairs but carefully planned encounters. Before you agree to do any interview, the following guidelines should be followed:

### Screening

- All media contacts should be first screened by a media relations staff, or failing that, by yourself.
- Get a clear understanding of why the reporter wants to interview you. What is the precise topic? Is it to your advantage to take part? Is it in your area of expertise or is someone else more suitable?
- Establish the reporter's deadline and how much of your time is required.

### Preparation

- An ill-prepared interview serves neither the reporter's nor your interests. Getting ready for an interview is as important as doing one.
- Make it clear to the reporter that you want to confine the questions to the prearranged topic. Set a time limit for the interview.
- If possible, send fact sheets, background information, and photographs to the reporter before the interview.
- Prepare for the interview. Plan your strategy. Write out your primary public health message and practice it. Draft some colorful quotes and anecdotes that illustrate your point.

### The interview

- When the reporter arrives, reconfirm the topic and the length of the interview.
- Give him or her your business card with the correct spelling of your name and organization.
- When you are both seated, ask the reporter, "How much do you know about (the interview topic)?" Since you are the expert, take control and lay out the situation as you see it—your SOCO.
- Briefly bridge through the negative or irrelevant questions and move the conversation back to your message. You can prevent "fishing expeditions" by reminding the reporter that you are prepared to be interviewed on the agreed-upon topic for that day. You are, of course, happy to set up an interview on another subject on another day.

- Stick to your agreed-upon time limit (you may want to have an assistant call you when the time limit has elapsed). Bring the interview to an orderly close with a summary, which should be a crisp and concise version of your message.
- Arrange a follow-up procedure so that any last-minute or verification questions can be handled.

### Post-interview

- Each interview, whether for the print or broadcast media, should be an opportunity to learn and improve.
- Keep an index card for every interview, jotting down the date, the reporter's name, the subject discussed, and where it appeared. Grade yourself on the interview. Did you get your SOCO in? Grade the reporters and file the card for future reference. Were they knowledgeable or uninformed? Are they friends or foes?
- If you discover you have given a reporter erroneous information, correct it immediately—even if the story has already appeared. If reporters have misstated facts, alert them so the story can be corrected. If your statements have been distorted, and you feel that the interview has been unfairly conducted, let the reporter know. If there is not a satisfactory response, inform the reporter that the issue will be brought to the attention of his or her editor.

There are not any prescribed formulas for the "correct" interview. However, there are some helpful hints in conducting yourself with each of the media. Below is listed some brief advice for each type of interview you may encounter.

## Print Interview

The print interview is probably the most common and perhaps the least threatening. It usually involves a one-to-one conversation with a newspaper reporter either in person or on the phone. Most of us are reasonably comfortable talking to another person about a subject in which we feel confident. The danger is in feeling too comfortable and saying too much. Make it clear to the reporter that you want to confine questions to the prearranged topic.

Reporters may tape the conversation to have exact quotes on hand, but they may simply note some important points. If the reporter calls on the phone (and you have already been cleared to speak with him or her), remember that you do not have to speak at that moment. It is perfectly acceptable to tell the reporter that you will call back in 10 minutes. Hang up, collect your thoughts, jot down some notes, get comfortable, and call back when *you* are ready to be interviewed.

Remember that there is no rule that says you must conduct a telephone interview sitting down. It's better to stand up, walk around the room, and gesture as you talk. It will bring a more natural tone to the conversation. Beware of inflections. Tongue-in-cheek remarks, a sarcastic tone, and even humor do not translate well into print. The exact opposite of what you meant may come through. In addition, your comments may be characterized: a statement with a condescending tone or with a smirk may be reported as such.

Try to speak in even, succinct, declarative sentences, but try to be natural and informative. Do not talk too fast. The reporter may be frantically trying to take down your message, so slow down and ask the reporter if you should repeat it more slowly. In today's world many reporters will transcribe their notes on a computer, which means you can hear them typing on their keyboards at the other end of the phone line. When you hear their clicking keyboard make certain you are articulating the message you want to see in their story. The print interview is the one place where you can use exact medical terms (if you explain them) because the reader can pause, reread, and study a word or phrase. The same is not true for the electronic media.

Remember that the interview is not over when the reporter stops the recorder or puts down the pen. Any comments you make during the time spent with the reporter are on-the-record. The interview is over when the reporter is out of earshot.

## Radio Interview

Here you must be sharply aware of inflections. The only thing the listener hears is your voice. Learn to modulate your voice in pitch, volume, and cadence. A deadpan monotone is as dreary and uninformative on the radio as it is from the podium. Use your hands and make facial gestures when expressing yourself on the radio. They will not appear themselves, but their effect will carry emotion and inflection to your voice. Use short, preferably monosyllabic words ("give" instead of administer, "make" instead of fabricate). They are easier to pronounce and easier to understand.

Many radio interviews are done by telephone. Again, do not engage in an interview either live or taped until you are ready. You are not required to carry out the interview while seated at your desk. It is permissible to stand up, walk around, do anything else that makes you comfortable (but do not tap your fingers on the desk or chew your pencil). Talk to your interviewer as you would talk to the people whom you meet on the street or someone you would meet in a supermarket— simply, directly, and interestingly.

## TV Interview

As with print and radio, television requires information and an articulate delivery. But additionally, TV interviews require two other vitally important factors— appearance and appeal. In particular, television has the peculiar property that it is far more important *how* you say something than *what* you say. This may seem heretical to some and "unprofessional" to others. But it is perhaps the most critical aspect of the television medium and one that must be understood and accepted, if you have any desire to transmit information through this medium.

This unique aspect of "seeing" is what also gives television its powerful impact, but if not used properly, results in the media manipulating the message-giver rather than the other way around. Television in the end does not deliver information, it gives perceptions; it does not deliver facts, it leaves impressions. As illogical as it may seem, your appearance and demeanor carry more weight than your command of information.

TV segments usually only contain a few 10–15-second quotes (called sound bites) from the interviewee. That means that you must be able to relate your entire message in a very short sentence and do it in an interesting and appealing way. You must also speak in short, easily understood words. If the viewers misunderstand you, they do not, as with newspapers, have the ability to go back and "reread" the story.

Even if what you say is technically correct, TV reporters are looking for catchy sound bites (like good one-liners). If your message is dull, but you also happen to make some other extraneous, but media-grabbing statement, you can imagine what will make the air. Your job is to make your message so exciting, the reporter is virtually obligated to put it on. The following, again, is a brief listing of tips to enhance your ability to get your message across on television:

- Be calm and relaxed. TV cameras and strange studio lights and microphones tend to make anyone uptight. Viewers will be turned off by what they perceive as stiffness and formality. This only comes with practice; there are no "secrets."
- Use natural eye contact. Unless told otherwise, always look at the person to whom you are speaking. That is a natural disposition. Do not look briefly at the cameras or studio monitors, it will give you a shifty appearance.
- Dress conservatively. For men, wear a dark jacket (gray or navy blue), and avoid checks and plaids. Wear a tie with small patterns of red (darker shades), whites, and blues. Shirts should be light colored (try to avoid bright white) with a straight collar (not buttoned down). Women should

wear a simple dress or business suit; stay away from large, brightly colored prints. Reflective and jingling gold jewelry, large distracting earrings, and bizarre hairdos will take the viewers' attention away from what you are saying.

- Facial expressions should be pleasant and natural. Avoid the natural tendency to look numb and stiff. *Smile!* It is not only all right, it is preferred—it gives your countenance a look of warmth and friendliness.

- Your body and posture should be straight but relaxed. Even a small slump looks terrible on TV (if you feel comfortable, you probably look bad). Feel free to move naturally, and use your hands when you talk (just stay away from wild gestures, especially in front of your face). Sitting forward toward your interviewer lends a sense of interest and confidence; leaning back, one of indifference and aversion.

- Speak in words of few syllables. They are less likely to be mispronounced, more likely to be understood, and you can get a lot more of them in the conversation in 15 seconds. Use those Anglo-Saxon words that carry emotion and add vitality to your speech: words like "live," "die," "love," "hate," "make," "save," "get," "find." People "get sick and have heart attacks." They do not "acquire illnesses and suffer myocardial infarctions."

- Speak in declarative sentences. Avoid answering questions with a simple yes or no.

- Do not quote exact figures from medical journals. Do not bother letting everyone know that exactly "53.2% of the case-patients taking 325 mg of aspirin daily significantly decreased their relative risk of suffering a re-infarction during the study period." Simply respond, "More than half the people taking an aspirin a day greatly reduced their chances of a second heart attack." Get used to using terms like "most of," "the majority," "almost all," "very few."

- Be a good listener. Nothing sounds worse than trying to answer what you thought was the question when the reporter actually asks something else. Do not assume you know what the reporter is getting at and jump over his or her lines. Hear the reporter out.

- Lastly, project conviction and confidence. Speak to your questioner with a real sense of interest and caring. It will come across to the viewer that way as well.

## EPIDEMIC MANAGEMENT

The best way to learn how to handle an epidemic is on-the-job training, but there is value in learning from those who have already been through the process.

Every epidemic is different; every local situation will have its own peculiarities; but the following may prove helpful:

- Stay away from the media. This advice may seem contradictory after talking about the importance of communicating with the public, but your number-one job on an investigation is to assist the local health officials, not appear on a morning talk show. If you are spending time before the cameras, you are not working up the problem.
- If accosted by the media as you arrive at the locale (and it is not uncommon to be met by a phalanx of reporters as you get off the plane), do not stop, but calmly keep walking to your destination. Answer any questions with a smile and the obvious response, "I'm here at the request of (the local authorities) to assist in their investigation. I'll be glad to talk to you after I have conferred with them." If pressed further, simply repeat your SOCO in any interesting way you wish, "As I said, I'm here to help, and I'll be happy to chat with you after I've gathered some information."
- Designate a single spokesperson. The underlying and inviolable rule is, "One messenger, one message." If the epidemic involves several agencies, attempt to have one person speak for the group effort. When differing viewpoints from competing agencies simultaneously appear in the media, it merely breeds confusion, and more damaging, signals to the public that those in charge of protecting their health are in disarray. Local and state health agencies have public relations specialists who are trained and get paid to talk to the press. Those communications experts probably know all the media people, have already established a good working relationship with them, and know the ins and outs of the local scene. Let them handle the press. They will have to do it anyway after you have gone.
- Try to have your spokesperson seek out the media first in a proactive, informational manner. It not only demonstrates responsibility but it also lets you set the agenda and control events. If the media find out first from another source, it becomes, "What did you know, and when did you know it?"
- Set a regular press briefing time. It establishes a routine; the media are not caught by surprise; and it offers you, again, the chance to make prepared statements and control events.
- Try to keep technologists and other allied people behind the scenes; they can give potentially confusing and contradictory information to the press. There must be one messenger delivering one cogent message. The press likes nothing better than controversy. Even something as simple as two different totals for the number of cases can give the media grist for

unnerving criticism. Along that line, try not to get into a numbers game with the press. Refrain from "upping" the numbers every day. Even with no news, an increasing number becomes in itself a news story and reason for headlines.

- Above all else, coordinate information with the local, state, and national officials. Not only will you keep the team players happy but you will also avoid creating controversies—since the press likes nothing better than to find that the state has facts that the local health department does not have, and vice versa. To paraphrase the late Mayor Richard J. Daley of Chicago, "The field epidemiologist is not there to create disorder, the field investigator is there to preserve disorder."

## PRESS CONFERENCES

The news conference increases your control in getting your message out to the media. But in the question-and-answer period that control can be snatched way by an aggressive reporter. Suddenly, a quiet give-and-take session can be turned into a feeding frenzy. To make sure that you do not end up with a negative situation, learn to shield yourself.

- Have a spokesperson open up the news conference by introducing the participants and stating the ground rules. Handouts should be distributed at the beginning of the conference. The spokesperson should tell the assembled reporters what areas will and will not be covered and for what reasons.
- Make sure you introduce yourself when you step to the microphone. Spell your name and give your position and affiliation.
- Your first sentence should be your key message (SOCO). Make it one that will be memorable and mentioned. If done well, it will be the first sound bite carried on all networks that night.
- Keep your opening statement brief and tightly focused. If it is concise, it reduces the chances that a reporter will misunderstand, interrupt, or even walk out. Speak in headlines; save the details and documentation for the handout.
- Do not just read your statement—communicate it. Look at the audience; speak with enthusiasm or concern; gesture.
- Set some ground rules for the question-and-answer session. For example, "Now I'd like to open it up briefly for a few questions. So that everyone gets a turn, I'll take one question from each of you. I'd appreciate it if you'd raise your hand when you have a question and identify yourself."

- If no questions arise, ask yourself the first question. That might break the ice and trigger other questions.
- Do not allow yourself to be bullied. When a reporter tries to interrupt you, tell him or her nicely that you would like to finish your answer. Use your hands—signaling to one reporter that you are ready to take his or her question, while gesturing with the other hand to tell another reporter that he or she is up next.
- Sum up. When you feel your topic has been sufficiently covered in the Q & A session, give notice that you will take one more question. Then do precisely that. Finally, briefly restate your key point, thank the audience, and leave.

## SPECIAL PROBLEMS

It is not possible to cover every twist and turn of dealing with the media, but several special situations often come up that require thinking about in advance.

- Personal opinion vs. local/state policy: If asked what the official local policy is on a certain subject, you should probably refer the question to the public information officer (unless in the rare instance you have been given the authority to be the spokesperson). You should feel free, in good conscience, to give your opinions on matters of science as a physician, veterinarian, nurse, or other health practioner. But policy matters are best left to those who know the policy and can take responsibility for it. If you feel foolish saying that you do not know the policy when you feel you should know it, simply say that you would like the reporter to meet with the person who can best answer that question.
- Press embargoes: Many releases of information to the press (including medical journal publications) have dates specified as to when that information can be disseminated to the public, the so-called press embargo date. The purpose of the embargo is to allow all media outlets to have an equal opportunity to cover the story. No one will have an edge due to the vagaries of the mail or access to the press release. If *everyone* has the written material in hand before the story is broadcast, then its health message can be disseminated in a coordinated, logical fashion.

Most medical reporters will receive the press release or medical journal before the release date and begin working with the story. If you are called before the release date, simply remind the reporter of the embargo and say that you are speaking with the understanding that the story will not be published before that time. If you have any particular questions, check with the publisher of the press release or journal's editorial office.

## SUMMARY

In contrast to past decades, the American public now gets most of its medical information from the media: newspapers, magazines, radio, television, and the Internet. You may be asked by the media to report and comment on your findings either during an investigation or afterward. Although your mission is to protect and maintain the public's health, the primary mission of the media is not public health but to sell their product or their time. Despite these somewhat opposite objectives, the media can and should be your ally. Learn how the media operate, and cultivate some simple practices of interviewing so you can communicate effectively with the public.

Be prepared for the interview, know what you are going to be asked about, and know the subject. Have a message to get across and do it simply, directly, and with conviction. Tell the truth, do not be afraid to say you do not know, and do not field questions in an area that is not yours. If possible, avoid the media in the field and refer them to the local health authorities. They, rather than you, should report the results of the investigation to their constituents. They, too, should comment on health policies and issues. Keep the appropriate media relations specialists informed of your press contacts. And, lastly, be sure that all levels of government have the same information. Nothing destroys confidence in our health structure more than conflicting facts.

## REFERENCES

1. Cline, R.J., Haynes, K.M. (2001) Consumer health information seeking on the Internet: the state of the art. *Health Education Research* Dec; 16(6):671–92.
2. Nielsen Media Research (2007). Available at: www.nielsenmedia.com/nc/portal/site/Public/menuitem.55dc65b4a7d5adff3f65936147a062a0/?vgnextoid=13280e5b2cea5110VgnVCM100000ac0a260aRCRD
3. Internet Health Resources. Pew Internet and American Life Project. October, 2006. Available at: www.pewinternet.org/PPF/r/190/report_display.asp
4. Jeffres, L.W. (1997). *Mass Media Effects*, 2nd ed., Prospect Heights, Ill.: Waveland Press.
5. Hughes, J.M., Gerberding, J.L. (2002) Anthrax Bioterrorsim: Lessons Learned and Future Directions. *Emerg Infect Dis.* Oct; 8(10):1015–1018. www.bt.cdc.gov/agent/anthrax/reference/eid.asp

# III

# SPECIAL CONSIDERATIONS

# 14

# LEGAL CONSIDERATIONS IN SURVEILLANCE AND FIELD EPIDEMIOLOGY

Verla S. Neslund
Richard A. Goodman
James L. Hadler
James G. Hodge, Jr.

Public health surveillance and field epidemiology—including investigation of disease outbreaks and clusters—are critical, basic functions carried out by public health agencies at local, state, and federal levels. Each of the 50 states operates and maintains public health surveillance systems, not only to monitor notifiable disease conditions caused primarily by infectious pathogens, but also to monitor noninfectious disease conditions and public health indicators, such as behavioral risk factors for injuries and chronic conditions.[1, 2] Along with the traditional collection and analysis of vital records, state-level surveillance forms the foundation for national-level surveillance systems, which may be coordinated by federal agencies such as the Centers for Disease Control and Prevention (CDC) and the National Institutes of Health.[1–3]

In addition to conducting surveillance, local, state, and federal public health agencies that are engaged in field epidemiology must be able to respond to disease threats by investigating the hundreds of outbreaks and disease clusters that occur in the United States each year. Outbreak response relies, not only on the legal authorities necessary for public health agencies to conduct surveillance and, therefore, to detect such problems, but also on the authorities and assurances required for carrying out the steps of an investigation and implementing appropriate control measures. Specifically, these legal authorities enable public health officials to obtain clinical specimens and data from persons affected by an outbreak; collect environmental samples; protect the privacy of information; conduct analytic studies (e.g., case-control or cohort studies) to test hypotheses about sources for pathogens and modes of spread; and implement and enforce control measures, such as vaccination, chemoprophylaxis, quarantine, or even seizure or destruction of property.

This chapter provides an overview of the legal issues relating to public health surveillance and field epidemiology. It discusses the general legal authorities for surveillance and public health investigations provided by the U.S. Constitution and by state laws; outbreak investigations and disease control in the United States; and legal issues related to the collection, analysis, and dissemination of surveillance data. In addition, the chapter presents information about new surveillance challenges beyond traditional infectious disease models, including the influence of bioterrorism preparedness on surveillance activities.

## GENERAL LEGAL AUTHORITIES FOR SURVEILLANCE AND PUBLIC HEALTH INVESTIGATIONS

### U.S. Constitution

Both federal and state governments have inherent powers to protect the public's health. Article 1, Section 8, of the U.S. Constitution authorizes Congress to impose taxes to "provide for the general [w]elfare of the United States" and to regulate interstate and foreign commerce. The Public Health Service (PHS) and CDC are examples of federal activities that may be generally supported by the authority of the welfare clause. Under the authority of the commerce clause of the Constitution, the federal government oversees such health-related activities as the licensing and regulation of drugs, biological products, and medical devices. Although the provisions in the federal Constitution are broad, the activities of the federal government relating to health and welfare nonetheless must fit within the enumerated powers.

By contrast, the public health powers of a state are extensive, rooted in its inherent powers to protect the peace, safety, health, and general welfare of its citizens. The Tenth Amendment to the U.S. Constitution specifically reserves all powers not expressly granted to the federal government nor otherwise prohibited by the Constitution to the states. Unlike the federal government, the states have vast, sovereign authority, including public health powers that are not limited to specific constitutional provisions. The states' police powers include the intrinsic right to pass laws and to take other measures necessary to protect the citizenry. In many instances, states have delegated their public health responsibilities to county or municipal governments, which likewise exercise the state's broad authority to examine, treat, and in the case of certain contagious diseases, even to quarantine citizens to protect the public health. The state's public health laws include not only the established statutes of the state but also regulations, executive orders, and other directives from health authorities that may have the force of law.

## State Police Powers and Public Health

The exercise of the states' police powers with respect to public health matters has limitations. The U.S. Constitution provides procedural safeguards to ensure the exercise of these powers is not excessive or unrestrained. The Fourth Amendment protects citizens from unlawful searches and seizures, and the Fifth Amendment prohibits the federal government from depriving any persons of life, liberty, or property without due process of law. The Fourteenth Amendment imposes similar due process obligations on states. Due process demands the government use even-handed and impartial procedures in exercising its police power. The basic elements of such due process include notice to the person involved, opportunity for a hearing or similar proceeding, and the right to representation by counsel. In addition, the exercise of the state's police power necessitates the principle of using the least restrictive alternative that would achieve the state's interest, particularly when the exercise involves limitations of the individual's personal liberty.

## MANDATORY REPORTING OF DISEASES AND CONDITIONS

Public health surveillance systems in the United States are established as an exercise of the states' police powers. These state-based systems are designed for reporting of diseases and conditions of public health interest by health-care professionals and laboratories. All states have laws and regulations that mandate the reporting of a list of diseases and conditions, as well as prescribing the timing and nature of information to be reported and the penalties for noncompliance with the reporting laws.[4] Required disease reporting varies greatly among states and territories. In some states, disease reporting is mandated by statutes that have not been reviewed by legislatures in decades. Other states have general statutes that empower the health commissioner or state boards of health to create, monitor, and revise the list of reportable diseases and conditions.[5] Some states require reports under both statutes and health department regulations.[6] Reporting may be required of a variety of professionals and organizational entities, including physicians and other health-care providers, diagnostic laboratories, clinical facilities, and schools and daycare centers.[7, 4, 8] Although state disease reporting generally is mandated by law or regulation, reporting of disease and death information by the state or territorial health department to CDC is voluntary.

The scope and nature of reporting requirements vary considerably by state; differing, for example, by the number of conditions required for reporting, time periods within which conditions must be reported, agencies to which reports must be submitted, and persons or sources required to report. Moreover, despite the legal requirements for reporting, adherence to and completeness of reporting also vary substantially by infectious disease agent, ranging from 6% to 90% for different common infectious conditions.[9] The deficiencies in reporting by physicians are accounted for, in part, by limitations in physicians' knowledge of reporting requirements and procedures, as well as the assumption that laboratories have reported cases of infectious diseases.[4, 10]

## CSTE's Role in Standardizing Reportable Diseases and Conditions

Since the early 1900s, PHS has attempted to collect disease information from all states about certain infectious diseases.[1, 11] Beginning in 1951, the Council of State and Territorial Epidemiologists (CSTE) was authorized by its parent body, the Association of State and Territorial Health Officials, to decide what diseases states should report to PHS and to recommend reporting procedures. CSTE meets annually and, in consultation with CDC, recommends additions and deletions to the list of diseases and conditions.

An assessment of state laws and regulations in 1989 highlighted an important impediment to the surveillance and control of infectious diseases—namely, variations in case definitions the states used for identifying and acting on reports of cases and the effect of lack of uniformity on limiting the ability to compare patterns of infectious disease occurrence between states. For example, some states required reporting of any person with a positive culture for *Salmonella*, whereas others required reporting of only culture-positive persons who were symptomatic.[4] To address these differences and to facilitate comparison of surveillance between states, CSTE and CDC developed and updated standardized case definitions for the nationally notifiable infectious diseases.[12] Implementation of uniform case definitions and related procedures was expected to provide for interstate reciprocal notification for cases of infectious disease when onset was in one state but the patient was hospitalized in or transferred to another state, and cases for which public health action (e.g., contact tracing) might be involved in different states. However, reporting requirements by state continue to differ: as of January 1999, of the 52 infectious conditions agreed on for national surveillance, only 19 were reportable in all states.[7]

In 1995 and 1996, CDC and CSTE expanded the list beyond the traditional collection of infectious diseases, recommending that elevated blood lead levels, silicosis, and acute pesticide poisoning be added.[7] The number of diseases and conditions on the list varies from year to year but is usually 65 to 75. The list of diseases and conditions under national surveillance is published each year in the annual summary of notifiable diseases in the CDC's *Morbidity and Mortality Weekly Report*. CSTE also keeps information about state disease and condition reporting requirements on its website, http://www.cste.org/NNDSSHome.htm.

## Enforcement of Reporting Laws

Even though few states choose to penalize physicians for not reporting notifiable conditions, disciplinary measures may be invoked in instances when failure to report has serious untoward effects. For example, the California Board of Medical Quality Assurance took action against a physician in that state for "gross negligence and incompetence, failure to report to local health authorities a suspected case of an infectious disease in a known food handler."[13] At that time, California law set forth legal responsibility of physicians, dentists, nurses, and others to notify local health authorities of persons ill with specified infectious diseases. In this instance, the physician had examined a patient he knew to be a food handler. Although the physician recognized the patient was jaundiced and possibly had hepatitis, he failed to report the patient's condition to local public health authorities. An outbreak of food-borne hepatitis followed in which at least 62 cases of hepatitis were associated with the food handler; one person died. In suspending the physician's license for one year (the suspension was stayed and the physician was placed on five years' probation), the California Board of Medical Quality Assurance declared that the "failure to report a suspected if not a known case of an infectious disease in a food handler was an extreme departure from the standard practice of medicine."[13] In the late 1980s, in Minnesota, a small proportion of physicians initially refused to report the identity of HIV-positive persons to the state health department as required, even though violation of any health department rule represented a misdemeanor.[14]

## EMERGING DEVELOPMENTS IN PUBLIC HEALTH SURVEILLANCE, INVESTIGATION, AND RESPONSE

Historically, public health surveillance was largely for infectious diseases and based on mandatory reporting of individual cases of disease. Increasingly, in the past decade, use of mandatory reporting as a surveillance method has been expanded through changes in state public health reporting statutes, regulations, or executive orders to include conditions and syndromes that fall outside more traditional infectious diseases. These especially include environmental and occupational health conditions, emerging infectious diseases, and diseases that may be due to bioterrorism.

In addition, through collaboration between the state epidemiologists and CDC, newer methods have been developed as a basis for state and national public health surveillance. These include use of the Behavioral Risk Factor Surveillance System to monitor prevalence of health risk behaviors such as tobacco smoking[15] and a variety of methods to monitor occupational disease, chronic conditions, and injuries. Methods range from telephone surveys (Behavioral Risk Factor Surveillance System) to the development and maintenance of cancer and birth defect registries to use of hospital discharge databases. Similar to updating the national list of notifiable infectious diseases and case definitions, a collaborative process exists to develop, define, and update a national list of chronic disease indicators.[16] CSTE maintains information on its website identifying indicators for chronic disease surveillance, including access to current data to assist public health practitioners assess indicators for their locales. In addition, publication of data on matters such as firearm-related injuries has significantly increased awareness of these public health issues, as well as the importance of surveillance to the consideration of law and policy interventions.

With the exceptions of tumor and birth defect registries, these newer surveillance methods do not use mandatory reporting and do not depend highly on state or federal law. They either use voluntary processes, such as willingness of the public to respond to a telephone survey, or employ existing databases from which individual identifier information usually is removed. However, their public health use is facilitated by the broad authority of state public health officials to obtain public health surveillance data.

## INTERPLAY OF FEDERAL AND STATE LAWS IN FIELD EPIDEMIOLOGY

### Legal Authorities of States in Epidemiologic Investigations

Similar to the public health activities discussed above, the states' inherent powers to protect the public's health provide the general authority for laws and regulations that empower health officials to conduct epidemiologic investigations.[17, 18] When an outbreak of disease or other event threatens public health, state or local public health authorities are responsible for investigating it because of their inherent police powers. In practice, institutions and individuals generally cooperate voluntarily in epidemiologic and outbreak investigations. However, if investigators meet with resistance, local or state public health officials can take legal actions, such as applying to a court with jurisdiction over the institution (or individual) for a subpoena or court order to compel the institution (or individual) to grant investigators access to the premises or records at issue. An individual can be compelled by court order to provide the information necessary to the public health investigation.

*Outbreaks* and *epidemics* are terms well known to the public, and problems for which the public expects aggressive responses. Regardless of the dimensions of any given outbreak, most health authorities employ a standard approach for investigating the problem. The elements of a typical outbreak investigation highlight many of the basic functional activities used more generally for the control and prevention of reportable conditions (see Chapter 5).

In addition to the legal authorities that both compel and enable health agencies to undertake such investigations, myriad related considerations exist regarding responsibilities and authorities for the individual elements of an investigation. Such considerations encompass the authorities necessary to obtain microbiological and other laboratory specimens from hospitals and private laboratories; review patients' medical records kept in the offices of physicians, dentists, and other health-care providers; administer questionnaires to and collect specimens from persons affected in the outbreak, as well as unaffected persons who may be important sources of information for solving the outbreak; retain information about medical histories and laboratory results; protect confidentiality; and implement a variety of measures intended to control the immediate problem and prevent recurrences. Such measures may include the ongoing collection of additional data, recall of an implicated product, closure of a business or restriction of activities relating to the source of an outbreak, isolation or other forms of restriction of activities of affected persons, quarantine of exposed persons, vaccination of or administration of antibiotics to exposed groups, and even compulsory treatment of some individuals or groups with antibiotics and other medications.

A measles outbreak in Iowa in 2004 illustrates several of the response and control measure options employed by state public health agencies, including some relying even more directly on specific legal instruments and procedures.[19] In that outbreak, in which large numbers of persons in an insular community with low vaccination rates were exposed to measles-infected patients, the public health response included voluntary isolation of the patients, as well as offering post-exposure vaccination prophylaxis to exposed community members who were deemed susceptible. In addition, when some of those who potentially had been exposed to measles first refused post-exposure prophylaxis and then were unwilling to comply with voluntary quarantine, those persons were served with state-issued involuntary home quarantine orders by the local public health nurse, in some instances with the assistance of local law enforcement officers.[20] The health department monitored compliance with quarantine orders through daily, unannounced home visits or telephone calls.

## Legal Authorities for Federal Intervention in Epidemiologic Investigations

By contrast to the broad state public health authorities, federal public health officials have limited statutory authorities to initiate independent epidemiologic investigations. For epidemiologists and public health officials employed by the federal government, the laws relating to the general powers and duties of PHS for research and investigation are found in Title III of the Public Health Service Act. The general statutory authority that applies to federal epidemiologic investigations is Section 301(a) of the Public Health Service Act, 42 U.S.C. Section 241(a):

> The Secretary shall conduct in the Service, and encourage, cooperate with, and render assistance to the other appropriate public authorities, scientific institutions, and scientists in the conduct of, and promote the coordination of, research, investigations, experiments, demonstrations, and studies relating to the causes, diagnosis, treatment, control, and prevention of physical and mental diseases and impairments of man.

In addition, subsection 6 of Section 301(a) indicates that the Secretary is authorized to "make available to health officials, scientists, and appropriate public health and other nonprofit institutions and organizations, technical advice and assistance on the application of statistical methods to experiments, studies, and surveys in health and medical fields." Although these provisions are broadly worded and are permissive rather than compulsory, they nonetheless give legal authority for intervention by federal epidemiologists in disease outbreaks and other instances in which such assistance is requested. In practice, local and state public health officials may request federal assistance in the epidemiologic or field investigation. Federal public health employees who collaborate with state and local public health authorities in such investigations generally are not exercising specific federal authority but rather are assisting the state or local investigation.

## LEGAL ISSUES RELATED TO DATA COLLECTION, ANALYSIS, AND DISSEMINATION

The processes of collecting data for public health surveillance, as part of an outbreak investigation or for other field epidemiology activities, may implicate numerous legal considerations, including (1) protection available under state or federal law during and after the investigation for records collected and generated in relation to the investigation; (2) privacy provisions for medical and other information; (3) required reporting of particular diseases or conditions; (4) status of information in investigative files under the federal Freedom of Information Act (FOIA) (5 U.S.C. §552) or state FOIA counterparts; and (5) the possible applicability of federal or state human-subjects research regulations, including the need for review of study protocols by institutional review boards and the need for informed consent for participation in the investigation or for procedures related to the investigation.

To determine what records will be kept or generated and where and how such records will be stored, federal, state, and local public health officials need to be familiar with legal protections applicable to documents and other records that will be examined, extracted, and compiled in association with the surveillance activity or outbreak investigation. Most states provide specific statutory and regulatory privacy protection over medical and public health records. In general, the privacy protection prevents disclosure of a name-identified record without the consent of the person on whom the record is maintained. Accordingly, state law generally protects such medical records in the hands of an investigator. Furthermore, such state laws frequently require that only certain authorized personnel have access to such private records and that such records be maintained in a secure manner. Public health investigators usually would be authorized access to such records for surveillance and related public health activities but would be bound to maintain the records in a manner that would protect the privacy of the identifiable information from unauthorized or inadvertent disclosure.

In the course of an outbreak investigation or surveillance activities, investigators may create or compile a variety of documents, including questionnaires, forms, investigative notes, copies or extractions of patient or other records, letters, reports, memoranda, drafts, manuscripts, and final reports. Depending on the nature of the records and the status of the investigation, these documents may not be protected from disclosure to the public by state or federal laws. Except for records afforded specific protection by state or federal laws (such as state laws protecting medical records), public health investigators should assume that all records collected may at some point be open to public scrutiny. This may include personal notes by the public health investigator, drafts of documents retained in the files, and other related information that is within the scope of the request.

## HEALTH INFORMATION PRIVACY IN EPIDEMIOLOGIC PRACTICE

An effective surveillance system includes both the capacity for data collection and the ability to disseminate the data to persons who can undertake prevention and control activities. The collection of vital records and other data for public health surveillance and during epidemic investigations may involve a variety of legal issues and considerations, which also are relevant to information gathering necessary for other basic disease-control activities (e.g., surveys, special studies, and categorical disease-control programs). Increasingly, surveillance is used for investigating the range of conditions affecting health; including, for example, injuries, chronic diseases, environmental exposures, and maternal and child health activities.[21] The underlying issues attendant to data collection in these situations are balancing the need for access to medical and other records against individuals' interests in privacy through the imposition of strict limits on access. These legal considerations, most of which are addressed by statutes or regulations, include protections available during and after investigations for records developed in relation to the investigation; special privacy provisions for medical and other information; and mandated reporting of specific infectious conditions, as noted above.

Protecting the privacy, confidentiality, and security of health data, whether in a research or public health activity, is fundamental to responsible data-sharing practices. Although often used interchangeably, the terms *privacy, confidentiality*, and *security* have distinct legal and ethical meanings with respect to identifiable health information.[22] *Health information privacy* broadly refers to the rights of individuals to control the acquisition, uses, or disclosures of their identifiable health data. The closely related concept of *confidentiality* refers to the obligations of those who receive information to respect the privacy interests of individuals who are the subjects of the data.

*Security* is different from confidentiality in that it refers to technological or administrative safeguards or tools to protect identifiable health data from unwarranted access or disclosure. Maintaining information security may become increasingly difficult in the modern area of digitized exchanges and large electronic health databases that can be hacked or infiltrated through unlawful invasions. However, electronic health systems also hold great promise for improving health care and public health efficiency as well as for protecting privacy and security.[23]

Varied privacy and security laws and policies for sharing health data reflect the fragmented nature of legal protections of health information privacy. Neither constitutional principles nor judicial decisions focused on common-law concepts of duties of confidentiality support an individual's broad expectation of health information privacy. Rather, federal and state statutes and regulations are the dominant basis for health information privacy protections in the United States.[22] An array of significant federal and state laws, discussed below, is intended to safeguard health information privacy.

## FEDERAL PUBLIC HEALTH INFORMATION PRIVACY LAWS

The federal **Privacy Act of 1974** applies whenever information is collected and maintained by a federal agency in a system of records in which the information is retrieved by an individual's name, identification number, or other identifier.[24]

The Privacy Act was the first national law to introduce fair information practices that allow individuals to access their own government-held information. A person also may seek amendments to information that is not accurate, relevant, or complete. Among other things, the Privacy Act protects individual privacy by (*1*) specifying the situations in which a person's health information may be disclosed without that person's consent, and requiring consent in other situations; (*2*) proscribing government maintenance of identifiable health information that is irrelevant and unnecessary to accomplish the agency's purposes; (*3*) requiring agencies to publish a notice about each record system describing its purpose and identifying disclosures outside the agency (e.g., "routine uses") that the agency has chosen administratively to make; and (*4*) requiring agencies to inform individuals of the statutory basis for collecting health information, purposes for which it is used, and consequences for not supplying the information.

The **Freedom of Information Act (FOIA)** of 1988 provides that agency records created or maintained by an agency and under its control are available to the public unless specifically exempted from disclosure.[25] The Act contains nine exemptions, several of which help protect the privacy of some public health data, including the following:

*Interagency and intra-agency communications.* Exemption (b)(5) permits the federal government to withhold from disclosure interagency and intra-agency memoranda or letters that would not be available "to a party other than an agency in litigation with the agency." This exemption may be used by the agency data holder, for example, to protect from disclosure a draft memorandum written by the investigator to his or her supervisor describing the early findings of an epidemiologic investigation.

*Personnel and medical records.* Exemption (b)(6) permits an agency data holder to withhold from mandatory disclosure "personnel and medical files and similar files the disclosure of which would constitute a clearly unwarranted invasion of personal privacy." This exemption may be invoked to protect confidential medical information about a person contained in an agency record.

*Information otherwise exempt from disclosure by statute.* Exemption (b)(3) provides that a federal agency may withhold from disclosure information "specifically exempted from disclosure by statute." For example, if a federal epidemiologic investigation is conducted under an assurance of confidentiality authorized by a federal statute (discussed below) the information collected pursuant to the confidentiality assurance may be exempted from disclosure under FOIA.

Additional privacy protections for research and other health data are found in the **Public Health Service Act (PHSA)**.[26] Sections 308(d) and 924(c) of the

PHSA provide strong protection for identifiable information collected respectively by CDC's National Center for Health Statistics and the U.S. Department of Health and Human Services' (DHHS) Agency for Healthcare Research and Quality.[27] Assurances of confidentiality under Section 308(d) can be used to protect individuals and institutions providing information. Section 308(d) provides that: "No [identifiable] information ... may be used for any purpose other than the purpose for which it was supplied unless such establishment or person has consented...."

Certificates of confidentiality, available to researchers within or outside government, are authorized under PHSA Section 301(d).[28] DHHS can grant these certificates to protect research participants from legally compelled disclosures of identifiable health information. Section 301(d) provides that health researchers may "protect the privacy of [research participants] by withholding from all persons not connected with the conduct of such research the names or other identifying characteristics of such [participants]." Researchers generally seek this confidentiality protection only when the health information collected is so sensitive (e.g., related to sexual practices or illegal conduct) that research subjects probably either would not participate or would provide inaccurate or incomplete responses without such protections.

Before the U.S. Department of Health and Human Services introduced the **Privacy Rule** promulgated pursuant to the Health Insurance Portability and Accountability Act (HIPAA) of 2000,[29] no comprehensive federal information privacy law existed. Rather, federal privacy laws generally applied to certain types of health information collected, maintained, or funded by the federal government through its specific agencies (e.g., Centers for Medicare and Medicaid Services, National Institutes of Health, and CDC). The HIPAA Privacy Rule was intended to give patients more control over their health information, set boundaries on use and release of health records, and establish safeguards that health care providers and others must achieve to protect the privacy of health information. The Rule holds violators accountable for improper disclosures of private patient information, but allows disclosure of certain data in patient records for public health purposes.

Specific provisions of the **E-Government Act of 2002** protect the confidentiality of federal government statistical collections of identifiable information, including health information.[30] The act restricts the use of information gathered for statistical uses to the purposes for which it is gathered and penalizes unauthorized disclosures. It also requires federal agencies to conduct "privacy assessments" before developing or procuring information technology that collects, maintains, or disseminates identifiable information.

Whereas the Privacy Act, FOIA, and E-Government Act apply to all federal agencies, other federal privacy laws and regulations relate to particular government programs or agencies. For example, a federal statute protects the privacy of health information generated in federally assisted, specialized substance-abuse facilities.

## State and Local Public Health Information Privacy Laws

Although many states have statutory laws similar to the federal Privacy Act and FOIA, and a few (e.g., California, Rhode Island, Maryland, Montana, and Washington) have passed additional privacy protections, most do not have comprehensive statutes regulating the acquisition, use, and disclosure of individual health data.[22] Rather, state privacy laws tend to regulate specific data recipients (e.g., public health agencies, health insurers); certain medical tests, diseases, or conditions (e.g., genetic tests, HIV status, mental disorders); or particular data sources (e.g., nursing or health-care facilities).

Significant additional privacy protections of public health data are featured in the **Model State Public Health Information Privacy Act of 1999**, and more recently, the **Turning Point Model State Public Health Act of 2003**.[31, 32] Both acts introduce modern privacy language to protect the privacy and security of identifiable health data acquired, used, disclosed, or stored by state public health agencies while preserving the ability of state and local health departments to use health data responsibly for the common good.

A significant development in the national protection of the privacy of medical information came in December 2000 with DHHS's publication of its **"Standards for Privacy of Individually Identifiable Health Information"** pursuant to HIPAA,[29] commonly referred to as the **Privacy Rule**. These regulations provide the first national standards for the protection of identifiable health information as applied to three types of covered entities: health, health-care clearinghouses, and health-care providers who conduct certain health-care transactions electronically.[33, 34] Although the Common Rule (see below) sets a national floor of privacy protections for many exchanges of identifiable health data, it does not preempt more stringent state and local privacy laws.[22] The Privacy Rule took effect on April 14, 2001, with compliance required for most covered entities by April 14, 2003 (and small health plans by April 14, 2004).[35]

In general, the Privacy Rule establishes standards for covered entities to use and disclose "protected health information" (PHI), which includes individually identifiable health information.[36] A covered entity may use or disclose PHI only as required or permitted by the Privacy Rule. It requires disclosures (without written authorization) in only two instances: to the individual and to DHHS for compliance investigations, reviews, or enforcement actions.

## LEGAL PROTECTIONS OF HUMAN SUBJECTS IN RESEARCH

As discussed above, substantial public health research activities involve the acquisition or use of identifiable health data. Unlike the constitutional norms that underlie public health data collections and corresponding privacy expectations, identifiable data for public health research are acquired under different legal and ethical structures.[37] In contrast to epidemiology and other public health activities, research is not always tied to grants of legislative authority and could operate unchecked absent legal protections. Unlike public health practitioners, public health researchers must adhere to regulations including advance written and informed consent of subjects (and sometimes their communities) that are codified in a series of federal regulations known collectively as the **Common Rule** (1993).[38] The Common Rule applies to virtually all research involving human subjects and federal funding. For most activities determined to be human-subjects research, the Common Rule requires a prospective review by an Institutional Review Board (IRB) or medical ethics board in compliance with various specifications.[39] IRBs review research proposals to assess the extent to which research subjects are protected during the course and aftermath of the research activities. The Common Rule requirements for IRB review are triggered only when an institution seeks federal funding to engage in human-subjects research or when it applies to the same requirements in reviewing all its human-subjects research pursuant to a multi-project or federal-wide assurance.

## FUNCTIONS AND RESPONSIBILITIES OF INSTITUTIONAL REVIEW BOARDS

As noted, the Common Rule vests authority within the IRBs to approve, disapprove, or require modifications of all federally funded human-subjects research. An IRB must approve human-subjects research before an investigator contacts human participants unless such research is specifically exempt by the regulations. In some state or local public health agencies, if uncertainty exists regarding whether an activity is research or practice, or whether it is exempt from the Common Rule, the IRBs may be asked to make the determination.

All IRBs comprise at least five members with diverse backgrounds, at least one of whom is a nonscientist and another of whom is not otherwise affiliated with the IRB's institution. IRBs review research proposals to assess the extent to which research subjects are protected during the course and aftermath of the research activities. They have a range of authority to approve research, require modifications to a research protocol, or disapprove of the proposed research entirely. Among other things, IRBs must examine whether:

- Individual or guardian consent for data collection appropriately meets all of the Common Rule requirements[40]
- The privacy of individuals and confidentiality of their identifiable information are protected[41]

- The research design is sound, safe, and effective[42]
- Research subjects are equitably selected[43]
- Data safety is appropriately monitored [44]
- Vulnerable populations (e.g., children, prisoners, mentally disabled persons) are protected[45]

Although IRBs must review active protocols at least annually, some of these protocols may be eligible for expedited review if the protocol previously was approved by the fully convened IRB. While the process of obtaining and confirming IRB approval may be time-consuming for investigators, it is grounded in the need to ensure adequate protection of participants.

## TERRORISM-RELATED SURVEILLANCE AND INVESTIGATION

Terrorism-related concerns have led to efforts to examine the adequacy of disease reporting laws and disease-specific surveillance to meet the challenge of detecting acts of bioterrorism as rapidly as possible, to minimize their health, social, and psychological consequences. In 2002, CDC reported on an examination of disease-reporting laws of 54 jurisdictions, including all 50 states, to determine how many had laws mandating the reporting of diseases caused by "critical biological agents"[46]—agents designated by CDC as having the potential for use in a bio-terrorist weapon. The study showed that particular deficiencies existed for the immediate reporting of diseases associated with Category A agents (i.e., anthrax, botulism, viral hemorrhagic fevers, plague, smallpox, and tularemia). Although anthrax, botulism, and plague were immediately reportable in most jurisdictions, tularemia was immediately reportable in fewer than half of the jurisdictions. The findings underscored the need for states and other jurisdictions to review existing disease-reporting laws to determine whether they include the most critical biological agents associated with bioterrorism,[46] an activity that has become a requirement of federal public health preparedness funding.[47]

To speed up reporting of some diseases and laboratory findings, use of electronic data captured from laboratories (electronic laboratory reporting) and Web-based clinical facility and provider reporting increasingly are replacing paper and mail-based reporting.[48–50] In some states, disease reporting regulations have been modified to provide a legal basis for such electronic reporting.[51]

In addition, syndromic surveillance—use of real-time data from existing systems that record events such as emergency department visits, 911 calls, and pharmacy purchases—is being explored at both the state and national levels to detect unusual disease activity up to several days before reporting of any specific diagnostic information by providers and to help monitor the scope and duration of outbreaks, including those detected by other means[52–54] (see Chapter 22). Although participation in these systems by health-care facilities and providers has been mostly voluntary, questions have been raised regarding whether state and local jurisdictions have the legal authority to obtain personal identifying information when necessary to investigate increases in any given syndrome.[55, 56] An analysis of statutes and regulations in New York City and New York State led to the conclusion that New York City had ample authority for its syndromic surveillance activities.[55] At least three states (Iowa, Nevada, and Arizona) have passed explicit statutory language authorizing syndromic surveillance.[57–59]

The anthrax attacks of 2001 and increased recognition of the potential for criminal behavior and other deliberate actions to cause disease outbreaks have crystallized the concept of "forensic epidemiology." Forensic epidemiology has been characterized as "the use of epidemiologic methods as part of an ongoing investigation of a health problem for which there is suspicion or evidence regarding possible intentional acts or criminal behavior as factors contributing to the health problem."[60] The operational challenges during joint public health and law enforcement investigations of such problems implicate several relatively new legal issues that, in turn, have stimulated development of new legal frameworks for interdisciplinary collaboration, such as the "agreement regarding joint field investigations following a suspected bioterrorist incident" entered into by the City of New York Department of Mental Health and Hygiene, the City of New York Police Department, and the Federal Bureau of Investigation field office in New York City.[61]

## STATE AND FEDERAL COOPERATION IN EMERGENCY RESPONSES

Beginning in 1999, federal government initiatives designed to improve national public health capabilities to respond to acts of terrorism raised questions about the adequacy of state quarantine, isolation, and other compulsory public health powers. Preliminary review of state quarantine, isolation, and other critical agent laws conducted informally by CDC in 2000 showed that most of these laws had not been revised since the 1940s—probably because voluntary cooperation of the public and advances in medical interventions used compulsory actions less frequently. However, in the context of public health threats related to potential bioterrorism events, the infrequent use of such actions also presented the possibility that public health officials were inexperienced or unfamiliar with the proper procedures for invoking the compulsory powers. Accordingly, CDC and other federal officials involved in terrorism preparedness have suggested that states examine public health laws—including quarantine and isolation powers—that affect their abilities to effectively respond to potential chemical and biological threats. Such assessments can help ensure that the laws enable public health officials to act promptly while providing adequate due process protections for individuals who may be detained as part of a terrorism response. In addition, terrorism initiatives increasingly focus on the need for advance coordination, planning, pharmaceutical stockpiling, and training that involves public health officials and officials from various law-enforcement, emergency-response, and other civilian agencies, as well as military intelligence experts.

The events following the September 11, 2001, attacks in New York City and Northern Virginia illustrate both the strengths of and challenges to traditional concepts of primary state and local responsibility for public health investigations. The catastrophic nature of the events rapidly taxed the ability of local and state public health officials to respond to the needs for surveillance of hospital and emergency department admissions, injuries, hospital-based syndromic surveillance,[52] and various environmental monitoring activities. Resources from CDC and other public health agencies had to be deployed to help gather this important surveillance information. Yet, the legal authority and oversight for most of these public health activities remained with local and state public health officials. The consistency in training, advance planning, and prior collaborative relationships between state, municipal, and local public health practitioners made possible an effective response during this emergency situation. In the aftermath of the events of September 11 and the anthrax attack in the United States, a draft model law (The Model State Emergency Health Powers Act) was created and made available for public review and use to strengthen preparedness.

You should understand that the basic authority of public health officials to conduct investigations of diseases or epidemics is the state's inherent police powers. Federal and state laws that govern the health and safety of the public are enacted pursuant to this broad authority. These laws provide, not only for the state to have access to medical and other records for purposes of public health investigations, but also for protection of the individual's interest in privacy by placing strict limits on access to medical, hospital, and public health records. While public health investigations and activities usually rely on the voluntary cooperation of individuals and institutions, federal and state laws provide authority for the use of compulsory measures when necessary for the protection of the public health and safety.

You are certainly not expected to know every facet of public health law. Yet you should have an appreciation of the legal issues that pertain to surveillance, to privacy of medical records, and to the legal responsibilities of both federal and state governments. The quality, quantity, and ease of collecting epidemiologic data can be enhanced materially by an awareness of these issues, and, if necessary, consultation with the legal profession.

ACKNOWLEDGMENT   We acknowledge David W. Fleming, whose work on a corollary chapter, "Frontline Public Health: Surveillance and Outbreak Investigations," in *Law in Public Health Practice* (New York: Oxford University Press, 2003, pp.143–59) contributed in part to this chapter.

## REFERENCES

1. CDC. Summary of notifiable diseases, United States, 2003. *Morb Mortal Wkly Rep* 2005;52:2–3.
2. CDC (2002). Surveillance for certain health behaviors among selected local areas—United States, Behavioral Risk Factor Surveillance System. *Morb Mortal Wkly Rep* 53 (SS05), 2–3.
3. Ries, L.A.G., Eisner, M.P., Kosary, C.L., et al. (eds.) (2004). *SEER Cancer Statistics Review, 1975–2001*. National Cancer Institute, Bethesda, Md. Available at http://seer. cancer.gov/csr/1975_2001. Accessed November 16, 2005.
4. Chorba, T.L., Berkelman, R.L., Safford, S.K., et al. (1989). The reportable diseases: I. Mandatory reporting of infectious diseases by clinicians. *JAMA* 262, 3018–26.
5. Gen Stat of Conn (revised to January 1, 2005), §19a-2a, Powers and duties, Volume 6, 787.
6. Public Health Code (revised through Sept. 21, 2004). Reportable Diseases and Laboratory Findings, §19a-36-A7, Diseases not enumerated, p. 529. Available at http://www.dph.state.ct.us/phc/phc.doc. Accessed November 16, 2005.
7. Rousch, S., Birkhead, G.S., Koo, D., (1999). Mandatory reporting of diseases and conditions by health care professionals and laboratorians. *JAMA* 282, 164–70.
8. Thacker, S.B. Surveillance. In: M.B. Gregg, R.C. Dicker, R.A. Goodman (eds.) (1996). *Field Epidemiology*, New York, Oxford University Press, pp. 16–32.
9. Thacker, S.B., Berkelman, R.L. (1988). Public health surveillance in the United States. *Epidemiol Rev* 10, 164–90.
10. Konowitz, P.M., Petrossian, G.A., Rose, D.N. (1984). The underreporting of disease and physicians' knowledge of reporting requirements. *Public Health Rep* 99, 31–5.
11. Thacker, S.B. Historical development. In: S.M. Teutsch, R.E. Churchill (eds.) (2000). *Principles and Practice of Public Health Surveillance*, 2nd ed., New York, Oxford University Press. pp. 1–16.
12. CDC (1997). Case definitions for infectious conditions under public health surveillance. *Morb Mortal Wkly Rep* 46(RR10), 1–64.
13. California Department of Health Services. Disciplinary action by Board of Medical Quality Assurance for failure to report a reportable infectious disease. *California Morbidity* 1978 (August 11).
14. Fidler, D.P., Heymann, D.L., Ostroff, S.M., et al. (1997). Emerging and reemerging infectious diseases: challenges for international, national, and state law. *International Lawyer* 31, 773–99.
15. CDC (1996). Addition of prevalence of cigarette smoking as a nationally notifiable condition—June 1996. *Morb Mortal Wkly Rep* 45, 537.
16. CDC (2004). Indicators for chronic disease surveillance. *Morb Mortal Wkly Rep* 53 (no RR11), 1–8.
17. Iowa Code, Title 4, Subtitle 2, Ch 139, §139A.3A (2005).
18. Conn Public Health Code §19a-36-A6 (2005).

19. CDC (2004). Postexposure prophylaxis, isolation, and quarantine to control an import-associated measles outbreak—Iowa, 2004. *Morb Mortal Wkly Rep* 53, 969–71.

20. Examples of Iowa's quarantine orders are available at http://ww.idph.state.ia.us/adper/cade.asp; see also Iowa Code §135.144 (2003 Suppl.), 139A.4, 139A.9, and 641 Iowa Administrative Code, Ch 1.

21. Birkhead, G.S., Maylahn, C.M. (2000). State and local public health surveillance In: S.M. Teutsch, R.E. Churchill (eds.), *Principles and Practice of Public Health Surveillance*, 2nd ed., New York, Oxford University Press. pp. 253–9.

22. Hodge, J.G., Jr. (2004). Health information privacy and public health. *J Law Med Ethics* 31:4, 663–71.

23. Hodge, J.G., Jr., Gostin, L.O., Jacobson, P. (1999). Legal issues concerning electronic health information. *JAMA* 282, 1466–71.

24. 5 USC 552(a) (1988).

25. 5 USC 552 (1988).

26. 42 USC 301, *et seq.*

27. 42 USCA 242m(d) and 299c-3 (2001).

28. 42 USCA 242m(d) (1997).

29. Pub L 104–191, 110 Stat 1936 (1996).

30. Pub L 107–347 (2002).

31. Gostin, L.O., Hodge, J.G., Jr. (1998). The "names" debate: the case for national HIV reporting in the United States. *Albany Law Rev* 61, 679–743.

32. Gostin, L.O., Lazzarini, Z., Neslund, V.S., Osterholm, M.T. (1996). The public health information infrastructure: a national review of the law on health information privacy. *JAMA* 275, 1921–7.

33. CDC (2003). HIPAA Privacy Rule and public health: guidance from the Centers for Disease Control and the Department of Health and Human Services. *Morb Mortal Wkly Rep* 52 (supp), 1–20.

34. 45 CFR 164.502(a)(2) (2003).

35. Gostin, L.O., Hodge, J.G., Jr. (2002). Personal privacy and common goods: a framework for balancing under the National Health Information Privacy Rule. *Minn Law Rev* 86, 1439–80.

36. DHHS, OCR Privacy Brief. *Summary of the HIPAA Privacy Rule: HIPAA Compliance Assistance*, 2003. Available at http://www.HHS.gov/ocr/privacy summary. Accessed September 12, 2005.

37. Hodge, J.G., Jr., Gostin, L.O. (2004). CSTE Advisory Committee. *Public Health Practice vs Research: A Report for Public Health Practitioners Including Case Studies and Guidance*. May 17, 2004. Available at http://www.cste.org/pdffiles/newpdfiles/CSTEPHResRpt HodgeFinal.5.24.04pdf. Accessed July 10, 2005.

38. 46 CFR 46 *et seq.* (1993).

39. 45 CFR 46.103 (1991).

40. 45 CFR 46.111(a)(4)-(5) (1991).

41. 45 CFR 46.111(a)(7) (1991).

42. 45 CFR 46.111(a)(1)-(2) (1991).

43. 45 CFR 46.111(a)(3) (1991).

44. 45 CFR 46.109(e) (1991); 45 CFR 46.111(a)(6) (1991)

45. 45 CFR 46.111(b) (1991); 45 CFR 46.201 (1991); 45 CFR 46.301 (1991) 45 CFR 46.401 (1991).

46. Horton, H., Misrahi, J.J., Matthews, G.W. et al. (2002). Critical biological agents: disease reporting as a tool for bioterrorism preparedness. *J Law Med Ethics* 30, 262–6.

47. CDC (2004). *Continuation Guidance—Budget Year 5. Attachment B. Focus B: Surveillance and Epidemiology Capacity.* June 14, 2004:1–8. Available at http://www. bt.cdc.gov/planning/continuationguidance/pdf/epidemiology_capacity_attachb.pdf. Accessed September 4, 2005.

48. Effler, P., Ching-Lee, M., Bogard, A., et al. (1999). Statewide system of electronic notifiable disease reporting from clinical laboratories. *JAMA* 282, 1845–50.

49. Backer, H.D., Bissel, S.R., Vugia, D.J. (2001). Disease reporting from automated laboratory-based reporting system to a state health department via local health departments. *Public Health Rep* 116, 257–65.

50. Jernigan, D.B. (2001). Electronic laboratory-based reporting: opportunities and challenges for surveillance. *Emerg Infect Dis* 7(3 Suppl), 538.

51. See, for example, 33 Pennsylvania Bulletin (Pa.B.) 2439 (effective Nov. 16, 2003) (under authority of 28 Pa.Code §27.4); 6 Code of Colorado Regulations (CCR) 1009–1, Reporting of Selected Cases of Morbidity and Mortality (effective September 30, 2004); Administrative Rules of South Dakota (ARDS) 44:20:02:06 (under authority of SDCL 34–22–9) (effective Dec. 7, 2003); Washington Administrative Code (WAC) 246–101–110(2) (effective Dec. 2004).

52. Henning, K. (2004). What is syndromic surveillance? *Morb Mortal Wkly Rep* 53(Suppl), 7–11.

53. CDC (2004). Framework for evaluating public health surveillance systems for early detection of outbreaks: recommendations from the CDC working group. *Morb Mortal Wkly Rep* 53(RR5), 2–3.

54. Loonsk, J. (2004). Biosense—a national initiative for early detection and quantification of public health emergencies. *Morb Mortal Wkly Rep* 53(Suppl), 53–5.

55. Lopez, W. (2003). New York City and state legal authorities related to syndromic surveillance. *J Urban Health* 80(2Suppl 1), i23–4.

56. Drociuk, D., Gibson, J., Hodge, J.G., Jr. (2004). Health information privacy and syndromic surveillance systems. *Morb Mortal Wkly Rep* 53(Suppl), 221–5.

57. Iowa Code, Title 4, Subtitle 2, Ch 139, §139A.3A (2005).

58. Nev Rev Stat, Ch 441A, §441 A.125 (2003).

59. Ariz Rev Stat, Title 36, §36–782 (2005).

60. Goodman, R.A., Munson, J.W., Dammers, K., et al. (2003a). Forensic epidemiology: law at the intersection of public health and criminal investigations. *J Law Med Ethics* 31, 684–700.

61. CDC, Public Health Law Program (2005). Agreement regarding joint field investigations following a suspected bioterrorist incident. Available at http://www2a.cdc.gov/ phlp/docs/Investigations.pdf. Accessed November 16, 2005.

# 15

## IMMUNIZATION PRACTICES FOR THE FIELD EPIDEMIOLOGIST

Harry F. Hull

Immunization is the most cost-effective public health prevention measure available. Effective immunization programs have essentially eliminated diphtheria, *H. influenzae* meningitis, measles, polio, rubella, and other diseases from the United States. These were once leading causes of death in young children as well as important causes of mental disability, blindness, deafness, lameness, and congenital heart defects. Still, some vaccine-preventable diseases continue to be transmitted at low levels. Others remain common elsewhere and can be imported into this country. Excellent field epidemiology is essential if immunization programs are to meet the challenges of controlling vaccine-preventable diseases in today's low-incidence environment.

## VACCINATION

While the terms *vaccination* and *immunization* are often used interchangeably, they have quite different meanings. Vaccination originally was the administration of the original smallpox vaccine containing vaccinia, the cowpox virus. The term now refers to the administration of any vaccine. *Immunization* means to activate the immune system against a disease by artificial means. *Immunization* is the preferred term in public health use. The term *vaccine-preventable diseases* (VPDs) refers to a subset of diseases for which a vaccine exists, which vaccine is routinely given to a high proportion of the population.

Vaccines are suspensions of modified live microorganisms, killed microorganisms, or processed or purified fragments of microorganisms. Toxoids—inactivated bacterial toxins—are not vaccines, but are immunizing agents often referred to as "vaccines" for convenience. Vaccines induce cell-mediated and humoral immunity to provide permanent or long-term protection against disease. Active immunization through vaccination is distinguished from passive immunization—administration of antibodies, typically in immune globulin, to provide temporary protection against disease.

Vaccinated persons are protected directly from disease by the response of their immune system to the vaccine. Many vaccines are more than 95% effective in reducing the risk of illness. Both vaccinated and unvaccinated persons are also protected indirectly from disease through herd immunity, the reduced chance that they will be exposed to microorganisms that cause disease. Simply put, most immune persons do not contract the disease and, hence, do not spread it on to others. Even if immunized persons do become ill, they often have milder symptoms and lower levels of pathogens in their secretions, a combination that reduces their potential to transmit. Immunization may also decrease carriage of microorganisms among healthy persons. An excellent example of herd immunity is the reduction in pneumococcal disease that occurred among unimmunized black infants[1] and the elderly[2] following the recent introduction of the 7-valent conjugated pneumococcal vaccine for infants.

## IMMUNIZATION PROGRAMS

The starting point for any epidemiologist in the field of vaccine-preventable diseases is to gain an understanding of immunization programs and how they are managed. You will find that every state's immunization program is unique. Even within a single state, local immunization programs may differ in their capacity or strategies for delivering vaccines. In the United States, most immunizations are administered in the private sector, paid for by private health insurance. The federal Vaccines for Children program buys vaccine for indigent children and Native American children. However, there are significant numbers of under-insured or uninsured children whose parents must either pay part or the full cost of having their children vaccinated. The Medicare program pays for most immunizations for adults aged 65 and older. Immunization of adults between 18 and 64 years of age is generally paid for either by health insurance or by individuals. Employers pay for immunization of workers in high-risk occupations. This patchwork payment system yields subpopulations that are un- or under-immunized and susceptible to disease.[3, 4]

## Immunization Schedules

Each state has a recommended immunization schedule. Most follow the harmonized immunization schedule of the U.S. Public Health Service's Advisory Committee on Immunization Practices (ACIP), the American Academy of Pediatrics, and the American Academy of Family Physicians. These recommended immunization schedules are based on a combination of science and feasibility.[5] Recommending bodies consider available data on the safety and effectiveness of vaccines as well as the epidemiology of disease and the economics of immunizing large populations. The age for immunization is critical, as immune response varies by age. Maternal antibodies passed to the fetus through the placenta may interfere with the immune response of infants. Infants and young children have immature immune systems that do not mount an adequate response to some vaccines. Older adults and persons with health conditions that affect the immune system may also have a suboptimal response to vaccination. Immunizations may be targeted to specific subpopulations, as the risk of complications varies with age and is increased by specific health conditions. People in certain occupations, particularly health professionals, may be at higher risk of contracting an infection. Duration of protection must be assessed to determine if and when additional doses are required to boost waning immunity. An important additional consideration is how a vaccine would fit into the current schedule, which already requires multiple visits, particularly in the first two years of life. New vaccines are merged into the existing schedule whenever possible because additional provider visits would decrease compliance and increase cost.

You will need to familiarize yourself with both the recommended and required immunization schedules in your state. Some study will be necessary because of the large number of vaccines included. All states have laws requiring that children be vaccinated against a list of specific diseases before they can attend school, be enrolled in day care, or, in some states, attend college. Children who are not vaccinated can be excluded from school or day care. These laws vary considerably from state to state, not only in the vaccines required, but also the conditions under which unvaccinated children may attend school. Some states permit only medical exemptions, others permit religious and/or philosophical exemptions to vaccination. Depending on the state, vaccination requirements are established either by an act of the legislature or by an administrative hearing process. Because both routes are cumbersome, several years may pass before a new vaccine is mandated. Requirements may also be influenced by the state resources available to support immunization programs as well as the philosophy of state governments.

## Immunization Records

Accurate records of a child's vaccination history are an essential component of every immunization program. Providers need to know which vaccines a child has already received to determine what vaccines are needed and avoid duplication of doses already administered. Schools, day care centers, and colleges need proof of vaccination to comply with immunization laws. Immunization programs use immunization records to measure how effectively children within their jurisdiction are being immunized, for planning and resource allocation. Immunization histories are also needed for children enrolled in the Women, Infants, and Children nutrition program and may be required for children to attend camp or participate in athletic programs. An accurate immunization history will contain the exact dates for each vaccination, the type of vaccine, and the lot number for each vaccination. This will ensure that the correct vaccines have been given at the recommended ages, and that sufficient time has elapsed between doses to achieve optimal immune response.

Although parental recall has been used to assess a child's immunization status, memory is often unreliable, particularly with today's complex schedules. A parental report that a child is "up to date" or "has all the shots they are supposed to" is not acceptable evidence of immunity. Immunizations are typically recorded on an immunization card held by a parent, but these records may be incomplete because the card was forgotten at the time of a clinic visit or lost. Federal law requires immunization providers to maintain records for every vaccination administered. Provider records are the standard for assessing immunization history, but may also be incomplete, particularly when a child has been treated by multiple providers. Many states have computerized immunization registries to provide accurate, complete, and permanent records to meet the needs of the multiple users of immunization data. An expanding number of states are able to share data with other registries so that records are available when families move or receive medical care in another state.[5]

## Immunization Coverage

Immunization programs may call upon the field epidemiologist to help assess immunization coverage—the percentage of the target populations that has received a specific vaccine. Since many vaccines are administered in the first 18 months of life, surveys of two-year-olds are most often used to provide an assessment of current program performance. For example, the National Immunization Survey is a telephone survey collecting the immunization history of randomly selected 19- to 35-month-old children. Parents are interviewed, and immunization histories validated in provider records.[6] Kindergarten-entry surveys use immunization histories to assess compliance with school entry requirements. They can also be used to assess the timeliness with which children are immunized prior to school entry.[7] CDC's national Behavioral Risk Factor Surveillance System, a random-digit-dialing telephone interview, is used for coverage data on adult immunizations.[8] Medicare claims data have also been used to assess annual influenza vaccination coverage in the elderly.

In the current high-coverage environment, a specific challenge that can be undertaken by you, as a field epidemiologist, is to define the demographic characteristics of under-immunized children in your jurisdiction and the reasons for their not being immunized. Your findings may be used to design outreach programs for immunizing these hardest-to-reach children.

## ROUTINE SURVEILLANCE

A key role for field epidemiologists interested in vaccine-preventable disease (VPD) control is routine surveillance. The principles of routine surveillance are discussed in Chapter 3. The goals of VPD surveillance are to provide data for evaluation of local and national immunization programs, as well as to detect outbreaks early to facilitate control efforts. In our low-incidence environment, a single case of certain vaccine-preventable diseases (e.g. polio, smallpox) constitutes a public health emergency. A challenge for VPD surveillance is that diseases that were once common are now so rare that physicians may not recognize the illness. Diagnosis may be difficult when the clinical presentation is atypical or the course of illness has been modified by prior vaccination. Family practitioners, internists, and OB/Gyn specialists need to be made aware of the changing epidemiology (see below) and the clinical presentations of illness in adults. You should encourage clinicians to have a high index of suspicion and to collect specimens for laboratory confirmation.

### Changing Epidemiology of Disease

Many VPDs were once considered childhood illnesses—a normal part of growing up. They were so infectious that virtually all children had contracted them before they completed primary school. Immunization has altered the epidemiology so that most children born in the United States are fully protected against these diseases before 18 months of age. The net effect is that vaccine-preventable diseases now appear in selected populations. A high percentage of cases are older adolescents and adults. For some diseases (e.g. pertussis), this shift in age has occurred because vaccine-induced immunity is no longer sufficient to prevent infection in these older age groups. This phenomenon occurs when vaccine-induced immunity wanes over time and is no longer boosted naturally through repeated exposure to disease. Another factor contributing to the age shift is that some age cohorts were incompletely vaccinated when a vaccine was first introduced. Because disease incidence fell rapidly, some unimmunized children grew up without contracting the illness and, hence, remain susceptible to infection. A third factor is changing immunization schedules. When it was recognized that there were unacceptably high rates of primary vaccine failure for measles and varicella vaccines, a second dose was added to the schedule. Many children did not receive a "catch-up" second dose, leaving a now-older cohort with suboptimal protection from a single immunization.[10] The occurrence of disease in adults and immunized persons presents the additional challenges. The clinical presentation of disease in adults may differ from that in children. For example, adolescents and adults with pertussis may have only a chronic cough without the characteristic whoop. Physicians may not consider the possibility of a "childhood illness" occurring in an adult. Disease in partially immune persons may also be milder than in unvaccinated persons. Vaccinated varicella cases have fewer lesions, for example. Both of these factors will hamper correct diagnosis and decrease the likelihood that cases will be recognized and reported.

Another change in the epidemiology of vaccine-preventable diseases is the contribution of imported disease. Strains endemic to the U.S. may have been eliminated, but vaccine-preventable diseases remain common elsewhere. Imported cases may occur in persons exposed outside the country, and these cases may result in sustained transmission here. Disease may be imported by visitors from other countries or Americans exposed to disease during their international travels. Persons traveling while ill can expose other passengers and initiate simultaneous chains of transmission in multiple locales. Immigrant populations can have significant numbers of non-immune individuals and may sustain transmission. Outbreaks involving undocumented populations may be particularly difficult to investigate and control.[11]

Among American children, under-vaccination and risk of disease cluster in two populations. One population has mothers of low economic and educational status, often single with multiple children in the household.[12] These families do not have the resources to devote the necessary time, money, and effort to get their children vaccinated on time. While such children are underimmunized in their preschool years, most are fully immunized at school entry. The other population has parents, often highly educated, who choose to not immunize their children because of fear of adverse reactions, a preference for more "natural" approaches to health care, or religious reasons. Many of these children are completely unvaccinated. These children are found at higher rates in states that permit philosophical exemptions to immunization. Unvaccinated children are often clustered socially, creating fertile ground for outbreaks.

## OUTBREAK INVESTIGATION AND CONTROL

Most outbreaks of vaccine-preventable disease involve person-to-person transmission. Respiratory spread predominates for the "childhood" illnesses, with true airborne spread occurring in some outbreaks. Fomites—shared drinking vessels or cigarettes, for example—may be implicated in meningococcal disease. Bloodborne spread and perinatal transmission may occur with hepatitis B. Hepatitis A may involve transmission through food, water, or sexual contact in addition to spreading among household contacts. Incubation periods for VPDs range from several days to several weeks, but may also extend to several months. Person-to-person transmission combined with longer incubation periods has the potential to produce outbreaks of long duration with multiple generations. Once an outbreak investigation begins, it is not unusual to find that several generations have occurred before the outbreak is uncovered (see Chapter 2).

As outlined in earlier chapters, your investigation of a vaccine-preventable disease outbreak will begin by searching for cases using an establishing case definition. You should devote considerable effort to finding the index case for the outbreak using dates of onset for the earliest known cases plus the probable incubation period of the disease to track their potential exposures. Searching for the index case is useful for determining the ultimate source of the outbreak, and may lead you to previously unrecognized chains of transmission.

You will also want to collect specimens for laboratory confirmation. Serologic specimens—either paired sera or a single specimen for IgM testing—are often sufficient to confirm the cause of illness. However, culturing the organism or identifying it by polymerase chain reaction will assist your investigation. For example, molecular epidemiology can be used to determine the geographic source of a measles virus. Strain typing will help guide your decisions on using vaccination and/or antibiotic prophylaxis to control a meningococcal or pneumococcal outbreak. Determining the antibiotic resistance profile of an outbreak strain will inform your choice of antibiotics for pertussis prophylaxis. Close consultation with your colleagues at the state laboratory and the CDC is essential so that correct specimens are collected with the correct technique. You must also store and transport specimens correctly to preserve the viability of the material. During weekends and holidays, special arrangements may be necessary to ensure proper handling (see Chapter 24).

Your investigation should collect demographics, symptoms, and complications for each case. You will want to explore thoroughly potential sources of exposure. Particular care needs to be paid to recording the immunization history, including the dates of *all* immunizations given, the type of vaccine, the lot number, and the manufacturer. Immunization history should be verified at the provider's office or in the state immunization registry, even when a parent has an immunization card. A recent study found that even school-based immunization records overestimated vaccination rates.[13] You should query all immunization providers that have cared for the case so that a history of non-vaccination is verifiable and duplicate doses are identified. Disease history should be collected, as cases and controls with prior disease are immune. Also, some states allow either a parental history of disease or a history of physician-diagnosed illness to substitute for vaccination for specific diseases, notably varicella. Cases and controls with a history of disease and/or an immunization history that cannot be verified are best excluded from the study.

As your outbreak investigation proceeds, you will be asked to define and implement a control strategy. VPD outbreaks are controlled by immunizing susceptible populations. For some diseases, vaccine will be supplemented by antibiotic or immune globulin prophylaxis. In order to limit transmission, control measures are often implemented early in the outbreak, well before an investigation is complete. Persons who may be incubating the disease or are beginning to become ill should be excluded from school or the workplace and isolated at home to reduce their opportunities to expose others. A plan for identifying and immunizing incompletely vaccinated persons in the outbreak population should be implemented as soon as possible. Your analysis should focus, not just on current cases, but on who has been potentially exposed and the populations where the next generations of cases are likely to occur. Mass clinics may be organized by state and local health departments if the situation warrants. In school outbreaks, children whose parents refuse to have them immunized are excluded from school until the end of the outbreak. As the investigation develops and the outbreak progresses, further control measures may be needed

The combination of highly effective vaccines, high immunization coverage, and herd immunity will, in an ideal world, reduce the incidence of vaccine-preventable diseases to zero. Consequently, outbreaks provide us with an opportunity to learn how and why the current immunization system is failing to meet that goal. Your initial case finding efforts will allow you to formulate hypotheses on the underlying causes of the outbreak and develop an investigation plan. A case control study is often warranted, but not always. For example, if a group of vaccine-refusers is the focus of the outbreak, the outbreak investigation may document complications of illness to help educate parents on dangers of vaccine-preventable disease.[14] Or it could focus on spread of disease within a community, so that all parents can better understand how unvaccinated children put other children at risk. Vaccine failure occurring in a single lot, from a single manufacturer or from a single clinic, could point to a failure to properly refrigerate vaccine or a manufacturing defect. An investigation of an outbreak in an ethnic minority or immigrant population could focus on the reasons why children did not receive the recommended vaccines.[15]

## Measuring Vaccine Efficacy

Vaccine efficacy—the percentage reduction in disease that occurs in vaccinated persons—is often part the investigation. Vaccine efficacy studies are essential for determining how vaccines perform in the field, as opposed to research studies. They are essential for evaluating immunization policy. For example, field studies showing that vaccine efficacy for a single dose of varicella vaccine was 72% to 85% were an important part of the ACIP decision to include a second dose of vaccine in the routine immunization schedule.[16]

A common error made by people unfamiliar with immunization programs is that if many of the cases give a history of vaccination, then there is a problem with the vaccine (i.e., vaccine efficacy is poor). However, no vaccine provides absolute protection, and small outbreaks can occur even when vaccine efficacy approaches 100%.[17]

Vaccine efficacy can be quickly estimated when vaccine coverage is known, using the curves developed by Orenstein et al.[18] (see Fig. 15–1). Using the 90% efficacy curve, an outbreak occurring in a population with 90% immunization coverage will have ~50% of cases that are vaccinated. Vaccine efficacy in percent is calculated by the following equation:

$$\text{Vaccine Efficacy} = 100 \times (1-(\text{Attack Rate Vaccinated}/\text{Attack Rate Unvaccinated}))$$

When conducting a case control study (Chapter 8) to measure vaccine efficacy, you will have to exercise care in choosing controls that have comparable chances of being exposed. For example, if most cases of a disease occur in a single grade, it may be better to match by grade, or even classroom, to ensure that controls have been involved in the same activities as cases. In outbreaks of many generations, children who become ill early in the outbreak may have different demographic characteristics or route and intensity of exposure than cases late in the outbreak. Your analysis would then include analyses of cases during defined phases of the outbreak as well as for the entire outbreak period.

For vaccines that require multiple doses, you will have to categorize cases and controls as being *unimmunized*, *partially immunized*, and *fully immunized*. Outbreaks in infants may also require you to create a category for those who have been immunized as appropriate for age, but have not yet received a complete primary series. For example, a four-month-old girl who has received two doses of diphtheria, pertussis, and tetanus vaccine is appropriate for age, but is not fully immunized. During outbreaks occurring in older children, adolescents, and/or adults, it may be valuable to analyze the time since their last vaccination as well as the total number of doses received during their lifetime.

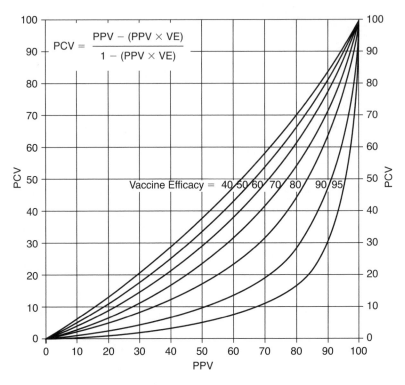

**Figure 15–1.** The relationship between the percentage of cases vaccinated (PCV) and the percentage of the population vaccinated (PPV) for seven different percentage values of vaccine efficacy (VE). [*Source:* Orenstein et al., 1985[18], with permission.]

Your analysis is likely to be complicated by vaccination of both cases and controls during outbreak control efforts As a result, some study subjects may be unimmunized for only part of the outbreak period. The immune response is usually not considered complete until at least two weeks have passed since vaccination. Notable exceptions to this are live vaccines, which provide immediate protection. When given shortly after exposure, a live vaccine may even abort an incubating infection. For example, measles vaccine prevents disease when given within 72 hours of exposure. Your study design will have to account for subjects' being immunized during the outbreak and have clear definitions of when a subject is considered immune after vaccination.

A final consideration regarding the effects that control efforts may have on your study pertains to vaccine reactions. Up to 5% of children may develop a rash and mild fever following the measles, mumps, or rubella vaccine. Live, attenuated influenza vaccine may produce symptoms of a mild respiratory infection that have to be differentiated from influenza. Your case classification system will need to distinguish adverse events following vaccination that may mimic disease, from the actual disease.

## Adverse Reactions

Everyone working with vaccines and vaccine-preventable diseases should be familiar with adverse events following immunization. All drugs and many foods can cause illness in small numbers of people caused by allergies or toxic effects. Similarly, vaccines have toxic side effects and may cause serious allergic reactions in a few individuals. Vaccines differ from other pharmaceuticals because they are given to large numbers of healthy people rather than smaller numbers of people who are ill. When, by happenstance, the onset of illness follows an immunization, these events may be falsely attributed to the vaccine. This is particularly true for infants, who receive many immunizations and may have hereditary neurological conditions that are not manifest until the brain is sufficiently mature. Major public controversies in the last 30 years include whether vaccines cause sudden infant death syndrome (SIDS), autism, encephalopathy, autoimmune diseases, and multiple sclerosis. Overall, the rates of serious adverse events following vaccination occur at rates that are several orders of magnitude less than the most severe complications of natural disease. For example, one to three children will die, and one child will develop acute encephalitis (often resulting in permanent brain damage) for every 1000 cases of measles in the U.S. This compares with less than one case of encephalopathy occurring for every *million* doses of measles administered.[19] Unfortunately, when disease is absent, reactions to vaccination become the focus of attention and are more feared than the disease. In addition to being familiar with the scientific data about specific adverse events, the field epidemiologist can help the public and decision makers understand the difference between events that are caused by a vaccine and those that occur randomly.

Before a vaccine is licensed, the Food and Drug Administration extensively reviews safety data provided by manufacturers. Vaccines that are found to have more than minor side effects and are judged to be insufficiently safe will not be licensed. However, the manufacturer's safety and efficacy data usually contain data from just several thousand subjects. Adverse events occurring at rates of less than one per 10,000 persons vaccinated cannot be detected reliably. Manufacturers conduct post-marketing surveillance for rare reactions and report them to the FDA and CDC. The Immunization Safety Office (ISO) at the Centers for Disease

Control and Prevention monitors reports of adverse events and conducts studies of the occurrence of specific health conditions after vaccination. If you are involved in the field with immunization programs, you need to be familiar with the Vaccine Adverse Events Reporting System (VAERS). Federal law requires all adverse events occurring after vaccination to be reported to VAERS. You will need to ensure that a VAERS report is filed on all adverse events that come to your attention. This includes both trivial, expected reactions, like redness at the injection site, and events clearly not related to the vaccination, like death of an infant in an automobile accident three days after vaccination. The VAERS database is monitored continuously by ISO for signals indicating rare events associated with vaccination. If a signal is detected, additional studies will be conducted. You may be asked to participate in a national or multistate case control study by searching for cases, reviewing medical records and conducting interviews. This approach was used to verify a signal of increased rates of intussusception occurring in infants who had received the first rotavirus vaccine.[20]

## THE FUTURE OF IMMUNIZATION PROGRAMS

The field epidemiologist interested in vaccines and vaccine-preventable disease will find exciting opportunities in the areas of new vaccines and international disease control. Human papilloma virus vaccine for the prevention of cervical cancer, herpes zoster vaccine, and a new rotavirus vaccine have been recently added to the recommended immunization schedules. Vaccines for respiratory syncytial virus, parainfluenza virus, human metapneumovirus, and streptococcus A and B are among the many vaccines in late-stage development. New technologies are being used to create novel delivery systems and offer the potential for vaccines to be used against noninfectious diseases in addition to infectious diseases.[21] Field epidemiologists are needed to study the background incidence of disease and evaluate the effectiveness of new vaccines in preventing disease. There will also be opportunities in academia and industry to conduct studies necessary for vaccines to be licensed.

Internationally, a 20-year effort to eradicate polio globally is nearing an end. Targets are being set in some areas of the world for the elimination of measles. The Gates Foundation and many other international donors are supporting efforts to introduce *H. influenza*, type b; Japanese encephalitis; pneumococcus; and other vaccines into the routine immunization schedule of many developing countries. As these efforts proceed, there will opportunities for experienced field epidemiologists to work in program development and evaluation. The introduction of an effective HIV vaccine will pose particularly exciting challenges for epidemiologists with vaccine-preventable disease expertise.

## REFERENCES

1. Talbot, T.R., Poehling, K.A., Hartert, T.V., et al. (2004). Elimination of racial differences in invasive pneumococcal disease in young children after introduction of the conjugate pneumococcal vaccine. *Pediatr Infect Dis J* 23(8), 726–31.
2. Kyaw, M.H., Lynfield, R., Schaffner, W., et al. (2006). Effect of introduction of the pneumococcal conjugate vaccine on drug-resistant *Streptococcus pneumoniae*. *N Engl J Med* 354(14), 1455–63.
3. Smith, P.J., Santoli, J.M., Chu, S.Y., et al. (2005). The association between having a medical home and vaccination coverage among children eligible for the Vaccines for Children program. *Pediatrics* 116(1), 130–9.
4. Smith, P.J., Stevenson, J., Chu, S.Y. (2006). Associations between childhood vaccination coverage, insurance type, and breaks in health insurance coverage. *Pediatrics* 117(6), 1972–8.
5. Kroger, A.T., Atkinson, W.L., Marcuse, E.K., et al. (2006). General recommendations on immunization: recommendations of the Advisory Committee on Immunization Practices (ACIP). *Morb Mortal Wkly Rep Recomm Rep.* 55(RR-15), 1–48.
6. Boom, J.A., Dragsbaek, A.C., Nelson, C.S.. (2007). The success of an immunization information system in the wake of Hurricane Katrina. *Pediatrics* 119(6), 1213–7.
7. Centers for Disease Control and Prevention (CDC) (2006). National, state, and urban area vaccination coverage among children aged 19–35 months—United States, 2005. *Morb Mortal Wkly Rep* 55(36), 988–93.
8. CDC (2006). Vaccination coverage among children entering school—United States, 2005–2006 School Year. *Morb Mortal Wkly Rep* 55(41), 1124–26.
9. CDC (2006). Influenza and pneumococcal vaccination coverage among persons aged >65 years—United States, 2004—2005. *Morb Mortal Wkly Rep* 55(39), 1065–68.
10. Lynn, T.V., Beller, M., Funk, E.A., et al. (2004). Incremental effectiveness of two doses of measles-containing vaccine compared with one dose among high school students during an outbreak. *J Infect Dis* 189(Suppl 1), S86–90.
11. CDC (1999). Rubella outbreak—Westchester County, New York, 1997–1998. *Morb Mortal Wkly Rep* 48(26), 560–3.
12. Smith, P.J., Chu, S.Y., Barker, L.E. (2004). Children who have received no vaccines: who are they and where do they live? *Pediatrics* 114(1), 187–95.
13. Stanwyck, C., Davila, J., Wake, L., et al. (2007). Assessment of kindergarten immunization rates in Colorado: school self-reports vs. health department audits, 2004–2005. *Pub Health Rep* 122(4), 461–5.
14. Rodgers, D.V., Gindler, J.S., Atkinson, W.L., et al. (1993). High attack rates and case fatality during a measles outbreak in groups with religious exemption to vaccination. *Pediatr Infect Dis J* 12(4), 288–92.
15. Hutchins, S.S., Escolan, J., Markowitz, L.E., et al. (1989). Measles outbreak among unvaccinated preschool-aged children: opportunities missed by health care providers to administer measles vaccine. *Pediatrics* 83(3), 369–74.
16. Marin, M., Guris, D., Chaves, S.S., et al. (2007). Prevention of varicella: recommendations of the Advisory Committee on Immunization Practices (ACIP). *Morb Mortal Wkly Rep Recomm Rep.* 56(RR-4), 1–40.
17. Yeung, L.F., Lurie, P., Dayan, G., et al. (2005). A limited measles outbreak in a highly vaccinated U.S. boarding school. *Pediatrics* 116(6), 1287–91.

18. Orenstein, W.A., Bernier, R.H., Dondero, T.J., et al. (1985). Field evaluation of vaccine efficacy. *Bull World Health Organ* 63(6), 1055–68.
19. American Academy of Pediatrics (2003). Measles. In: L.K. Pickering (ed.), *Red Book: 2003 Report of the Committee on Infectious Diseases*, 26th ed., American Academy of Pediatrics, Elk Grove Village, Ill. pp. 419–29.
20. Murphy, T.V., Gargiullo, P.M., Massoudi, M.S., et al. (2001). Intussusception among infants given an oral rotavirus vaccine. *N Engl J Med* 344(8), 564–72.
21. Plotkin, S.A. (2005). Vaccines: past, present and future. *Nat Med* 11(4 Suppl), S5–11.

# 16

# INVESTIGATIONS IN HEALTH-CARE SETTINGS

## William R. Jarvis

The term *health-care setting* refers to hospitals, rehabilitative centers, transitional care, ambulatory care, outpatient, private physicians' offices, free-standing clinics, dialysis centers, long-term acute care, long-term care facilities, and homes where health care is being delivered (Table 16–1). Investigations of outbreaks in these settings require special attention and differ from community outbreaks in several ways.

This chapter prepares you for field investigations in health-care settings. It highlights the differences between conducting a community investigation and one confined to a health-care facility or setting where health care is being delivered. The emphasis is on how to find the information you need and how to use data and resources that are generally readily available only in health-care settings.

## BACKGROUND CONSIDERATIONS

### Community versus Hospital-based Outbreaks

This section describes four of the most important and distinctive characteristics of infections in the hospital setting as compared to community acquired infections. First, hospital-acquired infections (e.g., bloodstream, respiratory tract, urinary tract, or surgical site infections are common, occurring in approximately 6% of hospitalized

**Table 16–1.**  Health-Care Facilities

Hospitals
Private physicians' offices
Freestanding clinics
Dialysis
Ambulatory surgery
Long-term-care facilities
Nursing homes
Rehabilitation centers
Institutions for the mentally or physically handicapped

patients or nearly 2 million infections per year in the United States.[1,2] Of these, urinary tract infections occur in an estimated 24 of every 1000 hospitalized patients; pneumonia in 6–10; bloodstream infections in 3; and surgical site infections are estimated to occur in 28 of every 1000 operations performed.[1,3] Although it has been estimated that approximately 32% of hospital-acquired infections may be preventable by fully implementing current recommendations, only 6% are actually being prevented.[3]

Most hospital or health-care-associated infections (HAIs) are endemic; epidemics of infection are infrequent.[4] When they do occur, outbreaks cover a wide range of infectious agents and sites—including outbreaks of noninfectious diseases. For example, recent outbreaks investigated by state health departments and the Centers for Disease Control and Prevention (CDC; www.cdc.gov) included such problems as infections associated with allograft implants[5], intrinsic contamination of contact lens solution, Severe Acute Respiratory Syndrome (SARS), *Curvularia* species infection in breast implant procedures,[6] vancomycin-resistant enterococci (VRE) in a community of acute and long-term care facilities,[7] vancomycin-intermediate resistant *Staphylococcus aureus* (VISA) infections in inpatients and a person on home therapy,[8] bloodstream infections in neonatal units in Colombia and Egypt,[9,10] and potential community acquisition of methicillin-resistant *S. aureus* (MRSA). Other examples include *Serratia marcescans* infections associated with narcotic use in a health care worker,[11] transmission of VRE and other multidrug-resistant pathogens in long-term care facilities, *Malassezia* or *Aspergillosis spp.* infections among immunosuppressed patients,[12] surgical site infections after cardiac surgery, establishment of endemnicity of VRE in a three-county region of California,[13] tuberculosis among patients and health-care-workers,[14] pyrogenic reactions in dialysis patients in Viet Nam, anaphylactic reactions to latex among pediatric surgery patients, and aluminum toxicity among dialysis patients.[15]

Second, patients receiving health care—for example, patients in acute or rehabilitative care settings, residents of long-term care settings, ambulatory care patients, and those receiving chronic hemodialysis or home care—have underlying diseases that make them significantly more susceptible to infection than their healthier community cohorts. Other risk factors for development of infection include invasive devices, such as intravenous catheters, indwelling urinary catheters, and endotracheal intubation; or invasive procedures, such as surgery. These numerous, interacting, intrinsic host and external exposure factors add complexity to the investigation and often require multivariate analyses to reduce or eliminate the effect of confounding variables and to identify the independent risk factor(s) for the adverse event.

Third, pathogens associated with health care, such as multidrug-resistant pathogens, *Mycobacterium tuberculosis*, MRSA, VRE, VISA; viral pathogens, such as hepatitis B and C viruses, respiratory syncytial virus, or rotavirus; fungal pathogens, such as *Malassezia, Aspergillus,* or *Candida spp*; and other microorganisms pose a much greater risk to patients and health-care workers in these settings than members of the surrounding community. Transmission of pathogens in health-care settings often is only appreciated after infections appear in patients or health-care workers, and the transmission of the pathogens causing colonization—the unrecognized iceberg effect—is not detected.

Finally, any outbreak in the health-care setting poses a risk for litigation against that facility. This adds to the pressure to rapidly identify the problem and institute effective control measures during the investigation.

## Overall Purposes and Methodology

As with community outbreak investigations, the primary purpose of your investigations in health-care settings is to determine the source of the outbreak and the mode of spread, to terminate the outbreak and to prevent further pathogen transmission. Investigation in these facilities also provides you with the opportunity to identify new or re-emerging agents or complications,[6, 7, 8, 13–15] previously unrecognized human or environmental sources, and new or unusual modes of transmission.[5, 6, 8, 11, 12] Furthermore, investigations in health-care settings may help determine risk factors for acquisition of disease in patients and health-care workers and facilitate development of prevention interventions.

## Pace and Commitment of the Field Investigation

Like all other epidemiologic investigations, your work must be conducted quickly, thoroughly, and responsibly. Pressure from a variety of sources may add to the sense of urgency to complete the investigation quickly. Health-care professionals will be looking to you for answers and recommendations to prevent further spread of disease to their "healthy" patients or to health-care workers (and in turn their concern for their family members). The hospital administrator(s) may already have closed the ward/unit/facility and stopped admissions to the affected unit; so every day that unit stays closed means loss of income for the hospital. Finally, the health-care industry is a common target of the media and lawyers, and outbreaks in a health-care facility may lead to adverse publicity and legal actions. However, these added pressures should not affect the conduct, thoroughness, or organization of your investigation. Although you can make preliminary recommendations based on sound infection control practices, such as patient isolation and hand hygiene, collect your data carefully; analyze it appropriately; and then make specific recommendations based on your findings. Whoever made control recommendations *before* you arrived, such as closing a certain ward to all admissions, discontinuing surgery, or relieving a health-care worker from duty, should be the one who reverses these decisions. On the other hand, if you make a decision to close a unit/ward, etc., you should before that decision determine what conditions must result for you to re-open them.

## RECOGNITION AND RESPONSE TO A REQUEST FOR ASSISTANCE

### The Report

There are a variety of ways you may learn of adverse events or outbreaks in the health care arena. First, the Joint Commission on Accreditation of Healthcare Organizations (JCAHO) requires that health-care settings maintain an active infection control program, including surveillance for health-care-associated infections, as a part of their standard for accreditation (www.jointcommission.org).[16] So routine prospective surveillance data can serve as a source for the identification of infectious disease (and noninfectious disease) outbreaks and as a measure of the intensity and efficacy of the facility's infection surveillance and control program. With caution (if similar definitions, surveillance methods, and numerator and denominator data are used for rate calculations), these data also can be used to monitor and benchmark infection rates by comparing the facility's rates to itself over time (intra-facility comparison) or with others in similar settings (inter-facility comparison). You must be sure that you are comparing your rates to others with a similar case-mix and distribution of underlying diseases and procedures.

Second, professionals trained in infection control techniques monitor infections in health care settings. These infection control professionals, or ICPs, also may work in free-standing clinics or long-term care settings and may work for home care companies. ICPs conduct routine surveillance for HAIs, usually using uniform definitions developed by CDC.[17] Patients with HAIs most frequently are found by review of medical records together with data from the microbiology laboratory; pharmacy, radiology, and Kardex records; nursing, surgical service, and physician reports; and discharge summaries. Detection of outbreaks in health-care settings often results from analyses of these surveillance data. Possible outbreaks also may be detected when an ICP calls a local or state health department or CDC for information on possible sources or modes of transmission of certain pathogens or for advice on prevention and control of infections. Reports of a possible outbreak also may come from the microbiology laboratory, physicians, the employee health department, or directly from employees, patients, patients' families, or the news media.

Lastly, an outbreak in a health-care facility may be recognized when laboratory support is requested from the state health department or CDC. When inquiring about the underlying problem you may identify an outbreak that the facility would like help investigating.

## The Request

Requests for epidemiologic assistance usually come from the ICP, the hospital epidemiologist, the facility's administrator, the company owning the facility or agency, or a private physician who has an outbreak in her or his practice. Health-care facility personnel may simply need laboratory support, such as culture confirmation, assessment of intrinsic product contamination, or molecular typing (e.g., pulsed-field gel electrophoresis or PFGE) of isolates to determine clonality. The laboratory may lack epidemiologic expertise or simply be too busy or understaffed to conduct an investigation on its own while still performing its usual duties. Inquiries about possible assistance may be guarded because of concern about potential future litigation or adverse publicity. This concern applies particularly if the federal government (e.g., CDC, Food and Drug Administration [FDA]; www.FDA.gov) is involved, where data obtained during the investigation are available through the Freedom of Information Act (FOIA). Patient-identifiable information is protected through the Privacy Act, but institutional identity and non-identifiable data on patients are not similarly protected by the Privacy Act. Thus, not infrequently, to protect privileged information, health-care personnel prefer on-site assistance from the local or state health department or a private consultant, rather than the federal government.

## The Response and the Responsibilities

Not all requests to investigate presumed outbreaks in a health-care setting require on-site visits. Because infections and other adverse events are so common in these settings and personnel resources are limited, you should obtain additional background information before agreeing to initiate an investigation. Quite frequently the problem can be solved by mail or telephone consultation. For example, if you receive a call requesting assistance to determine the source of surgical site infections among open-heart surgery patients during the previous two months, try to get additional information that may be useful in evaluating the need for assistance. This information might include current and background open-heart surgery-surgical site infection rates; the pathogens causing the infections; the antimicrobial susceptibility of bacterial pathogens; changes in personnel performing open-heart surgery or the surgical or other methods performed; and a line-listing of "cases" and their characteristics, exposures, and risk factors. Always ask if the "outbreak" isolates are available; this is particularly important to confirm the identity (e.g., genus and species) of the infecting strain(s) and to determine clonality of the strains (usually through genetic typing), both of which are essential laboratory components for conclusive epidemiologic investigations.

Next, ask the contact person to determine the open-heart surgery-surgical site infection rate among patients for several months to years before the suspected outbreak. From the background and current surgical site infection rates, determine if an outbreak may, indeed, be occurring or if the health-care facility actually has a high endemic rate. In other words, are background and current rates similar and are both above national median benchmark or published rates? Determine if the increased open-heart surgery-surgical site infection rate could be due to surveillance artifact. For example, has there been an increase in the surveillance staff or training of a new ICP? Have there been additions to the open-heart surgery staff or changes in open-heart surgery procedures or practices, such as new techniques, changes in procedures (like pre-operative shaving), changes in medical equipment, introduction of new techniques, or changes in antimicrobial prophylaxis? Are there any changes in the laboratory that would have increased recognition of the pathogen(s) (e.g., introduction of a new diagnostic test used on surgical specimens)? If an increase in the rate of these infections can be temporally linked to one or more of these factors, a full on-site investigation may not be necessary. Finally, ask the contact person about any interim infection control measures that may have been put into place. If good infection control practices have been implemented and the problem persists, an investigation may be warranted.

Before beginning an investigation, the participants need to discuss several critical issues, such as organization, personnel, resources, and responsibilities—all of which are discussed in Chapters 4 and 5.

## PREPARATION FOR THE FIELD INVESTIGATION

### Collaboration and Consultation

Investigations of outbreaks in health-care settings usually require substantial laboratory support. In addition to identifying the agent (if already done, confirmation is necessary), further typing of the organism may be necessary. For example, since many serotypes of *Pseudomonas aeruginosa* exist as common environmental organisms in hospitals, outbreaks of *P. aeruginosa* may require genotyping to link patient and environmental isolates. In addition, for some multidrug-resistant pathogens, such as MRSA, their prevalence in the facility may be so high that genetic typing, using PFGE or protein A sequencing, may be necessary to determine if the outbreak is caused by one or more strains. Also, serologic testing of numerous blood specimens may be required in outbreaks of health-care-associated viral infections, such as Hepatitis A, B, or C, or cytomegalovirus. Typing methods vary from organism to organism (see Table 16–2). Except for antimicrobial susceptibility testing, most genetic typing methods are available only in reference laboratories (university health-care setting, private, state health department, or CDC). Before accepting an invitation to start an on-site investigation, contact your reference laboratory to request their assistance; identify a contact person; ask what capabilities the laboratory has to assist this particular investigation; and determine what types of specimens should be collected and how they should be shipped. The laboratory personnel also should be able to estimate a time-frame for results. In some investigations, it may be warranted and more efficient for one or more laboratory personnel to join the on-site epidemiologic team. A more comprehensive discussion of the laboratory's role in investigating outbreaks can be found in Chapter 24. For outbreaks involving medical products, devices, biologics, or blood products, the FDA should be notified (http://www.FDA.Medwatch) and consulted for laws requiring the reporting of adverse effects. In addition, the FDA may know of a similar occurrence in other settings, indicating a problem of potentially greater scope. The FDA can help reduce the extent of the outbreak by issuing

**Table 16–2.** Types of Organisms for Which Typing Method Can Be Used

| TYPING METHODS | TYPES OF ORGANISMS |
| --- | --- |
| Antimicrobial susceptibility profiles | Bacteria (except *Pseudomonas cepacia* and *Staphylococcus epidermidis*), fungi, occasionally viruses |
| Serotyping | Some bacteria and viruses |
| Pulsed-field gel electrophoresis | Bacteria and fungi |
| Ribotyping | Bacteria |
| Phage typing | Bacteria (i.e., *Staphylococcus aureus*) |
| Polymerase chain reaction (PCR) | bacteria, viruses, and fungi |
| Plasmid analysis | Bacteria |
| Restriction fragment length polymorphism | *Mycobacterium tuberculosis* |

alerts or initiating a voluntary or non-voluntary recall. Similarly, for outbreaks primarily involving health-care workers or physical plant problems like potential toxic exposures, state agencies responsible for occupational health and/or CDC's National Institute for Occupational Safety and Health (NIOSH) can lend assistance with industrial engineering evaluations (see Chapter 19).

In some contrast to many community outbreak investigations, in a health-care facility you will often have assistance from personnel, such as ICPs and hospital epidemiologists, who are knowledgeable about the health-care facility and trained in infection control practices. These ICPs are an invaluable resource for background information about infection rates and implemented infection control practices in the facility and the location of other resources that may be available to you. In addition, the ICP staff may be available to be a part of the investigative team and assist you in the design of the study, the abstraction of data from medical records, the analyses, and the development and implementation of recommendations for prevention and control.

Personnel in the health-care facilities want to minimize the potentially negative impact that an investigation at those settings may generate. Often, disgruntled employees or those with a particular agenda may alert the media about the outbreak. You should anticipate public inquiries, and arrangements should be made early in the investigation—or even before the team arrives on-site—for such inquiries to be directed to and handled by administrative, public relations, or risk management personnel at the facility. In outbreaks that involve considerable media attention, it is essential that the media expert for the facility be included in frequent updates about the investigation. In this way, he or she will be knowledgeable and current and can determine what information to release to the media. In addition to permitting you to conduct the investigation unhindered by the media, this allows the facility to maintain control of this very delicate aspect of the investigation.

## THE FIELD INVESTIGATION

Health-care settings lend themselves to outbreak investigations because of easy access to many kinds of records (see above). Documentation is very important in these settings, but it varies; hospitals and free-standing clinics (surgery or dialysis centers) generally have more complete documentation than long-term care facilities or private physicians' offices. Computerized records are increasingly available and are very valuable; obtaining large amounts of data from a computer record is much more efficient than reviewing the medical records for this information. To the extent possible, attempt to obtain as much of the data as you can from the computerized records; however, before fully depending upon this source, be sure that the data are complete and valid. Often, the personnel recording such data are not familiar with the importance or the meaning of the information and incorrectly enter or misinterpret the data they are handling. Use your imagination to identify other sources of documentation, and do not be afraid to ask if other types of records exist. Outbreaks predominantly involving health-care workers often are more difficult to investigate because not all of the health-care workers will be treated at the health-care facility. Employee health department records can be used, although medical students, house officers, private physicians, outside agency personnel, volunteers, and other non-paid hospital personnel often are not included in hospital employee health programs. Time cards (to determine absenteeism possibly due to illness) and interviews with affected employees also are helpful.

Immediately upon your arrival at the health-care facility, arrange a meeting with all of the key personnel involved with the outbreak. This meeting should include the hospital administrator, chief of service, physicians who have patients involved in the outbreak, the hospital epidemiologist, the infection control staff, risk management personnel, appropriate public health authorities, and the field team. Also, invite any other key personnel who may be involved, such as the operating room manager, the head nurse from the affected unit(s), or the heads of the microbiology and medical records departments. At this meeting you should outline your initial plan for the investigation, indicate the time-frame this will require, and request any resources you need immediately, e.g., an office with a telephone, phone numbers of key personnel, a map of the facility, and directions to the laboratory and medical records department. If security is strict, request a temporary identification badge to allow freer movement around the facility. Also, ask for any additional information you may need to start the investigation, for example, policy and procedure manuals, any recent changes in them, and the opinion of the involved personnel about the potential cause of the outbreak. It also is important to confirm to all involved that you will maintain the strictest confidentiality for the patients and will work with all personnel to conduct the investigation quickly and efficiently with as little disruption of usual business as possible.

## Determine the Existence of an Epidemic

This step may have been started during the preparatory stages of the investigation. In the field, determine the background rate of the adverse event for yourself (see Chapter 5). Start with the appropriate records, often the microbiology and infection control records. Outbreaks involving blood products will require examination of transfusion reaction records; those involving dialysis patients require examination of dialysis session records. Be creative—what you need is not always computerized but often is systematically collected and recorded somewhere. You may have to look back at several years of data to calculate accurate background rates. If the data suggest a hyper-endemic rate rather than a true outbreak, the problem still may be worthy of investigation. Occasionally, only or no periodic surveillance will have been conducted in the "outbreak area." If this occurs, it may be very difficult, time consuming, or impossible to determine the background or current rate. In those instances, it may be necessary to estimate the rate of infection or adverse reaction using a sampling method.[18] Remember to look at other changes that may have occurred that will affect the rates you are calculating, for example, the ICP hired six new assistants one year, or four new surgeons or a new infectious disease specialist were added to the medical staff. New procedures may have been implemented before or during the outbreak, new diagnostic tests may have become available, or new units opened in the hospital—all of which might lead to an increased infection or illness rate (i.e., surveillance artifact).

At the same time, start looking closely at procedures around the patient care areas that are relevant to the outbreak. Look at everything and ask questions about every aspect of patient care no matter how seemingly trivial. See for yourself what is actually happening rather than relying on others. Written policies may or may not reflect what is really occurring on the patient care ward (policy often is not practice). Observe practices for yourself! After your initial review of the procedures occurring around the patients, create your initial case definition and determine what data you want to collect for each case. For example, patient demographic information, hospital locations, underlying diagnoses, date of onset of illness, and dates of invasive procedures should be collected. Other important data might include severity of illness indicators (e.g., the Acute Physiologic and Chronic Health Evaluation [APACHE] score, the Pediatric Risk of Mortality [PRISM] score, or the National Nosocomial Infections Surveillance [NNIS] surgical site infection risk index).[19–21] You very likely will want to get information on possible exposures such as operating rooms, surgeons, operating room team members, nursing and other patient contact personnel, and medications.

## Confirm the Diagnosis

In an infectious disease outbreak, contact all laboratories where the patient specimens initially are being processed and ask them to save all relevant isolates for possible further study. If the outbreak strains have been isolated or sent to an outside or private laboratory, obtain the isolates for possible confirmation or further testing. If possible, confirm that the cases are related by reviewing the microbiology laboratory data for species identification and/or antimicrobial sensitivity testing results. If you need typing of organisms beyond the capability of the microbiology department at the facility, consult a university or private laboratory, the state health department, or CDC. Remember, some typing techniques are research tools that may not be performed rapidly or may not be practical to apply to large numbers of isolates. Maintain communication with your laboratory colleagues to inform them of the progress of the investigation, what isolates are available and being sent to them, and to discuss what other specimens or samples they may want. At the same time, you can discuss with them the reasonable time-frame for notification of results.

## Define a Case and Count Cases

The case definition(s) should start with the clinical aspects of the disease. Try to include laboratory and clinical data in the case definition and inclusionary charac-teristics that relate to time, place, and person. For example, a case definition might include persons who developed a staphylococcal surgical site infection between November 1 and January 1; who were located on surgical floor, 3-West; and who had an orthopedic procedure. If the clinical case definition is confirmed by laboratory methods, you can call this a *Confirmed Case*. A patient with similar symptoms but lacking laboratory confirmation will then be called a *Possible Case*. This distinction may be useful later on when you analyze all your cases. Remember, start with a broad case definition; you can refine it as you continue the investigation. Remember, as you increase sensitivity you decrease specificity, and vice versa.

Methods for case-finding depend on the type of disease (infectious or non-infectious) causing the outbreak. Sources that may be useful include records from the infection control department (e.g., surveillance reports), microbiology labora-tory, clinic patients, emergency room, blood bank, or dialysis sessions. Case-finding can be done by reviewing the entire cohort of patient charts, if the cases are limited to a single ward or unit, or if the health-care facility has a reasonably manageable number of patients to review or has very complete electronic records. Dialysis outbreaks may require you to count each dialysis session, rather than counting each patient. This is because a patient may have more than one exposure at a single session, thus allowing each dialysis session to be treated as a single exposure.

At the same time you are ascertaining cases, collect the basic information you have already deemed important during your initial procedure review of the first identified cases. Again, after you have determined your case definition and found cases, compare the attack rate with the background rate to assure yourself that an outbreak is, indeed, occurring.

## Orient the Data in Terms of Time, Place, and Person

Descriptive epidemiology in health-care settings differs from that of community outbreak investigations only in that all of the cases are already hospitalized (in the healthcare facility or each patient has an available medical record (outpatient, dialysis, ambulatory, or home care). As with community outbreaks, organizing the data in terms of time, place, and person allows you to postulate who was at risk and who may still be at risk for developing the disease or adverse reaction.

### Time

The "epidemic curve" gives you a picture of the scope of the outbreak over time. It may give a clue as to whether the outbreak was due to a common source, person-to-person transmission, or another mode of transmission (see Chapters 2 and 5). For example, a common-source outbreak with subsequent person-to-person transmission is well illustrated by a food-borne outbreak in a retirement community (Fig. 16–1).[22] A high initial peak of onset of illness, suggestive of a single point source of infection, is followed by the continued occurrence of cases due to secondary person-to-person transmission, typical of outbreaks of viral gastroenteritis. The epidemic curve of an outbreak caused by contaminated patient equipment or poor infection control techniques also may span long periods of time until the recurring problem is corrected. For example, an *Acinetobacter baumannii* outbreak, traced to reuse of intravascular pressure transducers that were not adequately sterilized, continued for over a year until the problem was recognized and the decontamination/disinfection technique corrected (Fig. 16–2).[23] If health-care workers and patients are both affected by the outbreak, the date of onset of disease for patients and health-care workers should be plotted together and then separately to help determine how transmission may have occurred, that is,

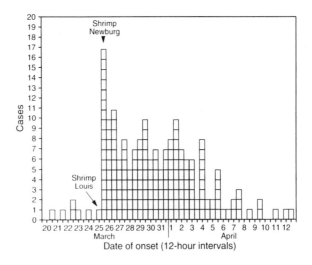

**Figure 16–1.** Cases of gastroenteritis originating from a common source with subsequent person-to-person transmission, by date of onset—California, March 20– April 12, 1988. [*Source:* Gordon et al., 1990.[22]]

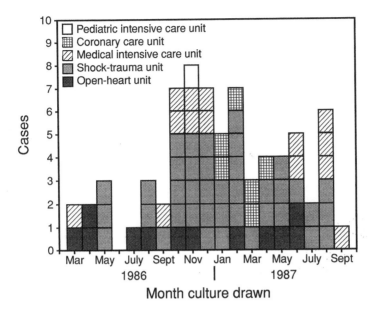

**Figure 16–2.** Cases of *Acinetobacter baumannii* bacteremia caused by contaminated patient-care equipment, by month that culture was drawn—New Jersey, March 1986–September 1987. [*Source:* Beck-Sague et al., 1990.[23]]

from patient to patient, patient to health-care worker, health-care worker to patient, or health-care worker to health-care worker.

### Place

At times, the location of the outbreak will be limited to a certain floor, unit, or operating room; at other times to a certain type of floor (e.g., all of the general surgical units because only surgical patients are being affected). The location of the outbreak may provide a clue to the mode of transmission or to certain risk factors due to patient placement or exposure. For example, during the initial phase of an investigation in a hospital of an outbreak of tuberculin skin test conversions among health-care workers and multidrug-resistant tuberculosis (TB) among patients, it was noted that most of the health-care workers worked and the patients had been treated in the outpatient human immunodeficiency virus (HIV) clinic. Further investigation documented that air in the examination rooms was at positive pressure to the central patient area and that the air from the examination rooms, where patients were receiving aerosol treatments, was recirculated to the central patient area and the nurses station. Thus, health-care workers and acquired immunodeficiency syndrome (AIDS) patients were being exposed to the air originating from rooms in which AIDS patients with active TB were being treated, and the infectious particles were being circulated via the ventilation system to areas where patients and health-care workers without TB were present.[24]

### Person

In investigating community-wide epidemics, you will often characterize the affected persons by many attributes such as age, gender, race, occupation, socio-economic level, etc.. In general, however, in health-care settings, you do not need to classify cases by so many variables. Most often, age, gender, and underlying disease are the most often used attributes that help you define the "at-risk" population. In contrast to community outbreaks, in many hospital outbreaks one must control for severity of illness or birth weight, because many exposures the patients have are linked to their age or how sick they are. Once one controls for severity of illness or birth weight, many factors that look important are no longer significant.

## Determine Who Is at Risk of Becoming Ill

As discussed in previous chapters (see Chapters 5 and 8), the purpose of charac-terizing the ill persons by time, place, and person is to give you an idea of who is at risk of disease and whom to study further. Therefore, in these settings you can either examine the entire population in a cohort study or you can randomly select controls from this population for a case control study (see Chapter 8). If, for example, you find that patients located on all general wards of the hospital over a period of one year developed pneumonia, you may want to take a random sample of all patients admitted to the hospital during that same year as controls for a case control study. If, however, you determine that the only patients in the facility who are at risk were located on a particular ward during a specific time interval and had a particular underlying diagnosis (e.g., appendectomy patients on a general surgi-cal ward during the months of April and May 2008), you may want to select *all* appendectomy patients located on that ward from March 1 through June 30, 2008, and review their charts as a "retrospective" cohort study.

Selection of controls is exceedingly important, because the wrong control group can easily lead to erroneous conclusions. For example, if, during case-finding, you discover that patients undergoing general anesthesia for a variety of surgical procedures developed surgical site and bloodstream infections, several possible control groups for a case control study could be selected, or several different cohorts.[25] If the study group (controls or the cohort) is selected from all patients undergoing surgery, there is a good chance that many of the non-ill patients will have undergone local, spinal, or epidural anesthesia, while all of the ill patients will have undergone only general anesthesia. Since the ill patients were previ-ously known to have undergone only general anesthesia, specific exposures related to general anesthesia (e.g., particular injectable anesthetics or intubation equipment) probably will not be identified with this group of controls. A better study group would include patients undergoing general anesthesia for surgical procedures during the correct time-frame. This will allow analysis of each individual inject-able and inhalational agent, respiratory equipment, anesthesiologist, and other possible risk factors.

## Developing and Testing Hypotheses

It is inefficient to test only one or two hypotheses at a time. You can test several hypotheses at once by collecting data on cases and controls, or the cohort, that examine a variety of risk factors. For example, if the disease is predominantly spread by the respiratory route, and all of the cases were intubated, you may want to examine all respiratory therapy practices and exposures, including the type of ventilator used, duration of ventilation, which respiratory therapist(s) took care of the cases each shift, which nurses suctioned the patients' endotracheal tubes, which medications were administered through the endotracheal tube and who prepared them, and how often the ventilator reservoirs were changed.

An excellent example of an outbreak investigation in a hospital is the investi-gation of surgical site infections caused by an unusual human pathogen, *Rhodococcus bronchialis*, after open-heart surgery.[26] This outbreak provided an opportunity to assess risk factors for infection with *R. bronchialis*, mode of transmission of the organism, and potential sources for this unusual nosocomial pathogen. Logical hypotheses for the source of surgical site infections after open-heart surgery included three possible exposures: pre-operative (e.g., nurses, physicians, wards), intra-operative (e.g., operating room environment or personnel), and post-operative (e.g., recovery room or intensive care unit personnel) exposures. By retrospective cohort analysis, the investigators analyzed a large number of variables as measures of potential risk for infection and possible exposures as the source of infection (Table 16–3). The only factor significantly associated with infection was the presence of one operating room nurse, Nurse A, during the operative procedure. Examination of Nurse A's intra-operative practices revealed that she could poten-tially contaminate the sterile field after performing an activated clotting-time test that involved the use of a water bath for incubation of a tube of the patient's blood. A revised hypothesis was that Nurse A contaminated the sterile operative field after performing the test; this would account for all of the cases of *R. bronchialis* surgical site infections during the epidemic period.

## Compare the Hypothesis with the Established Facts

Environmental and personnel cultures can help support the results of an epide-miologic investigation. Because many organisms are ubiquitous in health-care

**Table 16–3.**  Potential Risk Factors for Rhodococcus Sternal Wound Infection—
May 1 through December 31, 1988[a]

| | CASE | | | |
|---|---|---|---|---|
| PATIENTS | CONTROLS | ODDS P | | |
| POTENTIAL RISK FACTOR | (N = 7) | (N = 28) | RATIO | VALUES |
| Categorical Variables | | | | |
| Male sex | 7 (100) | 24 (86) | NC | 0.6 |
| Underlying conditions | 6 (86) | 22 (79) | 1.6 | 1.0 |
| Diabetes | 1 (14) | 6 (21) | 0.6 | 0.1 |
| Obesity | 3 (43) | 4 (14) | 4.5 | 0.1 |
| Smoking | 4 (57) | 9 (32) | 2.8 | 0.4 |
| Cancer | 1 (14) | 0 (0) | NC | 0.2 |
| Renal insufficiency | 0 (0) | 0 (0) | — | — |
| Treatment with steroids | 1 (14) | 1 (4) | 4.5 | 0.4 |
| Chronic lung disease | 2 (29) | 3 (11) | 3.3 | 0.3 |
| Presence of nurse A | 7 (100) | 6 (21) | NC | 0.0003 |
| Coronary artery bypass graft | 7 (100) | 28 (100) | — | — |
| Saphenous vein | 6 (86) | 26 (93) | 0.5 | 0.5 |
| Mammary artery | 6 (86) | 25 (89) | 0.7 | 1.0 |
| Transfusion | 4 (57) | 13 (46) | 2.2 | 1.0 |
| Continuous Variables | | | | |
| Preoperative stay (days) | 1.8±1.3 | 1.9±1.8 | — | 0.7 |
| Postoperative stay (days) | 6.2±1.3 | 7.5±3.7 | — | 0.4 |
| Age (years) | 59.4±5.4 | 58.5±11.0 | — | 0.9 |
| Number of underlying conditions | 2.2±1.9 | 1.1±0.9 | — | 0.2 |
| Duration of operation (min) | 284±64 | 292±87 | — | 0.9 |
| Duration of bypass (min) | 119±38 | 128±44 | — | 0.7 |
| Duration of aortic clamping (min) | 67±43 | 70±27 | — | 0.8 |
| Amount of blood reperfused (mL) | 903±236 | 901±317 | — | 1.0 |

**Table 16–3.** Potential Risk Factors for Rhodococcus Sternal Wound Infection—
May 1 through December 31, 1988ᵃ—Continued

| | CASE | | | |
|---|---|---|---|---|
| PATIENTS | CONTROLS | ODDS | P |
| POTENTIAL RISK FACTOR | ($N = 7$) | ($N = 28$) | RATIO | VALUE |
| Cardiac indexᵇ | 2.8±0.6 | 3.0±0.5 | — | 0.6 |
| Duration of treatment (days) | | | | |
| Stay in cardiac ICU | 2.2±0.4 | 2.9±2.2 | — | 0.8 |
| Swan Ganz catheter | 1.8±0.4 | 2.2±1.0 | — | 0.6 |
| Arterial line | 2±0 | 2.3±1.0 | — | 0.6 |
| Mediastinal drains | 2±0 | 2.2±0.8 | — | 0.6 |
| Pacer wires | 4.8±0.4 | 5.0±1.6 | — | 0.8 |
| Ventilation | 1±0 | 1.6±2.7 | — | 0.6 |
| Antimicrobial prophylaxis | 4.2±2.2 | 3.7±1.0 | — | 0.9 |

ᵃPlus-minus values are means ±SD. NC denotes not calculable; ICU, intensive care nit.
ᵇCardiac index was defined as cardiac output in liters per minute per square meter of body surface area.
[*Source*: Richet et al., 1991.[26]]

environments and are part of the normal environment or human flora, performing cultures of the environment or personnel without epidemiologic implications can be quite costly, waste precious time, and lead your investigation astray. However, when performed to determine if your epidemiologic data are pointing you in the right direction, environmental and personnel cultures can be very valuable.

To continue with the previous example, in order to establish that Nurse A was, indeed, responsible for all of the cases of *R. bronchialis* at the hospital, the investigators performed numerous cultures as indicated by the epidemiologic data. These included cultures of Nurse A's and Nurse B's hands before and after each performed the activated clotting-time test; nasal swabs from all cardiac surgery operating room personnel; swabs from Nurse A's scalp, pharynx, vagina, and rectum; swabs of Nurse A's operating room closet and its contents; her home; the neck-scruff skin, mouths, rectums, and paws of two of Nurse A's three dogs; and environmental swabs and air samples while Nurse A was present in or absent from the operating room. Only cultures of Nurse A's hands after performing the activated clotting test, Nurse A's nasal swab, settle plates from the operating room while Nurse A was present, Nurse A's scalp and vaginal cultures, and cultures of the neck-scruff skin of Nurse A's dogs were positive for *R. bronchialis*.

Antimicrobial sensitivity testing, plasmid analysis, and restriction fragment length polymorphism analysis showed that all of the outbreak isolates (patient, Nurse A, and Nurse A's dogs) were identical and distinct from non-outbreak stock *R. bronchialis* isolates.

The role of the water bath used to incubate blood samples for the activated clotting-time test was analyzed by using a colorless fluorescent dye. After simulating the beginning of an open-heart surgery procedure, eight out of eleven circulating nurses had "contaminated" the sterile field with fluorescent dye from the water bath. In addition, all of the nurses' hands; some of the nurses' wrists, forearms, and scrub suits; the outer surface of the water bath container; the table surface; and the floor around the water bath were "contaminated" with fluorescent dye. This experiment showed that, although the bath water was culture-negative for *R. bronchialis*, the water bath provided the mechanism for the organism to be spread from Nurse A's hands to the sterile field. Because Nurse A was epidemiologically implicated in the investigation, cultures were obtained from a variety of sources highly likely to yield positive results. Culturing of the operating room environment and other personnel earlier in the investigation would have been unfocused, increasing the work-load on the laboratory without significantly aiding the investigation and very likely missing the ultimate implicated source.

## Plan a More Systematic Study

Once the source and mode of transmission have been determined and you can make specific recommendations for control of the outbreak, you may want to perform additional studies. For example, after establishing by a case control study that a certain group is at risk, such as hematology–oncology patients at risk for bacteremia, you may want to analyze that group further for other risk factors. Using a cohort study model, for example, you could analyze the duration of chemotherapy, the specific chemotherapeutic agents, or the duration of neutropenia. You also might want to perform sero-surveys of patients and health-care workers to further define the population at risk after an outbreak of hepatitis B or anaphylactic reactions to certain drugs or products.

Evaluation of the efficacy of control measures that may have been undertaken before or during the investigation, and of recommendations that the field team makes to the hospital personnel, also should be conducted. It is imperative that you or members of the field team document that the implemented interventions terminate the outbreak and prevent further episodes of disease.

## Prepare a Written Report

Before departing from the field site, you should hold a meeting with staff of the health-care facility and local or state health department representatives to apprise them of what you did and your results. The health-care facility administrative director and infection control personnel are primarily interested in your recommendations for control measures. In fact, the legal department may ask you for recommendations from the first day of the investigation. As described earlier in this chapter, you can give preliminary recommendations based on previously documented guidelines for isolation, hand hygiene, hospital environmental control, and disease-specific prevention guidelines[27-43] at the beginning of or during the investigation. Additional recommendations based on the epidemiologic and laboratory data should be given to the facility at this debriefing. Your written report should describe any of the interim measures that were initiated and your final recommendations.

The written report for the facility, the state and local health department, and your supervisor should describe the problem as it was presented to you, the background information that you collected before and during the investigation, the methods and results of your investigation, and your final recommendations to the facility. The written report provides documentation of your investigation and, therefore, should thoroughly and accurately describe your approach or methods, your results, your recommendations, and any follow-up activities either you are planning or that you recommend that facility personnel conduct. Often, it is helpful to write the report (or at least keep detailed notes) as you do the investigation. For example, write the background information before you arrive at the outbreak site, document your methods as you decide each step of the process (this is extremely important for case definitions, which may change during the course of the investigation), and compile a file of results as they become available. You should be able to leave a brief written report, which includes your recommendations for control measures, with health-care facility personnel at your departure. This report should be clearly marked as a *Preliminary* or *Draft* document as it will become part of the permanent record that could be used in court. After returning to your home office, a final report with "clean" data, final laboratory results, and more sophisticated statistical analysis can be written.

## Medico-legal Aspects

Outbreaks of disease in health-care settings may lead to litigation against the facility. *Resist* all attempts by the facility administration to force you into making recommendations that your evidence and other relevant scientific data do not support. In addition, do not get caught up in interdepartmental politics and make recommendations without supporting data. The request for assistance in investigating an outbreak gives the health-care facility an excellent defense in court, especially if the recommended control measures were instituted and the problem stopped. By requesting assistance, the facility personnel have documented that they have taken the problem seriously and have sought a solution. Your final report may be one of the most important defense documents the facility may have for establishing that a thorough investigation was done and that recommendations by outside experts have been made. Furthermore, if the facility personnel can show that they fully implemented the recommendations with subsequent prevention of further diseases, they will have confirmed that they have controlled the outbreak.

Confidentiality and medical malpractice laws vary from state to state; therefore, conduct your investigation so that confidentiality of patients and employees is ensured (see Chapter 14). Therefore, you should not collect identifying data that are not absolutely essential; if you must collect identifying data to link records, a convenient method is the hospital identification number (if it differs from the patient's Social Security number) or the patient's birthdate and last four digits of the Social Security number. If possible, put this information on your data collection form where it can easily be removed by a paper cutter; that is, the top right-hand corner of the first page. This will also allow you to easily remove identifying data months later, if a litigant makes a request for your information. If an agency of the federal government conducts the investigation, the data obtained are available under the FOIA, as are the name of the institution and related correspondence. However, the Privacy Act prevents the release of patient or health-care worker names or other identifying information by U.S. government workers. If state health department personnel conduct the investigation, it is important for them and the facility personnel where the outbreak is occurring to know what data and information are recoverable during possible litigation.

## SUMMARY

Investigating outbreaks of disease in health-care settings is both similar to and different from investigating outbreaks in community settings. Both types of investigation involve a sick, frightened population who want immediate answers and solutions to the problem. Health-care settings have the advantage of multiple types of on-site records and a built-in professional staff of health-care workers, both of which are invaluable resources during an outbreak investigation. And, health-care settings provide the opportunity to study many aspects of disease in a closed, fairly well-controlled setting. Cases of disease in health-care settings involve complex patients, and multivariate analyses of data may be necessary to control for host and device-related risk factors. On the other hand, health-care settings have the disadvantage of a fairly stressful work environment due to the legal implications of outbreaks.

Each state health department has state-specific regulations with which health-care settings must comply. Also, the CDC has published guidelines relevant to the control of infectious diseases in health-care settings.[27–41] In addition, the Society for Healthcare Epidemiology of America (SHEA; www.shea-on-line.org) and the Association for Professionals in Infection Control and Epidemiology, Inc. (APIC; www.APIC.org) have published guidelines and position papers. For example, SHEA has published a position paper on controlling the most prevalent antimicrobial-resistant pathogens, MRSA and VRE.[42] All of these guidelines are meant to be a framework for individual health-care facility staff to use when writing policy and procedure manuals for the facility. The Occupational Safety and Health Administration (OSHA) writes the federal law that mandates certain practices in health-care settings (e.g., Blood-borne Pathogen Standard, Proposed TB Standard); many of these laws incorporate CDC guidelines. In addition, the CDC guidelines and OSHA regulations are references that should be used during the course of outbreak investigations in health-care settings.

## REFERENCES

1. Haley, R.W., Culver, D.H., White, J.W., et al. (1985). The nationwide nosocomial infection rate. *Am J Epidemiol* 121, 159–67.
2. Jarvis, W.R. (2001). Infection control and changing healthcare systems. *Emerg Infect J* 7, 170–3.
3. Haley, R.W., Culver, D.H., White, J.W., et al. (1985). The efficacy of infection surveillance and control programs in preventing nosocomial infections in U.S. hospitals. *Am J Epidemiol* 121, 182–205.
4. Haley, R.W., Tenney, J.H., Lindsey II, J.O., et al. (1985). How frequent are outbreaks of nosocomial infection in community hospitals? *Infect Control* 6, 233–6.
5. Kainer M.A., Linden J.V., Whaley D.N., et al. (2004). Clostridium infections: Associated with musculoskeletal-tissue allografts. *N Engl J Med* 350, 2564–71.
6. Kainer, M.A., Keshavarz, H., Jensen, B.J., et al. (2005). Saline-filled breast implant contamination with curvularia species among women who underwent cosmetic breast augmentation. *J Infect Dis* 192, 170–7.
7. Ostrowsky, B.E., Trick, W.E., Sohn, A., et al. (2001). Successful control of vancomycin-resistant enterococcus (VRE) colonization in acute and long-term care facility patients: working together as a community. *N Engl J Med* 344, 1427–33.
8. Smith, T.L., Pearson, M.L., Wilcox, K.R., et al. (1999). Emergence of vancomycin resistance in *Staphylococcus aureus*. *N Engl J Med* 340, 493–501.
9. Richards, C., Alonso-Echanove, J., Caicedo, Y., et al. (2004). *Klebsiella pneumoniae* bloodstream infections in a high-risk nursery in Cali, Colombia. *Infect Control Hosp Epidemiol* 25, 221–5.
10. Moore, K.L., Kainer, M.A., Badrawi, N., et al. (2005). Neonatal sepsis in Egypt associated with bacterial contamination of glucose-containing intravenous fluids. *Pediatr Infect Dis* 7, 590–4.
11. Ostrowsky, B.E., Whitener, C., Brendenberg, K.H., et al. (2002). *Serratia marcescens* bacteremia traced to an infused narcotic. *N Engl J Med* 346, 1529–37.
12. Chang, H.J., Miller, H.L., Watkin, N., et al. (1998). An epidemic of *Malassezia pachydermatis* in intensive care nursery associated with colonization of health-care worker pet dogs. *N Engl J Med* 338, 706–11.

13. Rosenberg, J., Jarvis, W.R., Reingold, A., et al. (2004). Emergence of vancomycin-resistant enterococci (VRE) in San Francisco Bay area hospitals, 1994–1998. *Infect Control Hosp Epidemiol* 25, 408–12.
14. Roth, V.R., Garrett, D.O., Laserson, K.F., et al. (2005). A multicenter evaluation of tuberculin skin test positivity and conversion among healthcare workers in Brazilian hospitals. *J Tuberc Lung Dis* 9, 1335–42.
15. Jarvis, W.R. (2004). Hospital Infections Program, Centers for Disease Control and Prevention On-site Outbreak Investigations, 1990–1999. In D.J. Weber and W.A. Rutala (eds.), *Seminars in Infection Control*, W.B. Saunders Co., Philadelphia.
16. Joint Commission on Accreditation of Healthcare Organizations (1990). Standards: infection control. In JCAHO, *Accreditation Manual for Hospitals*. Joint Commission on Accreditation of Healthcare Organizations, Chicago.
17. Garner, J.S., Jarvis, W.R., Emori, T.G., et al. (1988). CDC definitions for nosocomial infections, 1988. *Am J Infect Control* 16, 128–40.
18. Cookson, S.T., Ihrig, M., O'Mara, E., et al. (1998). Use of an estimation method to derive an appropriate denominator to calculate central venous catheter-associated bloodstream infection rates. *Infect Control Hosp Epidemiol* 19, 28–31.
19. Knaus, W.A., Draper, E.A., Wagner, D.P., et al. (1985). APACHE II: A severity of disease classification system. *Crit Care Med* 13, 818–29.
20. Pollack, M.M., Ruttimann, U.E., Getson, P.R. (1988). Pediatric risk of mortality (PRISM) score. *Crit Care Med* 16, 1110–6.
21. Culver, D.H., Horan, T.C., Gaynes, R.P., et al. (1991). Surgical wound infection rates by wound class, operative procedure, and patient risk index. *Am J Med* 91(suppl 3B), 152s–57s.
22. Gordon, S.M., Oshiro, L.S., Jarvis, W.R, et al. (1990). Food-borne snow mountain agent gastroenteritis with secondary person-to-person spread in a retirement community. *Am J Epidemiol* 131, 702–10.
23. Beck-Sague, C.M., Jarvis, W.R., Brook, J.H., et al. (1990). Epidemic bacteremia due to *Acinetobacter baumannii* in five intensive care units. *Am J Epidemiol* 132, 723–33.
24. CDC (1990). Nosocomial transmission of multidrug-resistant tuberculosis to health-care workers and HIV-infected patients in an urban hospital—Florida. *Morb Mortal Wkly Rep* 39, 718–22.
25. Bennett, S.N., McNeil, M.M., Bland, L.A., et al. (1995). Multiple outbreaks of post-operative infections traced to extrinsic contamination of an intravenous anesthetic, propofol. *N Engl J Med* 333, 147–54.
26. Richet, H., Craven, P.C., Brown, J.M., et al. (1991). A cluster of *Rhodococcus (Gordona) bronchialis* sternal-wound infections after coronary-artery bypass surgery. *N Engl J Med* 324, 104–9.
27. Garner, J.S., Hospital Infection Control Practices Advisory Committee (1996). Guideline for isolation precautions in hospitals. *Infect Control Hosp Epidemiol* 17, 53–80.
28. O'Grady, N.P., Alexander, M., Dellinger, E.P., et al. (2002). Healthcare Infection Control Practices Advisory Committee. Guidelines for the prevention of intravascular catheter-related infections. *Infect Control Hosp Epidemiol* 23, 759–69.
29. Mangram, A.J., Horan, T.C., Pearson, M.L., et al. (1999). Guideline for prevention of surgical site infection. *Infect Control Hosp Epidemiol* 20, 247–80.
30. Wong, E.S., Hooton, T.M. (1983). Guideline for prevention of urinary tract infections. *Am J Infect Control* 11, 28–33.

31. Tablan, O.C., Anderson, L.J., Besser, R., et al. (2004). Guidelines for prevention of healthcare-associated pneumonia, 2003. *Morb Mortal Wkly Rep* 26;53(RR-3), 1–36.

32. Bolyard, B.A., Tablan, O.C., Williams, W.W., et al. (1998). Guideline for infection control in health care personnel. *Infect Control Hosp Epidemiol* 19, 407–63.

33. CDC (1995). Recommendations for preventing the spread of vancomycin resistance. *Infect Control Hosp Epidemiol* 16, 105–13.

34. CDC (1997). Interim guidelines for prevention and control of staphylococcal infection associated with reduced susceptibility to vancomycin. *Morb Mortal Wkly Rep* 46, 626–8, 635.

35. CDC (1991). Recommendations for preventing transmission of human immuno-deficiency virus and hepatitis B virus to patients during exposure-prone invasive procedures. *Morb Mortal Wkly Rep* 40(RR-8), 1–9.

36. CDC (1997). Immunization of health-care workers. Recommendations of the Advisory Committee on Immunization Practices (ACIP) and the Hospital Infection Control Advisory Practices (HICPAC). *Morb Mortal Wkly Rep* 46(No. RR-18), 1–42.

37. CDC (1987). Recommendations for prevention of HIV transmission in health-care settings. *Morb Mortal Wkly Rep* 36(2S), 3–18.

38. Jensen, P.A., Lambert, L.A., Iademarco, M.F., et al. (2005) Guidelines for preventing the transmission of *Mycobacterium tuberculosis* in health-care settings. *Morb Mortal Wkly Rep* 30, 54(17), 1–141.

39. Mazurek, G.H., Jereb, J., Lobue, P., et al. (2005). Guidelines for using the QuantiFERON-TB. Gold test for detecting *Mycobacterium tuberculosis* infection, United States. *Morb Mortal Wkly Rep* 16, 54(RR-15), 49–55. Erratum in: *Morb Mortal Wkly Rep* (2005 Dec 23) 54(50), 1288.

40. Sehulster, L., Chinn, R.Y. (2003). Guidelines for environmental infection control in health-care facilities. Recommendations of CDC and the Healthcare Infection Control Practices Advisory Committee (HICPAC). *Morb Mortal Wkly Rep* 6, 52(RR-10), 1–42.

41. Boyce, J.M., Pittet, D. (2002). Guideline for Hand Hygiene in Health-Care Settings: recommendations of the Healthcare Infection Control Practices Advisory Committee and the HICPAC/SHEA/APIC/IDSA Hand Hygiene Task Force. *Infect Control Hosp Epidemiol* 23(12 Suppl), S3–40.

42. Siegel J.D., Rhinehart E., Jackson M., et al. (2006). Management of multidrug resistant organisms in healthcare settings. Available at: www.cdc.gov/ncidod/dhqp/pdf/ar/mdroGuideline2006.pdf (accessed April 21, 2008).

43. Siegel J.D., Rhinehart E., Jackson M., et al. (2007). Guideline for isolation precautions: Preventing transmission of infectious agents in healthcare settings. Available at: www.cdc.gov/ncidod/dhqp/pdf/guidelines/Isolation2007.pdf (accessed April 21, 2008).

44. Muto, C.A., Jernigan, J.H., Ostrowsky, B.E., et al. (2003). SHEA guideline for preventing nosocomial transmission of multidrug-resistant strains of *Staphylococcus aureus* and enterococcus. *Infect Control Hosp Epidemiol* 24(5), 362–86.

# 17

# INVESTIGATIONS IN OUT-OF-HOME CHILD CARE SETTINGS

Ralph L. Cordell
Jonathan Kotch
Michael Vernon

Each weekday morning in the United States, millions of adults go to work in offices, factories, and stores while their preschool children go to some form of out-of-home child care. These facilities range from child care homes, which may care for twelve or fewer children of various ages in one group, to chain-affiliated child care centers, where hundreds of children may be cared for in classes or secondary groups segregated on the basis of age. Regardless of their size or structure, these facilities all provide an opportunity for children to contribute the current strains of microbes circulating within their respective households to a microbial potluck and to acquire new infections that may be brought home and shared with other family members. One result of this process is that child care facilities amplify the prevalence of certain pathogens such as Giardia, Shigella, or hepatitis A within communities. Attempts to control this process by excluding obviously ill children from child care costs billions of dollars in lost productivity each year. Exclusion often drives parents to pressure health care providers to prescribe inappropriate antimicrobials, which contribute to increased antimicrobial resistance. Furthermore, a child excluded from one facility due to illness may be enrolled in another, thus spreading the infection to a new care center.

Nonetheless, there are very real, positive public health aspects to child care. High quality programs have the potential to improve social, cognitive, and behavioral development and prepare children for kindergarten. The enforcement of immunization requirements, especially at the center level, has resulted in higher immunization levels among children in out-of-home child care than among children cared for at home. Quality child care programs also provide training in hygiene and reinforce healthful behavior. Knowledgeable providers are important sources of information on child development and parenting skills, and providers are often the first to recognize developmental problems and to recommend further follow-up.

You and other professionals representing the local health department may interact with child care providers in a number of different capacities. Public health personnel frequently serve as resources for health recommendations and consultation for child care providers. Public health professionals often respond to questions about health and hygiene requirements and practices; assist in developing health and safety policies, programs, and strategies; interpret recommendations and regulations governing exclusion and communicable disease prevention; and provide training to child care staff on health and safety issues. Unfortunately, outbreaks of communicable diseases in child care facilities are a common reason for interactions between local health workers and child care providers. Because of this interaction and the epidemiologist's role in an investigation, you should be aware of some of the unique aspects of the child care environment. This chapter focuses on the detection, response, and control of outbreaks in this setting.

## SURVEILLANCE

As discussed in Chapter 3, surveillance is defined as the ongoing collection, collation, and analysis of information on illnesses in a given population, coupled with timely feedback to those who use it to guide policy and prevention strategies. One of the best descriptions of this system was written more than 50 years ago:

> Our system of notification of individual case reports is a haphazard complex of inter-dependence, cooperation and good will among physicians, nurses, county and State health officials, school teachers, sanitarians, laboratory technicians, secretaries, and clerks. It is a rambling system with variations as numerous as the individual diseases for which reports are requested and, as numerous as the interests and individual traits of the administrative health officers, epidemiologists and statisticians in the 48 States and several Federal agencies concerned with the data. It is a system that depends on persuasion, education, and, in some instances, alarm. *And the variables cannot be eliminated by regimentation and fiat* [emphasis added].[1]

Although those variables still have an impact to a greater or lesser degree—particularly in the child care setting—electronic surveillance systems such as the National Electronic Disease Surveillance System (NEDSS) and the Electronic

Surveillance System for the Early Notification of Community-based Epidemics (ESSENCE) have removed some of the variability in the system and contribute to enhancements in both timeliness and quality of information reported to local public health departments. Additionally, electronic surveillance systems have helped to reduce the reporting burden on providers. These systems have also been a major factor in improving the state and local health departments' abilities to identify and track emerging infectious diseases, outbreaks, disease trends, and potential bioterrorism attacks, and provide early warning and situational awareness of specific disease syndromes (e.g., respiratory, gastrointestinal, etc.) in the community to state and local public health authorities.

The most immediate local use for surveillance in child care facilities is the rapid identification of child care-associated outbreaks or clusters of illness; additionally, children in child care provide an important sentinel for the health of the community at large. A call from a child care center director concerned about the large number of cases of diarrheal illness among children in her facility was one of the earliest indications of the massive outbreak of milk-borne salmonellosis in northeastern Illinois in 1985 (see note 1). Calls from child care facilities also provide an important insight into the incidence of nonreportable conditions in the community, such as fifth disease, hand-foot-and-mouth disease, and respiratory infections.

## Kinds of Surveillance

Surveillance for illness in out-of-home child care facilities may be *indirect* (information about child care-associated illness is obtained from another source— usually through individual case investigations) or *direct* (child care facilities are part of the reporting system).

### Indirect reporting (notifiable disease case investigations)

In many areas, hospitals, laboratories, and other health care providers are required by law to report certain diseases or conditions to local health officials. Reporting requirements (e.g., who is to report and what is to be reported) for this passive reporting system vary by jurisdiction. Most areas require reporting by health care professionals; that is, physicians and other health care professionals. Some, but not all, require reporting by child care providers and schools. In most areas, reports lead to further investigations. These often take the form of telephone interviews of ill persons or, in the case of children, their parents. The purposes of these investigations are to collect basic demographic and descriptive information; identify sources of infection; provide indications for follow-up activities, including isolation or restriction of infected persons or prophylaxis of potentially exposed persons, such as household contacts; and provide health education.

Even in areas with excellent and detailed electronic reporting systems, these single-case investigations provide the opportunity to validate electronic data and are the cornerstone of effective public health surveillance and disease control activities within the child care environment. While they are usually conducted by well-trained staff at local health departments, we would offer the following observations. Parents may be reluctant to discuss specifics of child care arrangements with strangers over the telephone. These fears can often be reduced by explaining the reason for the information and how it will be used. Concerns about the interviewer's affiliation (e.g., "Are you really with the health department?") may be addressed by suggesting the person being interviewed call the health department and then asked to be transferred back to the investigator. Also, the structure and sequence of questions may minimize respondent discomfort and contribute to the accuracy of information. Appendix 17–1 is a composite script drawn from hundreds of interviews conducted by the authors over a period of years and illustrates a sequence and phrasing that we have found to be professional, nonthreatening, and productive in terms of obtaining sensitive information about child care arrangements.

Local health departments should develop a system for keeping track of information from these individual case investigations. This is especially important in programs where several persons are conducting investigations or where information is coming from multiple sources, such as complaints, case investigations, and relicensing inspections. The system should be simple, easy to maintain, readily accessible, and timely. If electronic systems are used, data should be accessible immediately after completion of interviews or investigations. Weekly data entry is of little use in detecting explosive outbreaks such as those caused by shigellosis in child care centers. We have found a note card system that lists the name and address of the facility, illness or problem involved (e.g., Giardia infection), and a record number that allows linkage with the complete case file to be useful. It is a good idea to follow facilities by both name and address as, in the case of chain centers, there may be multiple facilities with the same name and, as may be the case with child care homes, multiple names may be given for the same facility.

## Direct reporting (child care provider–based reporting)

While indirect surveillance involves information from sources other than child care facilities, direct surveillance involves reporting from facilities themselves. The key to effective direct surveillance is maintaining positive working relationships with child care providers and making sure that providers know what to report and how to report it. Child care providers may be concerned about reporting for a number of reasons, including the time constraints, potential loss of revenue, and possible adverse consequences for the reputation of their business. These issues and concerns should be addressed openly and frankly with providers at the outset and every effort made to make participation in the program a positive and rewarding experience. Studies have shown that child care providers are often unaware of reporting requirements and mechanisms.[2] Follow-up studies to this work found that provider knowledge of reporting requirements was greatest in those states where reporting to health departments was required by both public health and licensing statutes (RLC, unpublished data). Periodic contact through training programs (preferably conducted by health department staff and held either at the child care facility or during weekends or evenings), through mailings, or during contacts for other reasons (e.g., licensing inspections) is needed to ensure that providers are aware of the need to report.

Reporting requirements should be worded in language appropriate for child care providers. Vague terms such as "outbreaks" or "unusual occurrences" should be linked with specific examples such as "two or more children with diarrhea in the same classroom within a two-week time period." The average worker in an infant or toddler class probably has more contact with feces in a week than most pediatricians or public health workers experience in a year, and it may be useful to make sure that they realize "diarrhea" includes "the runs," "the loosies," "teething," "food allergies," and all the other euphemisms and explanations that are given for this condition. Time-based criteria such as "three or more loose stools in 24 hours" may be of little use as providers rarely observe children for 24 continuous hours. Two loose stools in the 10–12 hour period in child care may represent four or more loose stools in a 24-hour period. These definitions may also be misinterpreted or disregarded, and we have had at least one provider tell us that "diarrhea" was three or more loose stools in an hour.

Lists of notifiable diseases should include instructions on how and when to report specific conditions and include the telephone number of local and state health authorities who can provide information and assistance, if needed. Diseases should be identified by names familiar to laypersons as well as those used by health care providers. Child care staff often do not have access to specific diagnoses and may need to be encouraged and empowered to obtain this information from parents. However, parents do not always provide accurate information, and we know of more than one instance where health professionals with children admitted they intentionally gave their child care provider inaccurate information about a health condition involving their child.

## OUTBREAK INVESTIGATIONS

Probably the major reason to investigate outbreaks and clusters of illness involving children in child care facilities is to limit the spread of illness in the facility and among household contacts. Other reasons include gaining additional knowledge; training staff in skills and techniques of outbreak investigation; program evaluation and input; and public, political, or legal concerns. The nature and extent of investigative and control activities are also influenced by the severity of the illness, the risk to others, and the likelihood of meaningful intervention. Investigation and follow-up will always be necessary in outbreaks of severe illness such as shigellosis or *Escherichia coli* 0157:H7 infections. At the other extreme, investigating outbreaks of hand-foot-and-mouth disease may have little impact with respect to control but provides significant results in terms of understanding factors involved with the prevention and spread of this infection.

You should have a broad understanding of the variations of clinical expression of the more common diseases seen in child care settings as well as their mode of transmission. The most common organisms spread by the fecal-oral route are: Shigella, Salmonella, Giardia, hepatitis A, rotaviruses, noroviruses, and the enteroviruses. Rhinoviruses, influenza and parainfluenza viruses, *Haemophilus influenzae*, streptococci and, possibly, noroviruses are transmitted via respiratory secretions. Some conditions, like shigellosis, usually cause clinical signs and symptoms and spread easily to contacts in the facility as well as at home. Others, like hepatitis A in children, usually cause no or only mild clinical illness but more frequently cause overt disease in adults. Bacteria, such as *H. influenzae* and *Neisseria meningitidis*, can be carried by children in their nasopharynx, but only rarely will children develop overt disease.

Be aware that outbreak investigations can quickly become emotional, especially in those cases where children are being excluded or illness is severe. Parents of children who are not ill want assurance that their child will not be exposed, and parents of convalescing children want to return to work as soon as possible. Also, pediatricians may be giving conflicting advice, thus making providers feel they have lost control and, therefore, concerned about losing the confidence of the parents of children in their care. In such a setting, your arrival as a confident, competent public health official can easily seem like the cavalry coming over the hill to those in charge of the child care facility.

One of the best tools in your arsenal is a well-developed protocol for dealing with the situation. Although outbreaks are unique events, and it may be difficult to develop a detailed protocol for every possibility, there are a number of general features and considerations in outbreak investigations that benefit from the structure provided by an established protocol. Chapter 5 details a logical progression of investigative steps for most situations, and they are outlined below. However, local conditions will determine their relative importance and order. In some instances, considerable time and resources may be devoted to a particular phase of the investigation, while, in others, the same step may receive very little attention.

Mutual trust and respect is another important tool. Establishing prior relationships with providers through developing training and workshops and serving on advisory committees can promote an understanding of issues and challenges faced by each side in what might otherwise be an adversarial situation. Using standard protocols will give providers a sense of what to expect, ensure equality, and ease their concerns about being singled out for special treatment.

## Prepare for Fieldwork

Consider creating a general protocol that would specify those situations when field visits will definitely be made, situations where field visits may not be necessary, and the administrative personnel and process involved in making those decisions. The protocol should identify the tasks to be undertaken, personnel taking part in the field visit, their respective roles, and persons or groups to be notified prior to the visit. For initial visits involving outbreaks of significant infections, you may find it useful to include a public health nurse and a sanitarian besides yourself, as the epidemiologist, on the field team. Your role would be to interview the director and other staff to obtain the descriptive aspects of the problem—the time, place, and person information. The public health nurse should evaluate child care practices in classrooms involved in the outbreak; and the sanitarian should evaluate the environmental aspects, including food service and the physical plant. This approach focuses multiple talents and skills and allows staff to ask the same questions from different child care employees without seeming distrustful. Before the visit is completed, all three of you should meet, discuss your findings, and agree on follow-up activities. Representatives of child care licensing agencies should always be notified of potential field visits and invited to participate. Materials for specimen collection, sample notification letters for parents (see below), and educational materials for parents and staff should be assembled. It is a good practice to leave educational materials with the facility each time a field visit is made. Facilities do not always have photocopying capability; and misunderstanding can be reduced by using pressure-sensitive paper to document groups to be screened, follow-up activities, and recommendations.

## Establish the Existence of an Outbreak

If criteria for an outbreak have been previously defined in writing, this phase of the investigation would not likely be a major concern, as circumstances either will or will not meet the criteria. Examples of such criteria might include: two or more reports of children with a given illness (e.g., giardiasis) in the same classroom in a one-week period or more than 50% of children with a respiratory illness at any one time. However, it is often important to look for cases of similar disease in the patients' siblings, as child care cases may only represent intra-familial spread, not intra-facility transmission.

Generally, the best sources to help establish the existence of an outbreak include facility records and interviews with parents. While most child care facilities maintain records on attendance, they often do not give reasons for an absence and seldom indicate the nature of any illnesses involved. Information from parents is often unreliable, especially when it involves very mild illness or events more than one week prior to the interview. Moreover, despite the utility of having ready-made protocols and definitions, unusual situations or unpredictable circumstances are bound to arise. Perhaps you may have to create for yourself or others an epidemic curve to show that cases represent an unusual increase. Or you may have to inform parents and facility staff that a single case of a particular disease reflects just the tip of the iceberg and really represents many more unrecognized cases within the facility or possibly elsewhere. In such situations, creativity will be rewarded.

The creation of a clear, well-defined case definition is essential to demonstrating the existence of an outbreak and planning interventions. Case definitions should be written and included in the field notes and final report of every investigation. Case definitions should include time and population criteria as well as clinical or laboratory criteria. Molecular techniques, including determining resistance patterns, serotyping viruses and other isolates, and nucleic acid fingerprinting, can support links between cases and should be used whenever possible.

## Verify the Diagnosis

Verifying the clinical diagnosis of a child care-associated illness may be straightforward or may take considerable time and effort. Outbreaks identified through reports from health care providers usually involve at least one or two laboratory-confirmed cases of the illness in question. Your major task in this instance, then, is to implement effective control measures. Depending on a variety of factors unique to the outbreak, you may need to find and confirm additional cases, so that prevention and control measures can be extended to other groups or households. Outbreaks reported by child care providers and parents are often based only on symptoms. In these instances, determining a specific etiology can be labor-intensive and require specimen collection and laboratory support. The purpose and extent of laboratory testing (e.g., whether it will be restricted to particular classrooms or be facility-wide, or whether it will be restricted to children or include staff) and plans for follow-up of persons found to be infected need to be determined before the first specimen is collected. When the causative agent is not known, the laboratory may have to screen for multiple pathogens. In these instances, a two-stage scheme may be used to initially screen a small, representative group of no more than 10 cases for multiple pathogens to identify the responsible pathogen. Clinical data should be obtained concerning these same 10 children. A larger group can then be screened for the causative agent. Follow-up surveillance may be undertaken to evaluate the effectiveness of these measures.

Informed consent should be obtained before collecting specimens from children in child care settings. Sending consent forms home with children is usually nonproductive unless it is tied with a requirement that children be either screened, or excluded from child care. An alternative is to ask providers, often the director, to get consent from parents or to have field staff on-site get consent from parents during the morning when children are dropped off and in the evening when they are picked up.

Information on types of specimens to be collected, timing, transport media, and other parameters should also be included in the basic protocol. As has been emphasized before, consult the laboratory staff prior to specimen collection and give them information on clinical histories. Although providers can often collect stool specimens from very young children in diapers, specimens from older children may need to be collected by parents at home. In this instance, parents should be provided with written instructions and materials (e.g., specimen containers and swabs) for specimen collection and submission. While it is very difficult to collect blood specimens from children, the process can be made some-what easier with parental support and by using phlebotomists experienced in drawing blood from children. When available, molecular subtyping of isolates of bacterial pathogens may be helpful in defining links between illness in child care facilities and illness in the general community. Also, viruses undoubtedly play a major role in child care-associated outbreaks and, if laboratory expertise is available, viral testing should be considered in any testing requests.

## Orient the Data in Terms of Time, Place, and Person

You should be aware of some problems inherent to the child care setting that make history-taking difficult and that can compromise the validity of your data. Try to get clinical histories from at least a sample of children who are ill. When interviewing a parent about a child's food history or past activities, you may find it advantageous to have the child present during the interview because children have first hand knowledge of the historical events. Mothers are generally better historians than fathers when it comes to the health of children in the household. In instances involving teen mothers, grandmothers are often the best historians.

With respect to time, dates of onset are often difficult to determine. Facility records may not be detailed or accurate. Providers are often not aware of illnesses, because parents may keep ill children at home or illnesses may take place during weekends, vacations, or other periods when children are not scheduled to be in attendance. Precision is nice, but be flexible in your expectations. Onset dates by two- or three-day intervals or even by week, depicted on an epidemic curve, can help in assessing the magnitude of the outbreak and even the mode of transmission.

If there are distinctly different classrooms or locations where cohorts of children spend several hours or more, consider drawing a map, locating each ill child as a spot on the map to help identify areas of high or low risk. It is always a good idea to have a floor plan available so you can get a good idea of the location and movement of children. Even knowledge of airflow patterns can help explain illnesses easily transmitted via the airborne route.

As confounding as the issues just described can be, those relating to age, class, movement of children, and individual contact with cohorts of other children are additional key pieces of information for determining who is at risk. Data from child care-associated outbreaks are usually expressed in terms of classroom-specific attack rates, because age-specific rates will often include children from multiple groups and locations in the center and, thus, be a less useful epidemiologic marker. Groupings are often only loosely associated with age, and their structure depends on facility policies and licensing restrictions. For example, children in a 4-year-old classroom are probably not all 4 years old, and this group may also not include all 4-year-old children in the facility. Facilities commonly pool children from various classrooms early in the morning and late in the afternoon into "drop-off" groups. These groups need to be identified and their attack rates and group characteristics determined separately from classroom groups during regular operating periods. Sibling clusters may also be significant, as they may represent transmission outside the facility and provide a means for illness to spread from one classroom to another.

All these combinations and permutations of the children's attributes in the child care setting behoove you to "dig deep" for useful descriptive data and to be imaginative as well.

## Determine Who Is at Risk

At this time in the investigation you should have a firm diagnosis, a good idea of when and where illness occurred, and who were primarily involved. In the majority of outbreaks this information will give you ample evidence to identify the group primarily at risk of getting sick. The relatively straightforward review of the descriptive data will lead you to those you need to study more and to analyze. Only rarely will you have to resort to analytic methods to identify those at risk (see Chapter 8).

## Develop and Test a Hypothesis That Explains the Outbreak

With a good grasp of who is at risk and how the disease in question is normally transmitted, an epidemiologist should be able to create a scenario of how and why the outbreak occurred. In many instances the explanation is simply common sense and requires no further analysis or thought. Indeed, public health officials frequently act on common-sense hypotheses and limited descriptive data whenever control measures are implemented. However, there will be times when your hypothesis will require more analytic techniques. For example, an outbreak of *E. coli* 0157:H7 might be due to contaminated ground beef served at lunch, to exposure to a farm animal at a petting zoo, to spread of pathogens in a wading pool, or to fecal-oral spread from child to child. The control measures for each of these are obviously different. Analytic methods for most outbreaks are fairly straightforward and can easily be handled with spreadsheets or programs such as Epi Info (see Chapter 7). Staff should be familiar with whatever software packages or methods are used in tabulating or analyzing data. The white heat of a significant outbreak is no time to implement a new software package or data entry system.

Information on the risks associated with specific exposures can be useful in future outbreak investigations. Your hypotheses might include questions about which groups have the highest attack rates and the effectiveness of control measures. For example, it may be useful to compare attack rates among children in drop-off groups with those among children who are not in those groups. While infants and toddlers generally have higher attack rates than older children, comparisons of age-specific or group-specific rates may indicate where control activities should be focused.

## Evaluate the Hypotheses

Whenever possible, try to evaluate and/or confirm your hypotheses. Common-sense premises as well as hypotheses supported by statistical analyses in the field may all seem logical and persuasive; however, if practical, they should be evaluated by both observational and quantitative methods. The demonstration of higher attack rates in a particular classroom is enhanced by observations of inadequate equipment or poor hygiene practices. The importance of direct observation of child care practices cannot be overemphasized. Although caregivers may be especially careful when they know they are being observed, glaring problems can often be detected through observation. In the midst of a Giardia outbreak we have seen providers contaminate sinks with fecal material—sinks that were used for a variety of purposes besides washing diapers. Observations should include how equipment and facilities are actually being used rather than just what is present or absent. When observing operations in infant and toddler rooms, there is a tendency to focus on diaper-changing areas. While this is an obvious source of contamination, interactions among staff, children, and toys in other parts of the room may be more important and should receive as much if not more attention than the diapering table.

Post-intervention surveillance is probably the most critical evaluation of hypotheses generated and tested in conjunction with child care-associated outbreaks. Both parents and providers should be alerted to the need to maintain vigilance and be provided with information on how to report subsequent problems. Public health officials should make periodic contact with the facility for several weeks or months, depending on the nature of the problem, after the completion of interventions and other activities.

## Refine Hypotheses and Carry Out Additional Studies

Post-intervention surveillance may suggest other leads that need to be pursued. This activity may extend the scope of the current investigation by implicating family groups, other classrooms, or other facilities. In other instances, continued surveillance may suggest avenues to follow in future investigations of similar problems. For example, isolation of bacteria from fomites such as plastic toy foods may suggest that these be investigated in more detail in subsequent investigations. In the context of child care outbreak investigations, this step suggests that you should make use of experience and knowledge gained from past investigations and that emergent problems be viewed as opportunities to refine interventions and control strategies.

## Implement Control and Prevention Measures

Implementing control and prevention measures is the goal of a successful outbreak investigation. Most outbreaks resolve of their own accord once the number of susceptible children and staff has been reduced to the point where transmission no longer occurs. Your challenge is to end the outbreak before that point is reached. In many instances, how an intervention is implemented has as much impact on success as which intervention is implemented. Be sure to bring the providers into the decision-making process and keep the parents informed of the progress and findings. A summary list of control measures is presented in Appendix 17–2.

### Informing

*Control* measures are those steps undertaken in response to a particular problem, while *prevention* measures are those that should be in place at all times as part of normal operating conditions. Minimal control activities usually involve informing parents about the situation at the facility. While this is often done using posters or notices placed throughout the facility, a better method is through notices or letters given to parents. Also, these notices or letters often also serve as sources of information for health care providers who may be queried about the situation. These materials should identify the illness, indicate the dates of exposure and groups exposed, describe signs and symptoms of the illness, and give parents recommendations on follow-up activities. The latter may range from keeping ill children at home and notifying the facility to seeking immediate medical attention. Notices or letters should include phone numbers and names of individuals who may be contacted for additional information. In serious situations, specified in protocols, parents may be contacted by local health officials to verify that they were notified and are taking appropriate action.

### Educating

Control measures often include staff education, changes in policies and procedures, and modifications of the physical environment. Depending on the seriousness of the situation and available resources, health department staff may play a role in this training (e.g., by giving on-site training on hand washing or diapering). Specific examples of problem behaviors along with an explanation as to why such behaviors pose problems are useful training tools. Supervision and enforcement of existing policies and procedures are necessary follow-up activities, and post-intervention observation should demonstrate the effectiveness of training. Staff can be asked to explain changes in policies and procedures in order to determine their understanding as well as their implementation of changes. Observations can also verify that recommended physical changes have been made, such as moving diapering surfaces closer to hand washing sinks, installation of towel and soap dispensers, or elimination of wading pools or communal floor mats.

### Cohorting

Except for a few situations, such as those involving mild respiratory illnesses and fifth disease, symptomatic children are generally excluded from child care attendance. Criteria for readmission may range from resolution of symptoms to negative cultures. In situations where multiple children are involved, it may be possible to establish separate cohorts of infected and uninfected children. These are generally groups of children whose symptoms have resolved but who are still excreting a pathogen, most often an enteropathogen, and who are cared for in a group isolated from other children who are not excreting the pathogen. Although its effectiveness has only been systematically evaluated for giardiasis,[3] cohorting has been used to control outbreaks of other enteric illnesses, including shigellosis.[4,5] Guidelines for establishing cohorts should be part of the outbreak investigation protocol. One of the first steps in establishing cohorts is to determine the feasibility of dedicating staff and at least one classroom to the care of these children. Staff and rooms involved in the care of cohorts should not be used for noninfected children until the cohort is dissolved. Special attention should be given to care patterns early in the morning and late in the day when children are often pooled and to minimizing interactions between children in nonclassroom areas during the day. Screening is normally used to identify children infected with a pathogen. A goal should be to screen all children in the affected group and set up the cohorts in as short a period of time as possible. This can be extremely frustrating and requires cooperation from providers and parents. It may be helpful to collect samples on a Friday and have results available on the next Monday. One advantage to the cohort process, however, is that the facility can serve as a focal point for specimen collection and drop-off. Children are generally removed from the cohort and returned to their normal group one at a time once it has been demonstrated that they are no longer excreting the enteropathogen of interest. Eventually only a few children may remain in the cohort. Management of this situation needs to be discussed up front with providers and parents, as it will be difficult for providers to devote resources to one or two children.

There are several reasons why child care facilities are almost never closed by health officials during the course of an outbreak investigation and subsequent control measures. Parents of children in closed facilities may place their children, who may be incubating an infection or asymptomatically excreting a pathogen, in other facilities and thus spread the problem further. As long as they remain open, child care facilities can serve as foci for specimen collection, post-outbreak surveillance, and information dissemination. Once a facility has been closed, these activities become much more complicated and labor intensive. Lastly, we have found that child care providers and parents are much more cooperative and willing to provide information once they have been assured that public health officials are not likely to close their facility. Removal of this threat makes the whole process much more collaborative.

## Communicate the Findings

The last step to an outbreak investigation is to communicate the findings to those who have a need to know. A well-designed protocol should present a plan for communicating findings. At a minimum, a report documenting activities and results should be drafted for department files. The protocol should specify whether copies will be provided to the child care facility, licensing agency, or other governmental bodies. Parents should be considered in the flow of information. Unless there are extremely extenuating circumstances, the flow of information to parents should normally be through the director of the child care facility. However, confidentiality statutes may prohibit the release of medical information to persons other than parents or legal guardians. Therefore, it may be necessary to get permission to release information to the providers. In such instances it can be very helpful to have prior policies and procedures for this situation already in place.

Child care health consultants have been trained specifically to work with providers to develop such policies.

Depending on the seriousness of the situation, the media may take an interest in the investigation. Here again, a protocol can help identify communications pathways. If media attention becomes likely, it is a good idea to notify the child care facility ahead of time. While confidentiality statutes in many areas may prohibit release of information about a facility, parents may notify the media, and a bit of coordination and planning ahead of time may prevent major problems and embarrassment later on.

Lastly, a post-outbreak review of activities should be conducted. The purpose of this review is to determine what worked, what did not work, and how the process can be improved. The results of this review should be used to revise protocols and procedures.

Broader communication with child care facilities may be called for in response to a variety of public health events, such as community-wide outbreaks and emergency planning projects. Although lists from licensing agencies are useful in communicating with child care centers, they are generally incomplete or nonexistent for child care homes. A significant proportion of children in out-of-home child care are in these latter settings (exact numbers depend on definitions), and they need to be included in any communication scheme. Local resource and referral agencies are probably the best way to contact these smaller operations. Communication with the unlicensed, unregistered, informal child care arrangements often found in ethnic neighborhoods can be even more difficult. Messages to these groups may need to be transmitted through local churches or ethnic newspapers targeting these populations.

## SUMMARY

Although no two outbreaks are exactly alike, they all share a number of common aspects, and planning and preparation can make significant differences in the quality of investigations. The establishment and revision as needed of written protocols will help refine the investigative process and avoid many of the problems that arise when working in an emotional climate such as a child care facility in the midst of an outbreak of serious illness. This chapter provides a framework for protocol development. We would add that our society is such that out-of-home child care is a vital commodity that is often in short supply. The vast majority of child care providers take great pride in their work and are committed to the health and well-being of their charges. A collaborative approach to both surveillance and outbreak investigation in this setting is much more likely to be successful in both immediate and long-term goals than one based on authority and confrontation.

## NOTE

1. One of us (RLC) was working with the Cook County Department of Public Health and took this call during the last week of March 1985. The director of a local child care center expressed concern that several children in her facility had an illness diagnosed as "stomach flu" by local physicians. Stool cultures were collected from a sample of ill children. These came back positive for *Salmonella typhimurium*. The director later reported serving a contaminated lot of milk. Subsequent phone calls indicated that staff were also infected, and the facility director eventually voluntarily ceased operations temporarily because so many of her staff and children were ill.

## REFERENCES

1. Sherman, I.L., Langmuir, A.D. (1952). Usefulness of communicable disease reports. *Public Health Rep* 67, 1249–57.
2. Addiss, D.G., Sacks, J.J., Kresnow, M.J., et al. (1994). The compliance of licensed U.S. child care centers with National Health and Safety Performance Standards. *Am J Public Health* 84, 1161–4.
3. Bartlett, A.V., Englender, S.J., Jarvis, B.A., et al. (1991). Controlled trial of *Giardia lamblia:* control strategies in day care centers. *Am J Public Health* 81, 1001–6.
4. Tauxe, R.V., Johnson, K.E., Boase, J.C., et al. (1986). Control of day care shigellosis: a trial of convalescent day care in isolation. *Am J Public Health* 76, 627–30.
5. Mohle-Boetani, J.C., Stapleton, M., Finger, R., et al. (1995). Communitywide shigellosis: control of an outbreak and risk factors in child day-care centers. *Am J Public Health* 85, 812–6.

## APPENDIX 17–1. INTRODUCTORY SCRIPT FOR DISEASE INVESTIGATIONS CONDUCTED BY TELEPHONE INTERVIEWS

1. Verify whom you are speaking with, introduce yourself, and explain the purpose of your call.

   *Hello, is this the _____ residence? Am I speaking with Mrs._____? My name is _____ and I am with the County Health Department. I'm calling about your daughter's recent Giardia infection. Do you have a few minutes to talk with me about it?*

2. Start by asking about illness (e.g., onset, symptoms, etc.). (Interest and knowledge at this stage help validate the nature of your call in addition to confirming information from reporting sources—don't hesitate to ask about discrepancies)

   *Mrs. _____, our records indicate that your daughter became ill on the 10th yet you said she became ill on the 5th? I know it's tough to recall dates several weeks ago, but can you help us determine which is correct?*

3. Determine number of household members.

*Mrs. _____, counting yourself, how many people live in your household?*

4. Get names, ages, and occupations (including child care).

*Would you mind giving me the names and ages of these four people?*

*Do you work outside the home?*

*How about your husband Jim? Does he work outside the home?*

*Now you say Billy is 4 and Suzie is 18 months old. Are they in any sort of child care—baby sitter, or preschool, or other child care program?*

5. Clarify child care and set groundwork for communication with child care facility.

*Mrs. _____, you say Billy and Suzie aren't in day care, yet you and Jim both work. Who looks after the children while you two are at work? Does Ms. _____ come to your home or do you take your children to hers? I see. Does she care for any children other than your own? Does she know Suzie was ill? Do you know if any of the other children have been ill recently? Would you mind if we gave Ms. _____ a call? We may be able to help her keep the other children from becoming sick.*

## APPENDIX 17–2. EXAMPLES OF CONTROL METHODS

- Notify families of the situation at the child care facility.
- Recommend keeping symptomatic children at home.
- Initiate a program to cohort exposed, asymptomatic and convalescent children.
- Recommend that staff limit the number of children they work with and that they work with only a specific group of children.
- Improve hand washing in both staff and children. Supervise hand washing in children and give training on hand washing to staff.
- Clean and disinfect surfaces, toys, or other potential sources for disease transmission.
- Limit treats and snacks for children to those that are commercially prepared and individually wrapped.
- Eliminate potential sources for spread of disease such as wading pools, water tables, dress-up clothes, and communal floor mats.
- Eliminate communal play areas where all age groups congregate during early morning and late hours.
- Be cautious if the child care facility unilaterally implements control measures such as using only bottled water. The public may expect the health department to rescind these measures when there was no valid reason to start them in the first place.

# 18

# FIELD INVESTIGATIONS OF ENVIRONMENTAL EPIDEMICS

Ruth A. Etzel

Environmental epidemics are disease clusters linked to three main categories of agents: (a) pollutants and chemicals such as lead, mercury, and ozone, (b) useful commercial products that enter our environment and may have health implications, such as pesticides and herbicides, and (c) natural toxins that are part of our everyday life, such as toxins produced by molds and dust mites.[1]

Popular films such as *A Civil Action* (1998) and *Erin Brockovich* (1999) have highlighted concerns about environmental epidemics in American society. This chapter describes some of the key considerations when you conduct field investigations of environmental disease clusters. You may view such disease clusters as a bane or an opportunity. You must be able to apply a staged approach to investigation of clusters, spending the most effort on those that offer the greatest opportunity for prevention.

## OVERALL PURPOSES AND METHODOLOGY

The purpose of the field epidemiologist's investigation is to study the relationship between exposure to an environmental agent and health problems in order to determine the source of the disease and the method of spread, and to prevent further diseases from occurring. Environmental investigations allow one to identify new causes of disease, previously unrecognized environmental sources, and new or unusual modes of exposure. Also, investigations of environmental disease may

355

lead to the development of interventions to prevent additional cases of disease. But in some cases, they lead to a dead end. How can you best determine the level of investigation merited by a disease cluster?

## Recognition of a Problem

There are two primary ways that you may be asked to begin an environmental investigation. One is that an unusual environmental emission or measurement occurs, and this leads to a request for an investigation. The second is that an unusual cluster of disease prompts an epidemiologic investigation.

### Environmental release prompts a request for investigation

By far the most common situation that results in recognition of a problem is an event, such as a chemical leak or explosion, or the release of a monitoring result that is of concern to the community because they could be exposed to one or more contaminants. If a large amount of information has been published in the lay literature about the serious health effects from exposure to the contaminant, the public may be greatly concerned. Few things cause citizens to be more irate than the notion that their air, water, or food may be contaminated. At the outset, it may not be clear to you or the investigative team whether the citizens' concerns are appropriate. You or your colleagues might even want to dismiss the public's concerns as trivial. When environmental concerns are raised, commonly, the community starts to divide into two factions: those who consider the situation very dangerous and those who consider it otherwise. This community polarization, which usually occurs in the absence of data, is a serious threat to the investigation. The investigative team must meticulously avoid pretending to know the danger, or lack thereof, when it is still unknown. This may be particularly difficult to do, especially if you think you know the answer, but there is no more important step in gaining trust than admitting the extent of our collective ignorance about environmental hazards and their health effects. Failure to be honest about what we know and don't know may interfere with conducting a thorough assessment and obtaining an adequate history from the community. Just as in the clinical situation your diagnosis can usually made by doing a good history and physical examination, so in the community situation your preliminary assessment requires taking a good history, finding out as much as possible about the emission(s), and reviewing existing information. No prejudgments should be made, lest the community lose trust and decline to cooperate fully.

In emergency situations, the only data available to you may be from routine monitoring done by environmental agencies. An exposure index may have to be developed to guide the investigation. For example, the amount of contaminant in the dirt or the amount of particles in the air can be used as a proxy for actual internal exposure. When a trichlorophenol manufacturing plant near Seveso, in northern Italy, exploded in 1976, a large amount of dioxin was released. Nobody knew how much. Investigators developed models to predict how far the dioxin could have traveled under various wind and weather conditions, and proposed an exposure index. However, this exposure index gave an incomplete picture of the actual exposure, because it did not take into account individual variables such as where each person was at the time of the explosion, their age, the clothing they had on, their consumption of locally grown foods, their contact with soil, and their personal habits, including smoking. Figure 18–1 shows the pathway from chemical emission to potential health effect.

Note that one can conduct exposure assessment methods at every point from the agent to the individual.[2] Most commonly, only an estimate of the emission is available. Based on that estimate and knowledge of the wind speed and direction, one can identify the population at greatest risk and request, if necessary, that they take specific actions such as sheltering in their homes or evacuating the area.

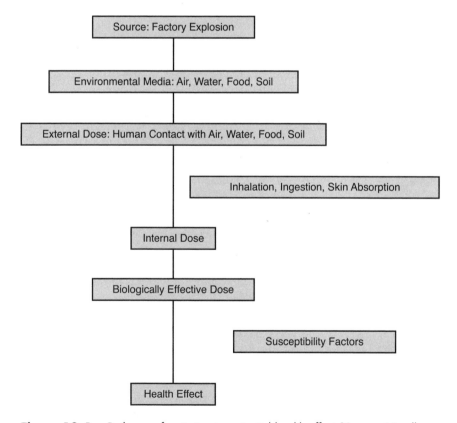

**Figure 18–1.**   Pathway of emission to potential health effect [*Source:* Needham, Gerthoux, et al., 1999.[2]]

Geographic information system (GIS) technology has advanced rapidly in the past decade, and can be useful in your initial assessment. Essentially, a GIS is a powerful computer mapping and analysis technology that allows large quantities of information to be viewed and analyzed within a geographic context.[3] One can estimate, for example, exposure levels to agricultural pesticides for individuals residing or working within defined geographic regions.

### Disease cluster prompts a request for investigation

A second way that the request for investigation may come to you is when a cluster of a disease is noticed by practicing doctors, health officials, community members, or citizens' groups. One of the most well-known requests for assistance in an environmental epidemic, portrayed in the movie *A Civil Action*, was to evaluate a high rate of childhood leukemia in the town of Woburn, Massachusetts. The request was made by a citizens' environmental group founded by a mother whose youngest son died of acute lymphoblastic leukemia. Often such groups are founded and led by parents of affected children or persons who are affected themselves. Citizens' groups may have previously requested assistance from the county or city health officials, to no avail. It is therefore important for you to assure that the county and state health officials are brought to the table to discuss if and how to conduct the field investigation. Because many local and state health departments receive dozens of calls about possible disease clusters each year, and because mounting extensive epidemiologic studies after each call is impractical, guidelines have been developed for investigating clusters.[4, 5]

## INVESTIGATING CLUSTERS OF DISEASE

An evaluation of a reported disease cluster includes four distinct stages. These stages, summarized below, have been extensively described in guidelines published by the New Zealand Ministry of Health.[6] The first stage is to collect preliminary information; the second stage is verification using preexisting records; the third stage is full case ascertainment; and the fourth stage is an epidemiologic study. At each successive stage one assesses more specific information and requires greater verification of the data. The boundaries between these stages are flexible. Depending on local judgment, |experience, and the available resources, you may choose to combine stages. At the end of each stage you must make a decision about whether to proceed further, and how to communicate the results of that decision to the community.

## Stage 1: Collection of Preliminary Information

When one is contacted about a possible disease cluster, detailed questions about the cluster should be asked. You should record the type of condition; the number of people reported to have the condition; the age, gender, and ethnicity of the affected people; the period during which they developed the condition; the location of the cluster; and whether the informant suspects a link to a specific environmental contaminant. After reviewing the preliminary information, a decision about whether to move to Stage 2 must be made. Some criteria for continuing the investigation and moving to Stage 2 include:

1. There are at least three cases of the same condition, or
2. A specific environmental contaminant is suspected as the cause of the cluster, it is biologically plausible, and there is a possible route of exposure.

If one decides not to continue the investigation, a short report should be written and communications made with the informant to advise them of the reasons for the decision.

## Stage 2: Verification Using Preexisting Records

The next step is to confirm the *existence of an epidemic*. Your goal at this stage is to get a quick, rough estimate of the likelihood that a statistically significant excess of the condition has occurred. Review the earlier records to assess whether the reported incidence is different from that in previous months or years, using such sources as existing hospital or clinic records to determine baseline incidence.

Develop an initial case definition and learn about the natural history of the condition, common risk factors, and background rates (if these are readily available). Ask the informant for assistance in gathering additional information. If you can confirm the diagnosis using readily available data, you should do so. *Verifying the diagnosis* may take a great deal of effort, but it is important. Review the records of all cases to confirm the diagnosis. It is ideal if the diagnosis can be pathologically confirmed. If this is not possible, however, one should assume that all reported cases are real. For example, in 1994, when a pediatric pulmonologist in Cleveland requested CDC's assistance to investigate a cluster of cases of acute pulmonary hemorrhage among infants, the diagnosis was confirmed by reviewing laboratory records for evidence of hemosiderin in alveolar macrophages (demonstrated in biopsy specimens or in bronchoalveolar lavage fluid three to six weeks after the initial hemorrhage). Hemosiderin results from the breakdown of red blood cells and is easily visible by light microscopy.

If a specific environmental contaminant is suspected, review the scientific literature and consult with other investigators who have studied that contaminant. Try to find evidence of biologic plausibility, strength, consistency, temporal association, and a dose–response gradient that would support a link between the reported contaminant and the condition. One should calculate preliminary observed vs. expected numbers or age-adjusted rates using preexisting records and community reports. Start by defining an appropriate geographic area and time period in which to study the cluster and determining the most appropriate reference population available using preexisting data. The geographic area and the reference population should be large enough to include all persons at risk of disease. Defining the reference population too narrowly can result in the false identification of a cluster.

For example, in the early 1980s, emergency room doctors in Barcelona, Spain, noticed that sudden increases in emergency room visits for acute severe asthma overwhelmed the emergency services on certain days. On those days, dozens of people appeared in the local emergency rooms with acute exacerbations of asthma. Some people died very suddenly: one man on the steps of the pharmacy where he was going to get his medications. Physicians were puzzled by their observations, so they contacted the local health officials, who were doubly concerned. First, because the city's residents were experiencing asthma attacks in large numbers, and second, because Barcelona had been selected as the venue for the 1992 summer Olympics and there was concern that the athletes and fans also might be felled by asthma attacks. It thus had the potential to become a political as well as a public health problem. To investigate further the impression of the emergency room physicians and to determine the existence of an "epidemic," the health authorities studied emergency room records for asthma visits at each of Barcelona's four large hospital emergency rooms. They documented the place, day, and time when each person seeking emergency room care experienced an asthma attack.

Figure 18–2 shows the daily number of asthma emergency room visits that occurred in Barcelona's hospitals in November and December 1984, by day of admission for persons 14 years and older and for persons under 14 years. This graph demonstrates that the number of visits on November 26 was far greater than expected, confirming the existence of an epidemic. In cluster reports where a specific potential contaminant is suspected, one should conduct a preliminary environmental health assessment. You should go to the site, review existing data including engineering and other land-use records, and review any existing environmental sampling data. At this early stage do not collect new data through environmental sampling, because such sampling is complicated and expensive. If you verify potential exposure sources, take time to consider exposure pathways and biological plausibility of the suspected contaminants. You also should review existing information regarding other risk factors for the condition (e.g., use of tobacco or alcohol). If the index cases cannot be verified or if there is clearly no possible source of exposure to the contaminant, you will probably decide to stop the investigation at this point. Moving to Stage 3 is indicated if you have verified at least five cases of the condition, there is a plausible source of the contaminant, and the investigation is likely to have a public health impact. A cluster linked to an environmental contaminant that has already been cleaned up may not require further study other than to confirm adequate clean-up. A cluster in which data suggest a persistent problem could indicate a need to proceed to Stage 3.

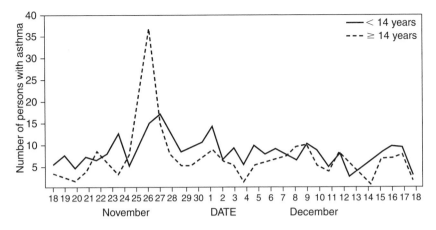

**Figure 18–2.** Daily number of persons treated in Barcelona hospital emergency rooms with acute asthma attacks by day, Barcelona, Spain, 1984. [Adapted from Antó, 1989⁹.]

## Stage 3: Full Case Ascertainment

In this stage one should look for additional unreported cases and verify that they meet the case definition. Review additional databases or medical records or contact the informant to obtain more information from the community. Conduct thorough histories and physical examinations of all the cases that have been identified. Bring a camera to record signs, such as rash that may be fleeting. Bring a variety of clear plastic bags to collect samples of substances that could be important to analyze (see chapter 24).

It is important to decide upon a *case definition* and to collect as many cases as possible. The case definition should be simple and easy to use. In the emergency epidemiologic investigation of acute pulmonary hemorrhage among infants in Cleveland, a *case* was defined as an infant younger than one year who had experienced an episode of acute, diffuse alveolar hemorrhage of unknown cause after discharge from the newborn nursery and who was hospitalized at Rainbow Babies and Children's Hospital during the period from January 1993 to January 1995. Cases were sought by reviewing all hospitalizations of infants under one year during that time and searching for evidence of pathologic confirmation of pulmonary hemosiderosis.

Spread your net very wide, to draw in as many possible cases as you can. This allows you to better assess the full spectrum of the illness. Later you can separate the "true" cases from the probable cases. If you narrow the case definition too soon, it will be very difficult to do any further studies. Note that local people can help spread the word about recruitment and can also help bring in affected people. You can ask state and county medical societies to advise physicians to report cases in their practices.

One should use standard analytic methods such as comparison of rates or the observed and expected number of cases to determine whether there is an excess of cases. "Cases" may be defined as days rather than individuals. For example, in the investigation of epidemic asthma in Barcelona, a day on which the number of admissions was far higher than would be expected by chance and hourly time clustering of cases occurred was called a "case day." Between 1981 and 1987, 1155 emergency department visits by 687 people occurred on 26 asthma "case days," or "epidemic days."

One can find additional analytic techniques in the Agency for Toxic Substances and Disease Registry's software program called CLUSTER Version 3.1. This software can help you determine if there is a statistically significant probability that a cluster occurred other than by chance. It includes 12 statistical methods that analyze the significance of a cluster using techniques that evaluate time, space, and both time and space clustering. Copies of the free software are available for download at http://www.atsdr.cdc.gov/HS/cluster.html. Remember to consider clinical significance as well as statistical significance in deciding how to interpret the results. When the analysis is completed, you must make a decision about undertaking an epidemiologic study or stopping the investigation. An epidemiologic study may not be merited if there is no excess of the condition and no documented exposure, or if there is excess of the condition and no biological plausibility that the excess rate is linked to an environmental contaminant. A full epidemiologic study may be warranted if there is an excess of cases of the condition and a biologically plausible link to an environmental contaminant.

## Stage 4: Epidemiologic Study

### The response team and the responsibilities

If you have gone through the first three stages and decided to conduct an epidemiologic study, you will need to assemble a study team. The team should include people with expertise in epidemiology, toxicology, statistics, laboratory science, and medicine. Depending on the problem under investigation, you may also need to consider industrial hygienists, hydrologists, and engineers. The team should also include representatives from any citizens' environmental groups who are involved, even if they are not professional scientists. A team leader should be designated at the beginning of the investigation. The team leader should be the single point of contact for all information that goes to state and local health officials, unless s/he delegates that responsibility to someone else. Communication with the media should be done by the state and local health department spokespersons. Whenever possible, invite medical students and other professional students to participate as part of their education in public health practice.

In *preparation* for the field investigation and to promote *collaboration*, try to develop strong working alliances with local practicing physicians, university faculty (if the community has a university) and key community groups such as religious and environmental groups. In Alaska Native or American Indian communities, it is important to meet with the tribal leaders and the tribal doctors to request permission to investigate and to discuss the appropriate conduct of the investigation. Because tribes are sovereign nations, if you are investigating an epidemic on reservation land, you must follow proper tribal protocol at all times. The tribe and other individuals in the community will be living with the issue long after you leave the scene, and it is absolutely crucial to engage with them during the initial days of the investigation and to build a relationship of mutual trust.

Requests for investigation of disease clusters may come from practicing doctors, county or city health officials, or state officials. When a practicing doctor calls, s/he may have done some preliminary work on the issue and may have an idea about the cause of the problem. When a pediatric pulmonologist in Cleveland noticed an unusually large number of cases of acute pulmonary hemorrhage admitted to the Rainbow Babies and Children's Hospital, he mapped out the locations of the infants' homes and noted that they were in an inner-city area of Cleveland (see Figure 18–3). He also spoke with parents and grandparents and learned that many of them reported using pesticides in their homes. He therefore developed the hypothesis that the cluster of cases of acute pulmonary hemorrhage was linked to pesticide use in the infants' homes.

Sometimes a community member may have a theory about the cause of the outbreak. This should be listened to respectfully. Discussions with community elders can provide important clues to the cause of the outbreak. In 1993, when a flu-like disease began striking down young, healthy people on and near the Four Corners region of Arizona and New Mexico, a Navajo physician consulted a Navajo medicine man about the apparently new disease. The medicine man told him that the illness was caused by an excess of rainfall, which had caused the pinon trees to bear too much fruit.[7] The medicine man also told him that many years ago such a sickness had occurred. He showed the physician an old photograph of a sand painting with a mouse painted into it and explained that the sand painting had been used by medicine men to treat the illness.[6] This historical information prompted investigators to consider mice and other rodents as possible disease vectors.

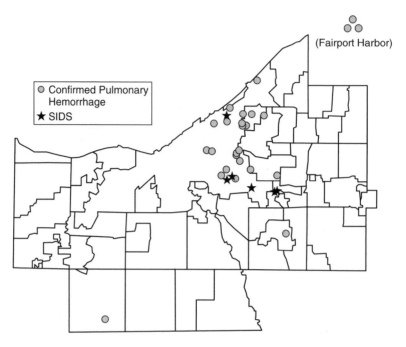

(Fairport Harbor)

○ Confirmed Pulmonary
   Hemorrhage
★ SIDS

**Figure 18-3.** Confirmed cases of pulmonary hemosiderosis and SIDS in infants, January 1993–May 1997, Cleveland metropolitan area and Fairport Harbor, Ohio. [*Source:* Northern Ohio Data & Information Service. The Urban Center, Maxine Goodman Levin College of Urban Affairs, Cleveland State University.]

In the initial days of the response, one may not be sure that the condition is associated with environmental contamination. At first glance, it might look to you and others as if the condition results from exposure to an infectious agent. Keep an open mind. Discuss the problem with infectious disease epidemiologists and environmental epidemiologists. Consider all possibilities in your differential diagnosis. In some cases, practitioners may think first of infectious diseases, only considering environmental contaminants after time has passed. This may be especially true with respect to environmental agents with delayed effects, such as radiation and some chemicals. For example, cases of paralysis may be brought to your attention because a local clinician is seeking botulinum toxin. Before providing botulinum toxin, you should consider chemical causes of paralysis such as acute exposure to thallium or diethylene glycol.

## The Field Investigation

In the investigation, one can get important clues to the cause of the outbreak by characterizing it in terms of time, place, and person. When all the cases have been identified, it is important to assess the *time course* over which they occurred.

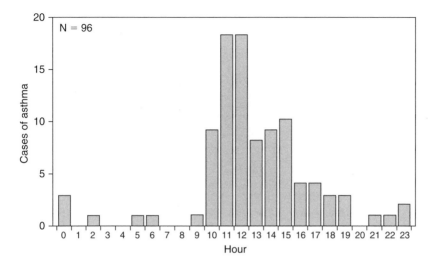

**Figure 18–4.** Number of persons aged 14 years and older treated at Barcelona hospital emergency rooms with acute asthma attacks, by hour, January 20, 1986, Barcelona, Spain. [*Source:* Antó, 1989[9].]

Characterizing the epidemic by drawing an epidemic curve can provide much useful information. Figure 18–4 shows the number of patients aged 14 years and older treated at Barcelona hospital emergency rooms with acute asthma attacks, by hour in Barcelona, Spain, on January 26, 1986. The epidemic curve illustrates that on "case days," most persons experienced their attacks in the middle of the day, primarily between 11:00 a.m. and 1:00 p.m.. This is a curious finding, because persons with asthma usually have attacks at night rather than during the day. This unusual finding prompted the investigators to wonder if people were being exposed to something that was present during the daytime. Additional review of the epidemics of asthma revealed that the "case days" occurred only on weekdays, never on weekends. The investigators hypothesized there might be something occurring during the day on weekdays that was not occurring on weekends.

Mapping the *location* where patients became ill can sometimes give you clues to the cause of the illness. This is especially fruitful when the illness is an acute respiratory condition such as asthma. In Barcelona, geographic mapping of the place where most persons who came to the emergency room with asthma on "epidemic days" experienced their attacks showed that cases were clustered in the city center of Barcelona, near the harbor and near an industrial area. Figure 18–5 shows a map of Barcelona's 12 districts and indicates the rate ratio of age-adjusted

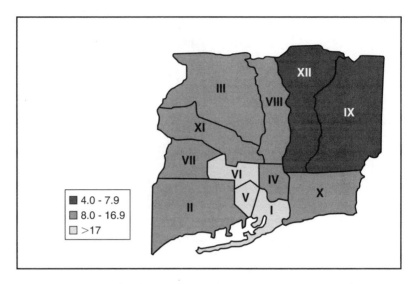

**Figure 18–5.** Map of rate ratio of age adjusted asthma attack rates for 12 asthma outbreaks, by district, Barcelona, Spain, 1984–1986. [*Source:* Antó, 1993[13].]

attack rates in each district. The rate ratio was highest in the three districts near the center of the city and the harbor.

Geographic mapping of asthma cases has been very useful in identifying other point-source asthma outbreaks. For example, in the late 1920s a cluster of asthma affecting 200 patients occurred in Toledo, Ohio.[8] Most affected patients lived within a one-mile radius of a castor bean mill, which also produced linseed oil. Many of the patients claimed that their attacks coincided with the odor of linseed oil from the mill when the wind was in the right direction. Figure 18–6 shows the location of the asthma cases and that of the linseed oil mill. When the health department staff investigated the possibility that linseed oil might be causing the asthma attacks, they found it unlikely because the seed was too heavy to become windborne. The mill, however, not only manufactured linseed oil but also expressed castor oil from castor beans. The castor beans produced a fine dust that was readily carried by the wind into the surrounding neighborhoods.

Even when the condition is not clearly linked to inhalation of air (like asthma), mapping can provide some clues for the astute epidemiologist. For example, when the cluster of cases of acute pulmonary hemorrhage occurred in Cleveland in 1993–1994, one of the first steps in the field investigation was to draw a map of the location of the cases. Figure 18–3 shows that there was a geographic cluster in the city center of Cleveland about three miles from Rainbow Babies and Children's Hospital. This was unusual, because the hospital's

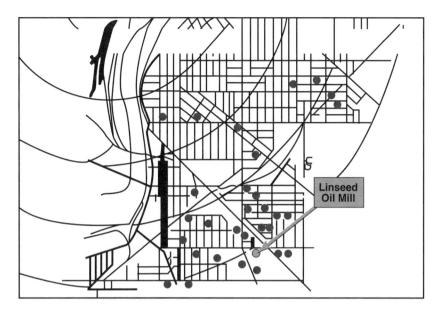

**Figure 18–6.** Map of West Toledo, Ohio, showing location of homes of persons with asthma attacks, West Toledo, Ohio, 1927. The dark dots indicate the location of homes with asthma attacks. [*Source:* Figley, 1928[8].]

catchment area was the entire state of Ohio, so one would have expected the infants' homes to have been scattered throughout the state. This geographic clustering led the investigators to ask additional questions about risk factors associated with the city center.

This geographic clustering was also extremely useful to the investigators in choosing the control group for the investigation. The researchers noted that case infants lived in areas of low socioeconomic status, so they decided to seek control infants only from the same areas. Matching by geographic area can be very important in environmental epidemiologic investigations because exposures to toxicants are usually higher in lower socioeconomic status areas. In studies that fail to match on socioeconomic status, poverty is often identified as a risk factor for the outcome of interest. In fact, poverty is often merely a confounding variable.

Finally, you must evaluate the characteristics of the *persons* affected by the disease. In Barcelona, careful review of Figure 18–2 showed that the asthma epidemic on November 26 occurred primarily among persons 14 years and older. This provided a lead as to the group at risk for the attacks and suggested those with greater opportunity for exposure to the inciting agent. The epidemiologists speculated that those less than 14 years old were likely to be in school, and there were few schools in the city center.

With respect to the 1994 investigation of the cluster of cases of acute pulmonary hemorrhage, a thorough description of the ill infants provided important epidemiologic information. All the case infants were African American and the average age was 10 weeks. This was useful to the investigators because such young infants are not ambulatory and may not spend much time outdoors. This prompted the investigative team to consider a thorough evaluation of the indoor environment.

When defining persons at risk, you should take special care to avoid stigmatizing persons or communities. During the epidemic of flu-like illness in the Four Corners region, some national newspapers began calling the illness the "Navajo plague." This resulted in unfortunate stereotyping of Navajo people, and a summer basketball camp for high school athletes at a nearby large university "disinvited" the contingent of Navajo teenage athletes who had already been invited.

## Assessing the Exposure

The purpose of environmental investigations is to study the relationship between exposure to an environmental agent and health problems. Many investigators go to great lengths to study the health problem but spend much less effort studying the environmental exposures. A major challenge facing you in conducting an environmental investigation is the difficulty and cost of obtaining accurate exposure information. Another challenge is that you may feel far more capable of assessing medical records and patient health status than of understanding environmental reports of chemical contaminant concentrations in air, water, or soil. Nonetheless, an adequate investigation demands that you partner with experts or develop enough proficiency to do a competent evaluation of such environmental data.

There are several ways to get a handle on environmental exposures. You can look at records of emissions from factories and other establishments. You can get a rough assessment of external dose by measuring air, water, food, or soil concentrations of the contaminant(s) to which people may be exposed. You should try to get measurements of contaminants in the environment, even though the time since the cases presented may be several weeks. This is because many environmental contaminants, such as dioxins, can persist in the environment for a long time, sometimes many years. You should attempt to get some biological measurement from blood, urine, or other tissues from cases and controls because this gives an assessment of internal dose of the contaminant. If, however, measures of contamination in human tissues cannot be obtained, then use whatever proxy measurements are available.

When unplanned chemical discharges or emissions occur, it is very important to collect specimens for future analyses. Shortly after the 1976 explosion near Seveso, for example, an Italian pathologist had the foresight to begin collecting extra samples of blood during medical examinations of people who were being evacuated from the affected area. At that time it was not possible to measure dioxins in serum. In the late 1980s, the technology to measure dioxins in small samples of serum became available, and the CDC laboratory was able to analyze the specimens collected during 1976–1977 and to validate the exposures that the pathologist and others had mapped out based on where people lived at the time of the release.[2]

If the suspected contaminant is airborne, industrial hygienists can help you develop methods to take samples of indoor air using table-top sampling and personal monitoring. In the 1994 investigation of infant pulmonary hemorrhage in Cleveland, a team of industrial hygienists and epidemiologists went to homes of case infants and controls to collect samples of the indoor air using Gillian personal sampling pumps, and to sample environmental surfaces for the presence of organophosphate, carbamate, and pyrethrin classes of insecticides. These persist in the indoor environment for months after application.

## Assessing Contaminants in Human Tissues

Chapter 24 describes laboratory support for the epidemiologist in the field, including descriptions of how to collect and send samples of human tissue for measurement of contaminants. Environmental health laboratories can analyze human samples for hundreds of contaminants, but the time to conduct the analyses may be lengthy and the cost of such analyses can be prohibitive. Sometimes exposure to contaminants can be rapidly assessed using simpler techniques such as light microscopy. For example, state health officials in Florida were notified of a family in which a woman and her two sons developed severe pain and paresthesias of the hands and paralysis of the lower extremities. The health department considered botulism, but noted that that the presentation was not classical, because botulism typically produces a descending paralysis. Two weeks later the patient developed alopecia. Could she have some other disease? Other possibilities needed to be considered. Thallium poisoning and diethylene glycol poisoning can each cause an ascending paralysis, but only thallium causes alopecia. To evaluate whether she might have thallium poisoning, the investigators suggested that a sample of the patient's hair be examined under a light microscope. Indeed, the root of the hair showed dense black coloration, a tell-tale sign of thallium poisoning. With chronic exposure, the root can look striped. This led investigators to refocus the investigations on ways that the patient might have ingested thallium.

Another inexpensive and useful clue to the possible role of environmental toxins is hemolysis on the peripheral blood smear. This tell-tale clue may disappear shortly after admission to a hospital because exposure to the toxin usually ceases at that time.

## DEVELOPING AND TESTING HYPOTHESES

When you have evaluated the data by time, place and person, you should develop and test a hypothesis. In situations where the disease is uncommon, the ideal approach is to test the hypothesis using a case control study design. Rarely is sufficient information available to conduct a historical cohort study, but when historical data can be obtained, you should conduct a cohort study (see Chapter 8). For example, as previously mentioned, the time–space clustering led the investigators in Barcelona to suspect that the asthma attacks might be linked to something being loaded or unloaded from ships in the harbor. They identified 26 asthma "epidemic days," and then performed a study in which "epidemic days" were days on which epidemics of asthma occurred in Barcelona, and "non-epidemic days" were days without epidemics of asthma. In this historical cohort study, they collected information about unloading of 26 products from ships in the Barcelona harbor and a variety of risk factors, including temperature and wind speed and direction. Barcelona has the second busiest harbor in the Mediterranean, and after studying each of the products loaded or unloaded from ships, they determined that the outbreaks of asthma were associated with the unloading of soybeans at the city harbor.[9] Table 18–1 shows a two-by-two table with the results.

The initial hypothesis to explain the cluster of infants with acute pulmonary hemorrhage in Cleveland was that insecticides were a factor associated with pulmonary hemorrhage. This hypothesis was generated by a local pediatric pulmonologist after taking careful environmental histories from many parents and grandparents of the affected infants. To test this hypothesis, a case control study was designed. In addition to measuring pesticides on bedroom surfaces, samples of urine from case and control infants were tested to look for organophosphate, carbamate, and pyrethrin pesticide residues.

**Table 18–1.** Two-by-Two Table Showing the Association Between Asthma "Epidemic Days" and Soybean Unloading in the Barcelona Harbor, 1985–1986

|  |  | UNLOADING SOYBEANS | | |
|---|---|---|---|---|
|  |  | YES | NO |  |
| Asthma | Yes | 13 | 0 | 13 |
| "Epidemic Day" | No | 249 | 468 | 717 |
|  | Total | 262 | 468 | 730 |

Odds Ratio: unquantifiably high
95% CI: 7.17—unquantifiably high
*Source:* Adapted from Antó, 1989.[9]

Examples such as the epidemic of asthma in Barcelona and the cluster of cases of infant pulmonary hemorrhage in Cleveland demonstrate the enormous advantage of having accurate and detailed information on time, place and person. Not all epidemics are as well characterized. This is particularly true of outbreaks that are not acute in nature, in which the numbers of cases are small, estimates of exposure in the cases and controls are crude and/or unknown, appearance of disease is delayed, and place of exposure is uncertain. When diseases with long latency periods are being studied, characterization of place may be complicated by the fact that the current residence may not be the same as the residence at time of diagnosis. If possible, you should collect data on the person's current residence and other residences for the past 20 years, as well as length of residence in each home or neighborhood. It might be necessary to collect environmental records from several different cities or neighborhoods to get a full picture of a person's exposures. Assessment of past exposures for studies of diseases with long latency can be facilitated by running analyses for contaminants in serum or tissue stored in existing specimen banks. Unfortunately, a specific etiologic agent cannot be identified in many non-infectious disease clusters. This may be because environmental samples and clinical specimens have not been collected at an appropriate time, have not been examined for the appropriate chemical or toxin, or have not been analyzed in a laboratory with the capability of assessing low levels of environmental contaminants in human tissue.

## Compare the Hypothesis with the Established Facts

The results of your statistical analysis will either support or fail to support your hypothesis. Beware of asserting that your hypothesis is "proven" or "disproven." Hypotheses are never "proven" or "disproven." Through hypotheses, theoretical propositions can be tested in the real world. The investigator can then advance scientific knowledge by supporting or failing to support the tested theory.

When you have collected your data, completed preliminary analyses, and formulated some ideas about how the condition might be linked to exposure to an environmental contaminant, step back and review whether it all hangs together in a way that makes sense. Do the route of exposure, the symptoms, and the time course make sense given what is known about the condition and the contaminant? In Barcelona, for example, health officials had to ask themselves whether a scenario that involved inhalation of soybean dust released from silos during unloading of ships at the harbor causing acute asthma attacks was plausible. Although few cases of soybean asthma had been previously reported, the association was deemed biologically plausible.

On the other hand, in the 1994 investigation of pulmonary hemorrhage in Cleveland, the sampling of indoor air and surfaces in homes did not demonstrate a significant difference between case and control infants with respect to levels of pesticides in the indoor air and surfaces of their homes.[10] Analyses of urine samples from case and control infants were at or below the level of detection. Thus, there was insufficient evidence to support the hypothesis that exposure to pesticides was linked to infant pulmonary hemorrhage. The researchers needed to step back and evaluate additional possible hypotheses for the problem.

## Plan a More Systematic Study

After the initial study, you may need to do more investigation to clarify the route of exposure or the risk factors identified in the field study. If your data support your hypothesis, you will want to do additional work to find out, for example, the mechanism by which the exposure relates to the condition under study. In Barcelona, to confirm the mechanism of disease, a case control study was undertaken. The investigators studied whether patients who came to emergency rooms on "epidemic days" had higher levels of anti-soybean immunoglobulin E (IgE) antibodies than individually matched controls who came to emergency rooms on "non-epidemic days." They found that 74.4% of those who came on "epidemic days" had a reaction with commercial soybean antigen extracts, compared with 4.6% of controls (odds ratio = 61, lower 95% confidence limit = 8.1). The statistical significance was greater for reactions with extracts of soybean dust taken from Barcelona harbor.[11] These results further supported the idea that there was an association between the release of dust during unloading of soybeans at the harbor and the occurrence of asthma outbreaks.

If your data do not support your hypothesis, more study is needed. For example, because the data did not support pesticide exposure as a risk factor for acute pulmonary hemorrhage in infants, a new hypothesis was suggested and tested in a second field study in Cleveland. The new hypothesis was that pulmonary hemorrhage was linked to exposures to *Stachybotrys* and other toxigenic fungi in water-damaged indoor environments. Data collected in a case control study supported this hypothesis.[12] In epidemiology, however, a single study is never definitive. Additional studies are needed to determine whether the association between infant pulmonary hemorrhage and exposure to toxigenic fungi is causal.

## IMPLEMENT CONTROL AND PREVENTION MEASURES

The ultimate reason that you undertake an investigation is to find a way to control the epidemic and prevent future disease from occurring. You must take appropriate action—depending on the type and degree of contamination and the estimated extent of the contamination—to stop the epidemic. Sometimes this involves taking immediate steps to close an establishment or alter its operations. The asthma outbreak in Toledo, for example, was documented to have been associated with the inhalation of castor bean grinding dust. After the factory stopped processing castor beans, the asthma epidemic disappeared. In Barcelona in 1997 health authorities required that bag filters be placed on the silos, reducing the amount of soybean dust emitted into the ambient air while soybeans were unloaded from ships. No further epidemics of asthma were reported in Barcelona.[13] In Cleveland, after pulmonary hemorrhage was linked to exposures to moldy home environments, health officials recommended that infants with pulmonary hemorrhage be removed from moldy homes. Before the recommendation to move, 5 of 7 infants had recurrent pulmonary hemorrhage; after the recommendation to move, 1 of 21 had recurrent pulmonary hemorrhage.[14]

If food is implicated in an epidemic, you may need to work with the manufacturer to recall the epidemiologically implicated lot(s). It may be necessary to stop distribution and hold the food in locked facilities until it is tested and released, or removed. For each product responsible for outbreaks, thoroughly evaluate the mode of transmission before reprocessing or converting to animal food. This is crucially important to insure that foods contaminated with toxins will not recur in the human food chain.

You may encounter problems when you try to implement measures to prevent additional cases because closing industries and recalling products puts an unexpected financial burden on the industry. If there is evidence of an association between exposure to an environmental contaminant and a disease, however, you should take applicable precautionary action to stop the spread of the contaminant. When contemplating precautionary action, consider the severity of the disease, the mechanism of contamination, and the availability of alternate sources of air, water, or food. The Precautionary Principle holds that "when an activity raises threat of harm to human health or the environment, precautionary measures should be taken even if some cause and effect relationships are not fully established." To quote Sir Austin Bradford Hill, "The evidence is there to be judged by its merits and the judgement (in that sense) should be utterly independent of what hangs upon it—or who hangs because of it."[15]

In *An Enemy of the People*, Henrik Ibsen described the dilemma faced by the doctor who discovers that his city's baths are contaminated; he is shunned by neighbors and colleagues and loses his job.[16] This scenario is not unfamiliar to environmental epidemiologists. While there is no lobby in support of asthma or arthritis, there are very powerful lobbies in support of lead, pesticides, and other chemical products. If your study implicates any of these products, you should be prepared to be raked over the coals by the industry-sponsored critics who will claim that your case is not yet proven and that action should be delayed. But as Sir Austin Bradford Hill stated, "all scientific work is incomplete—whether it be observational or experimental. All scientific work is liable to be upset or modified by advancing knowledge. This does not confer upon us a freedom to ignore the knowledge we already have, or to postpone the action that it appears to demand at a given time."[15]

## SUMMARY

Field investigations of environmental epidemics pose many difficulties for public health officials. This is particularly true of clusters of chronic diseases, in which the numbers of cases are small, estimates of exposure in the cases and controls are crude and/or unknown, appearance of disease is delayed, and place of exposure is uncertain. There are four distinct stages for evaluating such clusters. Environmental epidemics allow you to identify new causes of disease, previously unrecognized environmental sources, and new or unusual modes of exposure. Also, investigations of environmental disease may lead to the development of interventions to prevent additional cases of disease.

## REFERENCES

1. National Institute for Environmental Health Sciences (2006). 2006–2011 Strategic Plan: New Frontiers in Environmental Sciences and Human Health, p. 4. http://www.niehs.nih.gov/external/plan2006
2. Needham, L.L., Gerthoux, P.M., et al. (1999) Exposure assessment: Serum levels of TCDD in Sereso, Italy. *Environmental Research* Section A 80, S200–S206.
3. Vine, M.F., Degnan, D., Hanchette, C. (1997). Geographic information systems: their use in environmental epidemiologic research. *Environmental Health Perspectives* 105(6), 598–605
4. Washington State Department of Health (2001). Guidelines for investigating clusters of chronic disease and adverse birth outcomes. Washington State Department of Health, Olympia, Washington.
5. Alexander, F.E., Boyle, P. (eds). (1996). Methods for investigating localized clustering of disease. *IARC Scientific Publications* No.135. International Agency for Research on Cancer, Lyon, France.
6. New Zealand Ministry of Health (1997). Investigating Clusters of Non-Communicable Disease: Guidelines for Public Health Services. Wellington, New Zealand.
7. Arviso Alvord, L., Cohen Van Pelt, E. (1999). *The Scalpel and the Silver Bear: The First Navajo Women Surgeon Combines Western Medicine and Traditional Healing* Bantam Books, New York.
8. Figley, K.L., Elrod, R.H. (1928). Epidemic asthma due to castor bean dust. *J Am Med Assoc* 90, 79–82.
9. Antó, J.M., Sunyer, J., Rodriguez-Roisin, R., et al. (1989). Community outbreaks of asthma associated with inhalation of soybean dust. *N Engl J Med* 320, 1097–102.

10. Montaña, E., Etzel, R.A., Allan, T., et al. (1997). Environmental risk factors associated with pediatric idiopathic pulmonary hemorrhage and hemosiderosis in a Cleveland community. *Pediatrics* 99(1). http://www.pediatrics.org/cgi/content/full/99/1/e5.
11. Sunyer, J., Antó, J.M., Modrigo, M.J., et al. (1989). Case-control study of serum immunoglobulin-E antibodies reactive with soybean in epidemic asthma. *Lancet* 1(8631), 179–82.
12. Etzel, R.A., Montaña, E., Sorenson, W.G., et al. (1998). Acute pulmonary hemorrhage in infants associated with exposure to *Stachybotrys atra* and other fungi. *Arch Pediatr Adolesc Med*; 152: 757–62.
13. Antó, J.M., Sunyer, J., Reed, C.E., et al. (1993). Preventing asthma epidemics due to soybeans by dust-control measures. *N Engl J Med* 329, 1760–3.
14. Dearborn, D.G., Smith, P.G., Dahms, B.B., et al. (2002). Clinical profile of 30 infants with acute pulmonary hemorrhage in Cleveland. *Pediatrics* 110, 627–37.
15. Hill, A.B. (1965). The environment and disease: association or causation? *Proc R Soc Med* 58, 295–300.
16. Ibsen, H. (1977) *An Enemy of the People*, adapted by Arthur Miller. Penguin Plays: New York.

# 19

## FIELD INVESTIGATIONS OF OCCUPATIONAL DISEASE AND INJURY

William Halperin
Douglas Trout

In earlier chapters of this book the majority of discussion has concentrated on field investigations of acute and mostly infectious disease problems. For the most part, the operational and epidemiological tools and methods that have been described are relatively simple, straightforward, and complementary: the request for help; the local social and political scene; and the "players" involved generally seem logical, understandable, predictable, and cooperative. Moreover, you, the field investigator, will usually know or have a good idea of the clinical, laboratory, and epidemiological characteristics of the disease under study. To be sure, in some instances you will not. But this simply makes the investigation more challenging and frequently more difficult.

Imagine now an industrial setting where you may never have set foot before, where you have few or no technical skills and little understanding of the manufacturing process, where there are often many social "agendas" playing off of each other and you, and where your investigation may be subsequently faulted as biased because of real or perceived allegiances. Furthermore, very often in this scenario you will not know what is the responsible agent; whether it is an agent used in production, a contaminant, or a product; where it came from, how workers were exposed; or other critical clinical and epidemiological aspects of the condition. Lastly, your performance of operational and epidemiologic functions may be significantly compromised because their conflicting forces can limit studies, muddy interpretation, and jeopardize valid conclusions.

Welcome, then, to the arena of occupational disease and injury—a highly challenging and difficult world, a world requiring not only great operational and technical skills, but, in may ways, for the field epidemiologist, a very different mindset.

## PREPARATIONS FOR THE INVESTIGATIONS

### The Request for Assistance

The request for assistance may come from a variety of sources and entail several different kinds of investigations. State and local health officials may be notified of a possible problem by health care providers; by one or more workers, who feel there is a health problem in the workplace; by management requesting an evaluation; by union representatives; or by a federal agency that needs support from local sources. Because of statutory and legal considerations, particularly at the federal level, agencies such as the Occupational Safety and Health Administration (OSHA) and the National Institute for Occupational Safety and Health (NIOSH) can and do perform investigations independently of other health agencies. Regardless of the source of the request and even your possible involvement in the field investigation, you, as a field epidemiologist, should have a good understanding of both the operational and epidemiological imperatives for a successful investigation in the workplace.

### The Right of Entry

You must know the legal basis for conducting a study in the workplace, otherwise known as the *right of entry*. Right of entry concerns one's ability to review records, to conduct interviews, to examine workers, to measure levels of exposure, and to perform all other aspects of a field investigation. A successful challenge to your right of entry will not only prevent completing an investigation, but may also result in a great deal of lost time and effort, as the legal challenge may only come after the groundwork and preparation for the site visit has been completed.

Right of entry is idiosyncratic to the auspices under which the investigation is being conducted. State health departments may or may not have specialized regulations for investigations of the worksite or may base their actions on general rights and responsibilities incurred in protecting the public's health. NIOSH's right of entry for responding to requests from workers or management is spelled out in federal regulations. An epidemiologist working for OSHA would also have a legal foundation for entry.

The auspices under which the investigation is conducted will determine whether workers have a right to be interviewed and examined in private, whether the information will be kept confidential, whether the workers will be compensated when away from their jobs, and whether there is a basis for preventing possible retribution for participation.

Epidemiologists who are not working under a governmental umbrella may find that they have no legal basis for investigation at the worksite and are dependent on a commitment of all parties to do what is necessary for the goal of prevention or on a negotiated agreement between management and labor.

## Trade Secrets

Maintaining trade secrets is a serious consideration when conducting studies in the workplace. Trade secrets include such things as ingredients, processes, or other intellectual material developed by a company that provide it a legitimate advantage over commercial competitors not privy to that information. You have two quite different considerations concerning trade secrets. One consideration is to protect against purposefully or inadvertently divulging a legitimate trade secret. The best thing to do here is to ask the company to identify any trade secret information when and if it is provided to you. The second consideration is how to respond to an intransigent company that claims that everything up to and including the names of management officials are trade secrets. These issues are often better dealt with by those who specialize in the law, rather than in epidemiology. However, you should be forewarned so as not to enter into agreements that can not be undone.

## Signing Contracts

It is not unusual for you to be asked to sign contractual documents before entering the workplace. Some documents will concern issues of liability regarding possible injury to you and your obligation to comply with health and safety requirements like wearing personal protective equipment such as hard hats and eye protectors. Other documents may concern the dissemination of results contingent upon review and approval. Earnest investigators have sometimes found themselves precluded from publishing information of public health value because of restrictions to which they agreed.

## Comportment in the Field: Maintaining a Tripartite Relationship

Success in field epidemiology depends in part on technical skills and part on social and interpersonal skills. You should not assume that the interests of the workers in the local workforce are consistent with local management, or that local interests are consistent with national management of either the union, if there is one, or the employer, if they are a national or international company. Similarly, interests of the medical department or the engineering department, may be quite different from the legal department which in turn may have different motivations from the insurers. All industries and unions are complex organizations that you, the epidemiologist, a newcomer to the scene, have very little chance of truly understanding.

One effective approach to working with a diverse set of partners in the workplace is to establish early on a tripartite group consisting of the investigative team, representatives of labor, and representatives of management. All of them should be openly informed about all aspects of the study from design through interpretation and conveyance of results to the affected workers. In addition, in more controversial situations, you may want to establish a professional advisory panel of experts in epidemiology, exposure assessment, or toxicology, for example, who can offer technical advice on the conduct of the study. Your overriding commitment must be the protection of the health of the workforce. While this sounds fairly reasonable, be forewarned that epidemiologic questions in the workplace often have huge economic consequences, and one side or the other may have disproportionate resources to offer (e.g., participation by expert consultant epidemiologists and the like) making it difficult to maintain either the perception or the reality of evenhandedness between labor and management. Needless to say, evenhandedness in dealing with labor and management should not be equated to evenhandedness in protection of workers' health versus protection of commerce, because your role, as a health professional, is protection of health.

## Be Realistic and Open about the Consequences of an Epidemiological Investigation

The realistic and experienced epidemiologist understands that investigations often do not provide satisfying answers to the basic questions of whether there is a problem of occupational etiology in the workforce. This is particularly true of cluster investigations, but it is also true of preplanned large-scale cohort studies searching for an association between exposure and outcome. It is best to communicate the possibility of both success and failure to labor and management throughout the investigation so that expectations are not unreasonable when a final report is delivered. Labor and management can contribute by helping to provide or facilitate your realistic communication to the workforce throughout the investigation.

You should also not contribute to the misconception that management or labor leadership may have about the consequences of epidemiologic studies. While it is immutable that the goal of epidemiology is prevention, the consequences of learning the epidemiologic truth may result in adverse consequences for labor and/or management. In the short term, regulatory or enforcement actions may be initiated and lawsuits may well be generated. There may be additional production costs such as re-engineering of the manufacturing process or altering the architecture of the workplace. However, in the long term, there may be reduced morbidity and reduced operating expenses as the newer processes become safer and more efficient. Industrial processes that lose feedstock chemicals or the products of the manufacturing process into the work environment are wasting money for the employer as well as endangering the workers.

## Participation of Company, Union, Newspaper, or Voluntary Organizations in Data Collection

Tight budgets for field research, limited availability of skilled personnel, and other limitations make it very attractive to accept help in conducting an investigation. The help may come in the form of assistance such as collecting and copying company records or abstracting records for histories of exposure. Many employers and unions may have epidemiologists who are willing to contribute their efforts by helping in the review of records, analysis of data, and the formulation of reports. You need to exert strict control of the data and analysis in order to insure that bias and the appearance of bias are prevented. The introduction of bias can be subtle. For example, enthusiastic employees or volunteers using open-ended questions about exposure and disease may exert added effort to elicit responses consistent with their preconceived assessment of the likely association.

## Notification of Results

Those preparing for an investigation should be aware of the need to protect the rights of individuals who might be involved in the investigation (see Chapter 14). Among the important issues considered by human subject review boards (HSRBs) or institutional review boards (IRBs) are issues related to informed consent and notification of results. Consider the issue of notification of employees of the results of epidemiologic studies early in the planning phase for the study. In this context there are two types of notification, personal and group. Individuals who participate in medical studies such as blood tests and pulmonary function tests should receive an individualized explanation of their results. How the results of epidemiologic analyses are handled depends upon the importance of these findings to the study subjects, who then have personal decisions to make. On the other hand, you are also obliged to inform other cohort subjects of more ambiguous results, even if they were not voluntary participants in a study, but only members of a historical cohort that was the subject of an epidemiologic study in which there was no contact between the investigator and the cohort member. At a minimum, study results that have little if any practical impact on any conceivable decision making by the cohort member could be communicated through town meetings, local newspapers, or company newsletters. An example would be communicating via the news media of the completion of a cohort mortality study in which no excess risk of mortality was observed. At the other extreme, substantial effort should be made to contact and inform persons who could take effective preventive action, if they had access to the new information that your studies provide. For example, workers appropriately notified of an excess risk of bladder cancer, associated with a previously unrecognized bladder carcinogen, should be personally notified, as they may benefit from clinical intervention.

## KINDS OF STUDIES IN THE WORKPLACE

There are four main circumstances in which an epidemiologist will be asked to conduct an investigation in a workplace. These are:

1. Investigation of one or more cases of previously recognized occupational disease or injury
2. Investigation of one, few, or many cases of disease or injury that are not well recognized as occupationally related
3. Determination of whether exposure is associated with an adverse health outcome
4. Evaluation of the effectiveness of an intervention.

### Investigation of Cases of Known Occupational Etiology

#### Case study

A nurse epidemiologist conducting surveillance in hospital emergency departments for cases of occupational agricultural disease and injury found several cases of carbon monoxide poisoning among farmers who used gas-powered high-pressure water sprayers for cleaning hog pens. Carbon monoxide poisoning is a well-recognized preventable occupational disease; however, its relationship to hog farming was not initially apparent. Investigation revealed that farmers kept their hogs indoors in cold weather and cleaned the barns of offal with gas-powered high-pressure water sprayers. Case finding led to the identification of other cases in hog farmers and later to the recognition of the carbon monoxide hazard of water sprayers when used indoors, particularly after flooding from heavy rains. An experiment in a typical home car garage in which a water sprayer was operated indoors showed that no degree of ventilation through windows and doors—even using fans—could prevent accumulation of dangerous levels of carbon monoxide.

Information on the hazards of indoor use of gas-powered water sprayers and other gas-powered equipment is now circulated periodically by NIOSH, the Consumer Product Safety Commission, and other groups. Also special public service announcements warning of these hazards are made after regional flooding.

The framework for investigation of cases of known occupational etiology was established in the 1980s by David Rutstein, Professor Emeritus at Harvard Medical School and colleagues at NIOSH. They developed the concept of the Sentinel Health Event (Occupational), SHE(O).[1] A SHE(O) is defined as an unnecessary disease, disability, or untimely death that is occupationally related and whose occurrence provides evidence that there has been a failure of prevention. These failures can be used to characterize the magnitude and trends of a problem such as industrial lead poisoning. They can also be used on a case-by-case basis as an impetus for defining what failures are responsible for a particular case and for developing interventions to remedy those particular failures. For example, an adult case of lead poisoning is a SHE(O) because the case represents a failure of prevention. The failure may have been because of inadequate use of substitute materials, inadequate ventilation, inappropriate personal protective equipment (e.g., a respirator), or inappropriate medical management (e.g., failure of medical monitoring and medical removal from exposure). Your role, as an epidemiologist in investigations of sentinel health events, is to assist in the recognition of such events; to participate in their evaluation, usually with the aid of an industrial hygienist; to arrange for appropriate interventions; and to summarize and disseminate appropriate information to prevent similar cases elsewhere. Examples of SHE(O) include lead encephalopathy in workers exposed to lead in radiator repair or battery reclamation; leukemia in workers exposed to benzene; and silicosis among workers in foundries. A SHE(O) list for occupational injuries, work-related musculoskeletal syndromes, and psychological outcomes has not yet been developed. The concept of sentinel health events is not limited to occupational exposures, but characterizes much of what field epidemiologists and public health professionals do; namely, investigate individual cases and small clusters of other preventable conditions. This is in considerable contrast to performing analytic studies in much larger populations.

A pragmatic framework for investigation of one or more cases of a SHE(O) is an appreciation that in the workplace, effective prevention is based upon the implementation of a *hierarchy of prevention*.[2] The essential three elements of the hierarchy are primary, secondary, and tertiary prevention. Primary prevention includes techniques aimed at preventing the disease or injury process before there is a pathological effect. Secondary prevention entails early detection of disease or injury before signs and/or symptoms appear, when it is presumably more easily treated. Tertiary prevention involves application of clinical care and rehabilitation.

Assessing the hierarchy of prevention is important to you, as the investigator, to determine if there has been a failure in prevention and to ascertain if you have successfully communicated to both the workers and the employers the greater effectiveness of primary over secondary over tertiary prevention.

The cascade of techniques in the hierarchy of prevention for occupational disease includes the following examples: (*1*) Primary: pre-market testing of feedstock chemicals; substitution of less for more toxic feedstock chemicals; engineering controls, such as enclosed systems; environmental monitoring to insure engineering effectiveness; and personal protective devices if engineering controls are not adequate. (*2*) Secondary: periodic biological monitoring for absorption of toxins, periodic medical examination for early signs or symptoms of intoxication, and early medical diagnosis of disease. (*3*) Tertiary: appropriate therapy and rehabilitation. The more effective primary techniques for prevention are largely in the venue of the industrial hygiene and safety engineering staff.

## Investigation of Cases of Unknown Etiology

### Case study

In 1988, union representatives of a chemical plant in upstate New York requested that NIOSH investigate a perceived excess of bladder cancer and cardiovascular disease among workers manufacturing chemicals for the rubber industry.[3] Case ascertainment was conducted via discussion with labor representatives and management. A rough estimate of the population potentially at risk was made by actual physical measurement of several sample personnel file drawers using a yardstick and an extrapolation to the total number of personnel file drawers. Initial assessment suggested that the number of known bladder tumors was more than would be expected based on this crude estimate of total numbers of current and former employees. A walkthrough of the plant by an industrial hygienist identified in the worksite the presence of and the real potential for worker exposure to a number of chemicals, including ortho-toluidine—a suspected carcinogen—based upon published experimental animal studies. A retrospective cohort study was done in which all former and current employees were identified. Thirteen incident bladder tumors were diagnosed between 1979 and 1989 among 1749 current and former workers compared to an expected number of 3.6 tumors. This yielded an incidence ratio of 3.6. Seven of the cases occurred in workers who worked primarily in the chemical production department, giving a department-specific incidence ratio of 6.5. The initial estimate of excess risk on the initial site visit led to efforts to reduce exposure. In part based on the more refined study that took several years to complete, ortho-toluidine has been recognized as a human carcinogen.

The scenario of investigation of cases of unknown etiology differs from the investigation of a SHE(O) where there is a well established relationship between occupational exposure and disease. The motivation for investigation of a SHE(O) is identification of a failure of prevention. The motivation for investigation of cases of unknown etiology is, in addition, the early identification of a heretofore unrecognized or unaccepted association between exposure and outcome. Clearly the difficulty here is distinguishing between a chance occurrence of an unrelated case of disease and the first signal of the occurrence of a new disease–exposure relationship.

Most clusters result from coincidence and chance, but that does not mean that clusters are not useful sources of information. There are many examples of investigations of small numbers of occupational cases that led to the discovery of a new disease–exposure relationship. These include the investigation of cases of angiosarcoma of the liver associated with vinyl chloride in plastics manufacturing, the association of oat cell carcinoma of the lung with bis-chlorl-methyl-ether exposure in chemical production, the association of azospermia with dibromo-chloro-propane, and many more.

As in all other realms of field epidemiology, the successful investigation requires, not only technical expertise in methodology, but judgment in differentiating the presence of a real causal association from happenstance. The United States is so large, composed of such a magnitude of workplaces that, by happenstance, even rare events will cluster. There are attributes of cases and case clusters that suggest a cause-and-effect relationship with exposure rather than a random occurrence. Some of these attributes include pathological or patho-physiological aspects of the cases; multiple similar cases; unusual or distinctive pathology; many years of exposure in the case of carcinogens, suggesting an effect of a higher dose; many years since first exposure, suggesting sufficient latency or time since first exposure for carcinogens; a common unique exposure shared by the cases; a chemical relationship between a suspect intoxicant and a structurally similar known hazard; and, of course, biological plausibility based on prior toxicologic studies in experimental animals. Clearly the more signposts of a real causal association, the less astute need be the epidemiologist.

## Investigative Team

The scope of the workplace investigations frequently requires expertise beyond that of the epidemiologist, necessitating the **work of a team**. Industrial hygienists are trained to understand industrial processes as well as measurements of exposure. If you attempt a field investigation without the benefit of an industrial hygienist, you run two major risks of failure. On one hand, most industrial processes to some degree look and sound frightening, but in reality have been made reasonably safe through engineering controls, including ventilation, use of environmental monitoring, use of personal protective equipment, and other controls. Without the benefit of an industrial hygienist, you may easily overreact to innocuous exposures and processes. Similarly, without training or experience in exposure assessment or industrial processes, it is unlikely that you would recognize real hazards. While an industrial toxicologist would be a very effective third member of a field team, in reality, toxicologists are usually consultants rather than primary field investigators. A toxicologist plays an instrumental role in identifying possible hazards among the many chemicals that are either used; produced in normal operations; or inadvertently generated when, for instance, there are changes of temperature or pressure in the manufacturing process.

## Does Exposure Cause Disease?

### Case study

TCDD or tetrachloro-dibenzo-dioxin has been described by toxicologists as the most potent manmade toxin. It is a contaminant in the manufacturing of herbicides and other industrial processes. The concern about TCDD is based on exposure studies in experimental animals and mechanistic studies that have demonstrated a molecular basis for toxicity involving binding to subcellular receptors. Starting in the late 1970s, NIOSH investigators identified over 6000 workers, exposed to TCDD in the manufacture of herbicides, who were exposed at quantifiable levels decades before and at substantially higher levels than would be found from normal environmental exposure.[4] These workers were followed through time to see if their cancer mortality differed from what would be expected in the general population—which has low-level exposure. Some cancers of interest were specified *a priori*, based upon animal experimental studies or cluster investigations in humans. The study took about a decade to complete and has provided some of the best data on the human experience with high-level TCDD exposure. The study documented a significant increase in all cancers combined and a specific increase in a rare tumor: soft tissue sarcoma.

There are usually two typical situations in which the question is asked whether exposure can cause disease. In one situation, workers themselves or their employers have become aware of a potentially hazardous exposure. For example, a feedstock chemical may have been recently found to cause cancer in animal feeding studies. In the other situation, researchers have become aware of the potential toxicity of a chemical and are actively searching for an occupational group to study. In either situation, for an epidemiologic study to adequately answer the question of whether an exposure is related to a disease outcome, it must clear many hurdles. If these hurdles are not cleared, you can be fairly well guaranteed an inconclusive study—after a substantial amount of effort and time has been expended and expectations have been raised.

There are two ways, neither easy, of going about answering whether an exposure is related to a disease outcome. One way involves *risk assessment*. There are two essential ingredients here. First, the quantitative relationship between exposure and adverse effect must be known either from experimental studies, usually in laboratory animals, or much less frequently, from human data. Second, the exposure in the workplace must be characterized quantitatively. Based upon the level of exposure and the dose–response relationship, predictions of adverse effects can be attempted. Predictions of risk are very difficult for numerous reasons. Among the difficulties are inaccuracy in estimating exposure; extrapolation across species from experimental animal to humans; extrapolation beyond, usually below, the level of exposure even in human studies, to lower levels of actual exposure; and idiosyncrasies of susceptibility and differences in metabolism and pathological reaction among experimental animals and humans.

The alternative approach to answering the question of whether exposure in a workplace is associated with a disease outcome is to *conduct a study*. Before raising expectations that a study will address this question, you must consider whether a study will lead to an accurate or a biased assessment. Numerous questions must be posed. Is the population large enough to avoid a falsely negative study? Has the population been exposed long enough to allow for expression of disease if it were going to occur? Were the exposures high enough to expect that cases would occur? There are even more pragmatic questions such as whether records of exposure exist, whether membership in the worker population over time is known, and whether there would be cooperation among management and workers in estimating exposure or ascertaining if disease or death has occurred.

Three study designs fit this situation. The first design is *cross-sectional*. This is the easiest design to carry out. The cross-sectional investigation studies workers who are presently at the workplace and do not need to be located. The workers can be questioned and examined, and exposures can be measured at the same time. There are major limitations to this approach. The current population may represent healthy *survivors*. *Cases* may be long gone along with other sick and well *leavers*. A cross-sectional study of survivors will falsely underestimate the adverse effect of exposure. Second, exposure measured at this point in time is only relevant if the interval or *latency* between exposure and outcome is short, as you would see with a short-acting poison. With carcinogens and other agents that require chronic exposure, the expected latency between exposure and outcome may be decades.

An alternate approach is a *cohort design* in which considerable effort is expended to acquire a complete worker roster over decades and to follow them through time to determine their disease or mortality incidence (see Chapter 8).

There are two ways that a cohort can be followed through time. One is the *historical*, otherwise known as *retrospective* cohort study, and the other is the *prospective* cohort study. In the retrospective study, you identify a group or cohort of workers who were exposed to a potential hazardous agent many years in the past. Membership in the cohort is dependent upon their having a potential for exposure. The cohort is then followed through time to the present time or some other arbitrary recent date. Their mortality experience, for example, between 1940 and the present, is then compared with a nonexposed and otherwise comparable worker population or to the mortality experience of the general population.

Virtually all cohort studies of occupational disease are of the retrospective or historical type. However, in a purely prospective cohort study, membership of the cohort and determination of their current exposure is made in the present time, and the cohort is followed in time into the future to determine if their future disease experience is comparable to a nonexposed worker population or the general population. Cohort studies can be partially retrospective and followed into the future as well, and hence partially prospective. A further complication is that exposure can have ceased in the past, continued through the present, or persist into the future.

There are overwhelming problems with the purely prospective approach in which exposure persists into the future. First, if there is sufficient cause for concern about the adverse effect of the exposure, precaution would argue for diminution of the exposure now. Second, even with a strong adverse effect, it usually takes a fairly sizable multi-plant cohort to detect the adverse effect during decades of observation during which worrisome exposure persists. It may take an even longer period of observation for a smaller cohort from a single plant. There is an ethical problem of conducting a prospective cohort study when you suspect that the effect of current levels of exposure will be deleterious.

We should emphasize that the role of the epidemiologist cannot be limited to statistical analysis alone, but must consider the toxicity of the agent of interest, the projected risk to the study population, if exposure persists; and the ethics of observation with or without intervention. Clearly an essential element of conducting occupational studies is estimation of the exposure for cohort members. The cohort design is preferable to the cross-sectional approach because the cohort contains cases and survivors whether they currently work at the plant site or not. In practice, the cohort approach is usually limited to retrospective studies of mortality rather than morbidity. Death certificates are readily available, whereas it is very difficult to locate, question, and examine all cohort members to determine rates of non-fatal disease, especially among those already deceased from other causes.

A third approach is the *case referent* or *case control* design (see Chapter 8). The prerequisite here—since you are starting with cases rather than exposure— is for you to know specifically what disease is associated with the exposure.

Often case control studies can be performed by selecting all cases from a previously conducted cohort study and comparing them with a random sample of non-cases—a so-called nesting approach. Finding all cases, rather than a potentially biased sample of cases, can take as much effort as identifying all cohort members and their death and disease status in a cohort design. However, considerable time can be saved by this method because you only have to estimate exposures in cases and a sample of the others. But this approach also requires that there be variation in exposure, otherwise you will find that cases and referents are equally exposed.

As a field investigator you may be asked the more challenging open-ended question of whether the workplace is safe, rather than the more specific question of whether a known outcome is associated with a workplace exposure, or whether a specific exposure is associated with an adverse outcome. Answering this question is not a simple task. A knowledgeable industrial hygienist should be able to supply a generic list of potential exposures for generic occupations and industries. However, a thorough assessment of potential exposures will require a site visit by an industrial hygienist to assess, as examples, an industrial process, the feedstock chemicals used in the process, or the potential for the process to generate new chemical products. This can be a very sophisticated undertaking, as changes in manufacturing processes, such as changes in temperature and pressure, will produce different products than expected. The workplace should have a file of Material Safety Data Sheets (MSDS) required by OSHA for products that are in use. Your role in this situation, particularly if you are a physician, is primarily to see if there is a health concern that is motivating the inquiry. You are likely to be humbled if you are working with an insightful industrial hygienist, toxicologist, or ergonomist, because they may well find potential hazards that are otherwise not evident to the untrained eye. If you are asked to evaluate whether a workplace is healthful, attempt to have the question and your response also address issues of safety from injury as well.

When confronted with the question of whether exposure leads to disease, your major challenge is to recognize that it is the exception when this question can be answered in a specific workplace. The observational studies discussed all have advantages and disadvantages to be considered. In general, cohort studies are considered the strongest type of observational study in assessing the association of workplace exposure and health outcome. Further, a large-scale study is necessary to avoid a falsely negative study. Large studies are very expensive in time and effort. Even if the circumstances are adequate to launch an epidemiologic study, including exposure assessment, you must consider whether embarking on a demanding, multi-year investigation may inadvertently delay practical actions that could be taken much sooner to reduce exposure, the so called "paralysis through analysis." Feasibility assessments can be conducted by the investigative team to assess available data and to make a determination concerning the usefulness of embarking on a large-scale study.

## Evaluation of an Intervention

### Case study

Many states conduct surveillance of occupational lead poisoning by requiring that laboratories report cases with elevated blood leads to the state health department. States vary in their use of the information: some analyze and disseminate the data, others offer consultation, and some states refer companies that do not accept consultation to OSHA, so that OSHA may conduct formal investigations into whether the workplace is in compliance with applicable regulations for worker protection.

Rosenman, in Michigan, used epidemiological analyses to evaluate the effectiveness of referral by a state health department of workplaces with excessive blood lead levels to OSHA.[5] A comparison population consisted of companies using lead where blood lead levels were not in excess. Inspection by OSHA found more remediable problems in companies with workers with elevated blood lead levels than among companies where workers' blood lead levels were not in excess—demonstrating the effectiveness of the referral program.

Field epidemiology goes beyond investigation of epidemics and can be applied to the evaluation of interventions as shown in the above examples. There is a *continuum of techniques* used for the prevention of occupational disease and injury. These are described above in the *hierarchy of prevention*. You may be requested to evaluate the effectiveness of these interventions. For example, industry may invest substantial resources in campaigns to increase the use of seat belts. A reasonable question might be whether the campaign approach is effective in increasing seatbelt use. Epidemiologic approaches may be utilized ranging from establishing a surveillance program for seat belt use before, during, and after initiation of the educational intervention, to even conducting a trial in which alternative interventions might be instituted in various plants of a large company.

### Case study

In 2001, NIOSH received a request for a health hazard evaluation from a label printing company that used several amine compounds in its manufacturing process. The request stated that employees in the plant were experiencing intermittently blurred vision. Although visual changes associated with occupational exposure to selected tertiary amines has been reported in a variety of workplaces in the past, accurate measurement of amine compounds in the air had been difficult. Exposure assessment and medical evaluation by NIOSH investigators found that employees had work-related vision problems associated primarily with exposure to the tertiary amine dimethylisopropanolamine (DMIPA); these health effects posed an immediate safety hazard.[6] NIOSH investigators provided recommendations to reduce workers' exposure to the amine, and subsequently the company altered its manufacturing process and ultimately discontinued use of that amine. Follow-up evaluation by NIOSH investigators revealed markedly reduced exposure to DMIPA and resolution of all visual symptoms among the workers.[7]

## Other Considerations in Conducting Occupational Investigations

### Wearing blinders

Think logically when you are studying the nature of an epidemic. An epidemic in the workplace *may or may not* be of occupational etiology. For example, gastrointestinal symptoms may be related to a food product served in the cafeteria or in the community. The workplace may be a window through which a problem in the greater community can be observed. On the other hand, occupational epidemics may not be restricted to the workplace. As examples, community residents may be affected either by toxins carried home by workers on their clothes or vehicles, or by toxins emitted from the plant carried by air or water,.

### Consider outcomes other than cancer

The focus of occupational epidemiology for the latter half of the twentieth century was in two areas: occupational cancer and pulmonary disease. In the latter half of the century there was growth in interest in neurotoxicity, adverse reproductive effects, and musculoskeletal disorders. The change in focus was usually precipitated by the advent of a major epidemic and epidemiologic investigation. Future directions are somewhat unpredictable but will probably include several long-standing problems that have been ignored regardless of their substantial toll on mortality (e.g., occupational injury) and morbidity (e.g., dermatitis). New areas of focus will undoubtedly reflect development of new technology, such as personal use of video display terminals and cellular telephones; new advances in biological science, genomics that will provide opportunities to understand subcellular risk factors and mechanisms of disease; and greater interest in social and psychological factors, such as job stress and fatigue.

### A special word on Years of Potential Life Lost (YPLL)

A YPLL is a year of potential life lost. Simply put, a death at 75 years rather than at an arbitrary expected age of 85 years results in (or costs) 10 years of life lost. A death at age 25 costs 60 years of life lost. Unfortunately, occupational epidemiologists have focused their interest mostly on relative risks as a measure of public health impact. For example, if one case of some disease or injury is expected and four occur, then the relative risk is four. However, four deaths of disease A at age 75 cost a total of 40 YPLL and four deaths of disease B at age 25 cost a total of 240 YPLL. Occupational cancer that usually occurs in older age, and occupational injury that usually occurs in younger age might have the same excess relative risk but will cause far different losses of life. A corollary to this is: given deaths from a common disease and deaths from a rare disease, much more YPLL will result from the common disease than the rare one, *provided* all deaths occur at the same age and the relative risks are the same for both groups. **Quantifying exposure.** There is a saying in toxicology that "the dose makes the poison," meaning the greater the dose, the more toxic the effect. Quantifying the relationship between dose and effect is essential to modern quantitative epidemiology and risk assessment. Demonstrating a greater adverse outcome with a higher dose adds to the weight of the evidence for causality. Therefore, in designing a study, you might logically limit the cohort to workers with the most years of exposure. This should increase the probability of your finding an adverse effect among the workers related to exposure and increase the efficiency of your study by permitting you to study fewer persons. The downside of this restriction is that the comparison group for the worker cohort is external to the worker population thus limiting the possibility of demonstrating a dose-related effect. A second problem in using a comparison population external to the worksite is the *healthy worker effect*. Studies of workers usually find them to be healthier than the general population, especially for cardiovascular disease. This healthy worker effect probably derives from the selection process workers go through to qualify for a job and from the social and economic benefits of employment.

Years of employment is a crude measure of exposure. More sophisticated measures include estimates of probability of exposure based on knowledge of the job. Even more sophisticated measures can include incorporation of environmental measurements that were made over time. Thus, workers can be characterized by levels of exposure-days which, in turn, can be described as parts per million of exposure times days of exposure. Even more sophisticated measures may go beyond total dose and provide dose rates. Using progressively more sophisticated measures of exposure in an occupational study often provides more and more accurate views of the actual dose–response relationship. The cost of these dose characterizations, however, is substantial. You can limit the cost by using a fairly crude measure of dose, such as years of employment in the cohort analysis, then do a *nested case control* study within the cohort (see above) using the most sophisticated measures possible to describe exposure of the cases and referents.

## SOURCES OF INFORMATION

At the start of the investigation, you will benefit from two types of information: (1) information specific to the worksite and (2) more general knowledge about the industry, occupation, exposure, or disease that has motivated the investigation. Every workplace that is under the jurisdiction of OSHA keeps a log, called the "OSHA 300 Log of Work-Related Injuries and Illnesses." Cases of injury and illness requiring more than first aid that occur in that particular workplace are supposed to be recorded on the log, which is kept for five years and is accessible at the worksite. This source is usually not a complete roster of cases of illness or disease, but it is a helpful starting point. The roster is a line listing of cases, not a statistical analysis of the injury or illness experience of the workplace. The Bureau of Labor Statistics of the Department of Labor collects a national sample of OSHA 300 logs and from this provides an Annual Survey, which is a statistical analysis of illness and injury by industry. This information is helpful in comparing the experience of particular industries with the general experience of all industries and can also serve as a point of comparison for a particular workplace. The other sources of information about a worksite are the Material Safety Data Sheets, MSDS, which should be available in the plant office for every commercial product that is being used at the plant site.

The other types of knowledge are more general. While there are myriad sources and texts, the following are starting points:

### Texts on Industrial Processes

Burgess, William. *Recognition of health hazards in industry. A review of materials and processes*. John Wiley and Sons. New York. 1995, 2nd Edition. ISBN 0–471–06339–8.[8]

DiNardi, Salvatore R. Editor. *The occupational environment: evaluation, control and management*. American Industrial Hygiene Association, Fairfax, Virginia, 2003, 2nd Edition. ISBN 0–932627–82–X.[9]

Cralley Lester V., Cralley Lewis J. Industrial hygiene aspects of plant operations. Volume 1 Process Flows; Volume 2 Unit operations and product fabrication. Macmillan Publishing Co. New York, 1982. ISBN 0–02–949350–1.[10]

### Help from NIOSH

Assistance from the Centers for Disease Control and Prevention (CDC) and NIOSH can be accessed via a toll free number that provides access to CDC and NIOSH technical information resources: 1-800-CDC-INFO (1-800-232-4636).

The NIOSH web site (http://www.cdc.gov/niosh/homepage.html) provides an excellent portal to information on chemicals and toxicity.

**Table 19-1.** Selected Field Investigations of Occupational Disease and Injury

| DESCRIPTION/PROBLEM | METHODS | REFERENCE |
|---|---|---|
| Eight former workers at a microwave-popcorn production plant were reported to have severe lung disease. Study indicates that they probably had occupational bronchiolitis obliterans caused by the inhalation of volatile butter-flavoring ingredients. | Cross sectional survey among workers at the facility, with findings compared with data from the third National Health and Nutrition Examination Survey. | Kreiss, K., Gomaa, A., Kullman, G., et al. (2002). Clinical bronchiolitis obliterans in workers at a microwave-popcorn plant. *N Engl J Med* 347(5), 330–8. |
| The role of airborne transmission of SARS has been unclear. This study provides the first experimental confirmation of viral aerosol generation by a patient with SARS, indicating the possibility of airborne droplet transmission. | Exposure assessment in a hospital unit where patients with SARS were cared for. | Booth, T.F., et al. (2005). Detection of airborne severe acute respiratory syndrome (SARS) coronavirus and environmental contamination in SARS outbreak units. *J Inf Dis* 191 (9), 1472–7. |
| Healthcare workers incur frequent injuries resulting from patient transfer and handling tasks. This study found that implementation of patient lifts can be effective in reducing occupational musculoskeletal injuries to nursing personnel in both long term and acute care settings. | Pre- and post-intervention study taking place at four hospitals and five long-term care facilities. | Evanoff, B., Wolf, L., Aton, E., et al. (2003). Reduction in injury rates in nursing personnel through introduction of mechanical lifts in the workplace. *Am J Ind Med* 44, 451–7. |

**Table 19–1.** Selected Field Investigations of Occupational Disease and Injury—continued

| DESCRIPTION/PROBLEM | METHODS | REFERENCE |
|---|---|---|
| Silica is one of the most common occupational exposures worldwide. Results of this study support the decision by the International Agency for Research on Cancer to classify inhaled silica in occupational settings as a carcinogen | Pooled cohort study (including 65,980 workers) to investigate lung cancer. | Steenland, K. et al. (2001). Pooled exposure–response analyses and risk assessment for lung cancer in 10 cohorts of silica-exposed workers: an IARC multicentre study. Cancer Causes and Control 12 (9), 773–84. |
| Bricklayers and craft workers may be occupationally exposed to a variety of substances including several lung carcinogens. This study suggests the need for intervention activities to prevent a number of cancers and other respiratory diseases. | Proportionate mortality ratio analysis based on the underlying cause of death was conducted to evaluate the mortality patterns of union members. | Salg, J., Alterman, T. (2005). A proportionate mortality study of bricklayers and allied craftworkers. *J Ind Med* 47(1), 10–9. |
| Information concerning risk factors for infection with SARS are needed for prevention. This study found that activities related to intubation increase SARS risk and use of a mask (particularly a N95 mask) is protective. | A retrospective cohort study was conducted to determine risk factors for SARS among nurses who worked in two critical care units in a Toronto hospital. | Loeb, M., McGeer, A., Henry, B., et al. (2006). SARS among critical care nurses, Toronto. *Emerg Infect Dis* [serial online] 2004 Jul. Available from: http://www.cdc. gov/ncidod/EID/vol10no2/03–0838.htm |

## Help from colleagues

The Occupational and Environmental Medicine List provides a vibrant daily forum for professionals. Participants include clinicians, public health experts, and hygiene and safety professionals from 60 nations. Members seem ready and capable to offer information and technical expertise to professional colleagues on a broad range of subjects. See their web site: http://occhealthnews.com.

## CONCLUSION

Field investigations in the workplace, like all other epidemiologic endeavors, share a reliance on basic methods of epidemiology used wisely as part of logical problem-solving. While one would like to conclude that one only needs professional capability in epidemiology to work successfully in workplace investigations, that would be naïve. Little in medical training and probably less in academic epidemiologic training prepare the investigator with a sufficient understanding of chemical toxicities, mechanisms of toxicity, industrial processes and their failures, personal protective devices and their deficiencies, and complex social and political organizations. At a minimum, to work in the occupational arena, one should form a team with an industrial hygienist. Expertise on interpretation of the social and economic complexities of the workplace is more difficult to find. You should avoid advice to stay neutral between the interests of labor and industry. Rather, you should stay dedicated to the goal of prevention. In doing so you will find allies among both labor and industry and probably do an effective job in the epidemiologic investigation. Several recent field epidemiologic investigations are summarized in Table 19–1.

## REFERENCES

1. Rutstein, D., Mullan, R., Frazier, T., et al. (1983). The sentinel health event (occupational): a framework for occupational health surveillance and education, *J Am Public Health Assoc* 73, 1054-62.
2. Halperin, W.E. (1996). The role of surveillance in the hierarchy of prevention. *Am J Ind Med* 29, 321–3.3. Ward, E., Carpenter, A., Markowitz, S., et al. (1991). Excess bladder cancer in workers exposed to ortho-toluidine and aniline. *J Nat Cancer Inst* 83, 501–6.
4. Fingerhut, M., Halperin, W., Marlow, D., et al. (1991). Mortality among U.S. workers employed in the production of chemicals contaminated with 2,3,7,8-tetrachlorodibenzo-p-dioxin (TCDD). *N Engl J Med* 324, 212–8.
5. Rosenman, K. (2000). Evaluation of the effectiveness of following up laboratory reports of elevated blood leads in adults. In press. *American Journal of Industrial Hygiene.*

6. Page, E.H., Cook, C.K., Hater, M.A., et al. (2003). Visual and ocular changes associated with exposure to two tertiary amines. *Occup Environ Med* 60, 69–75.
7. NIOSH. (2003). Health Hazard Evaluation Report 2002–0379–2901 Superior Label Systems, Mason, Ohio. Available at: http://www.cdc.gov/niosh/hhe/reports/pdfs/2002–0379–2901.pdf
8. Burgess, William (1995). *Recognition of Health Hazards in Industry. A Review of Materials and Processes,* John Wiley and Sons, New York, 2nd ed. ISBN 0–471–06339–8.
9. DiNardi, Salvatore R. (ed.) (2003). *The Occupational Environment: Evaluation Control and Management.* American Industrial Hygiene Association, Fairfax, Virginia, 2nd ed. ISBN 0–932627–82-X.
10. Cralley, Lester V., Cralley, Lewis J. (1982). Industrial Hygiene Aspects of Plant Operations. Volume 1, Process Flows; Volume 2, Unit Operations and Product Fabrication. Macmillan, New York. ISBN 0–02–949350–1.

# 20

# FIELD INVESTIGATIONS FROM THE STATE AND LOCAL HEALTH DEPARTMENT PERSPECTIVE

Jeffrey P. Davis
Guthrie S. Birkhead

The underpinnings of state and local public health practice involve disease surveillance and epidemic field investigations, both of which can occur virtually anywhere and any time. The frequency and breadth of these activities throughout the United States far exceed what is done at the federal level. For example, in New York State several hundred outbreaks or "events" are reported each year that require some level of investigation, often by a local health unit. These range from relatively mundane and routine to highly charged and compelling. When new diseases or routes of transmission are discovered, this often grows out of an investigation beginning at the local level. You can never know, when the first call arrives, how big or important the investigation will become.

Working and networking diligently with colleagues and appropriately communicating ideas and information across jurisdictional lines and between scientific disciplines are key to the success of state and local field epidemiologic activities. However, you should be aware of certain critical factors that can provide new insights into the conduct of even the most routine investigations and related activities. The following framework for investigations in this field and discussion of issues in state and local surveillance are not intended to be comprehensive, but they should give you some insight into this area and help you focus on the realities of conducting these activities in the early 2000s. We have also selected some examples among the many consequential field investigations conducted by state and local field epidemiologists and their partners to illustrate the issues. Although we use the words *state* and *federal* throughout the chapter, they are completely interchangeable with *provincial* and *national*. Many of the issues discussed here apply, to a greater or lesser degree, to other countries and jurisdictions and their various constituents.

## THE FRAMEWORK FOR FIELD EPIDEMIOLOGY

### Statutes, Regulations, Codes and Ordinances

In the United States, the Constitution does not designate protection of health as one of the powers and responsibilities assigned to the federal government. These matters are left to the states. States thus have substantial powers and duties with regard to public health matters. Each state and some cities have a code of public health laws and regulations that charges the state or local government with the responsibility of protecting the public's health[1] (see Chapter 14).

In brief, the following factors relating to statutes, regulations, health codes, and ordinances are always determinants of public health practice at the state and local level: responsibility, authority, powers, the balance of public health actions with what is necessary and justifiable (from which arises the need for good data) to avoid abuse of powers, and the need to maintain the cooperation of all involved.

Laws and regulations provide state and local health authorities with specific powers to collect health-related data, to investigate health events or disease occurrences, and to take actions to protect health. These powers can sometimes be extraordinary, and they may overcome individual rights to privacy by giving health departments the ability to collect disease reports with personally identifying information. These laws and regulations can also abridge putative personal freedoms by providing health departments the power to quarantine or to close or restrict a place of business (e.g., a restaurant) that may be a source of disease.

If you are working under the power of these statutes and regulations, you must respect and protect confidentiality or risk losing cooperation of health care providers and the public—both essential to the success of your efforts. For example, the Minnesota Department of Health has a long history of reading a carefully worded statement to potential respondents during telephone interviews that states cooperation is voluntary and information will not be released in identified form.[*]

---

[*] K. Moore, personal communication.

You should be frequently reminded that your primary goal in a field investigation at the state or local level is to facilitate and permit application of control measures. Research is only a secondary purpose within the context of the state or local legal framework. Nevertheless, consent from individuals to provide information about themselves is an important principle. Generally, consent is not needed for basic field investigations, although responses to questionnaires are voluntary. However, you may reach a critical point in your investigation where the line into research is crossed, thus requiring a formal consent. This situation will typically involve approval of an investigational review board.

In sum, always have a clear understanding of the legal framework in which you are collecting information and conducting investigations. In addition, you should be aware that the results of your investigation may be used to take legal action, making it important that the data are correctly collected, analyzed, and interpreted.

## Fiscal and Personnel Infrastructure

The size of a health department, population served, funding opportunities, and eagerness of staff to seek resources all have a bearing on the scope of field investigations. Even in a country as rich as the United States, it is fair to say that many local and state health departments are strapped for resources (money, people, and technology) because of a chronic lack of support. In many local settings the "field investigator" is a public health nurse, sanitarian, or college graduate—all without specialized training—who often has a full-time job doing something else. Furthermore, there generally is substantial turnover of personnel at the state and local level, and it is difficult to recruit specialized staff (e.g., information systems specialists) owing in part to relatively low public-sector pay scales. This creates a constant need for training. Currently, Epidemic Intelligence Service (EIS) officers from the CDC, former EIS officers, preventive medicine residents, and persons with master's degrees in public health or comparable training are key to maintaining and strengthening the epidemiologic workforce at the state and local levels.

Much field investigation capability at the state and, to lesser extent, the local level is funded by federal dollars.[2] So state and local agencies need to be able to "pounce" when funding becomes available. In recent years, categorical federal funds, focused on emerging infectious diseases, bioterrorism and public health preparedness, have provided much-needed support to many state and local health departments to enhance their investigative capabilities. Therefore, field epidemiologists need to take advantage of outbreaks or other events to help justify funding appropriate infrastructures at the state and local level. A well-known example is the provision of funds from federal, state, and local governments to state and local health departments for surveillance and vector control following the emergence in 1999 of the West Nile virus.

## Effectiveness of Collaboration

A team effort is critical at state and local levels to conduct successful field investigations. The members of the team typically include epidemiologists, laboratory workers, sanitary engineers, environmental experts, information systems specialists, statisticians, media relations staff, attorneys or legal advisors, and additional support staff depending on the type of problem being investigated. In large or potentially important outbreaks, team members may include representatives from state and local health jurisdictions; other state/local agencies, such as those responsible for natural resources, the environment, conservation, or agriculture; and, as needed, police agencies and the Federal Bureau of Investigation.

You need to be comfortable working as part of the team and communicating with your counterparts to explain the strengths and weaknesses of the epidemiologic data. This often involves both learning the vernacular of different disciplines on the team and teaching the epidemiologic principles involved.

## Networking and Information Sharing

Networking at the local level follows from the need for teamwork. Also, because many public health problems cross jurisdictional boundaries, good communication across city, county, regional, and state borders is necessary. Historically, state health departments have these responsibilities within states, and the CDC and other federal agencies (the Food and Drug Administration, the Department of Agriculture, and the Environmental Protection Agency) have these responsibilities at the national level. The CDC may become directly involved in state or local investigations at the invitation of the state epidemiologist and is often relied upon to provide technical and laboratory assistance even without direct investigative involvement. Because of complex networks, increasing sources of relevant information, and templates (e.g., standard questionnaires) that are readily available to field investigators, some information sharing and organizing tools are essential to enhancing networking processes—particularly those that are Internet related. These include the Epi Info[3] computer software for outbreak investigation (latest version: Epi Info™ version 3.3.2, release date: February 9, 2005) and the Epi-X system[4] developed by the CDC to improve communication about currently active outbreak investigations (see Chapter 7). Electronic mail list-serves such as *Promed* provide a valuable communication forum on emerging public health threats.

## Information Transfer and the Rapidity of Technological Advances

### Health-care systems

Economic trends and pressures within the health-care system, such as the emergence of managed care in the private and public sectors, have created the need for state and local field epidemiologists to find, understand, and use the resulting databases and information. Furthermore, computers, data transmission, and data storage technology coupled with standard software analytic packages have facilitated the increasing use of large databases (e.g., hospital discharge) by state and local epidemiologists. One use of these databases has been to evaluate the surveillance of a wide variety of diseases. For example, New York State was able to measure the completeness of meningococcal disease reporting by comparing traditional disease reports with computerized hospital discharge records.[5] Hospital charts were reviewed to confirm the diagnosis of meningococcal disease and to match surveillance records for one calendar year. Using methods for comparing reports of the same disease events from different, independent data systems (the Chadra–Sekar–Deming, or capture–recapture, method), the completeness of surveillance reporting of meningococcal disease in the state was found to be 93%.

There can be pitfalls, however, when you use large electronic databases. Coding issues, for example, can challenge you, depending on the underlying purpose for which the data were gathered. Merging and integrating data from different sources are difficult to do and require complementary database design and trained staff, who may not be available at the state or local level. Examples of both the potential promise and the pitfalls of electronic data for field epidemiologic investigations are described later in this chapter.

### Other data sources and technologies

Standard field-tested instruments are of great value in fieldwork. Many state and large local health departments have developed a standard format for field questionnaires. Excellent examples are found in the Epi Info[3] package and the comprehensive and user-friendly Minnesota Standard Foodborne Disease Exposure Questionnaire that has been widely used and can be readily customized for use in the field.* A standardized questionnaire is also found in the *Foodborne Disease Handbook*.[6]

You should also be aware of a number of available resources regarding late-breaking health issues. Many state and local health departments disseminate weekly, biweekly, or monthly reports that contain descriptions of important local

---

* K. Smith, personal communication.

health events. The CDC, in *The Morbidity and Mortality Weekly Report* (*MMWR*) and in the *MMWR Recommendations and Reports* series, publishes a wide variety of health-related information from local to international jurisdictions on late-breaking issues, secular trends, and recommendations related to prevention and control of many health concerns. The *MMWR* can be accessed at http://www.cdc.gov/mmwr. The *Emerging Infectious Disease* journal published by the CDC and accessible at http://www.cdc.gov/eid is another source, an on-line journal for field epidemiologists who want to keep up with the latest investigations in the emerging infectious disease world. *Promed* is an electronic mail list-serve for exchange of information or posing questions, again in the emerging infectious disease area. The *Epidemiology Monitor Newsletter* is a good source of information on available software, job openings, and other issues of interest.

The state or local public health laboratory is also a data source and an important partner. The rapid advances in DNA-based technology, such as pulsed-field gel electrophoresis (PFGE) and gene sequencing, and the emergence of networks to share data electronically (PulseNet, FoodNet, and OutbreakNet), have provided state health departments with much-improved opportunities to prevent and control recently identified infections, keep up with new technologies, and communicate disease-related information. Concomitantly, these advances provide new challenges to respond promptly and adequately to field investigation and surveillance findings.

## Politics: Local, State, Federal

Politics is omnipresent, particularly at the state and local level, because most authorities responsible for public health (commissioners) report to political leaders. Nevertheless, objective data and information generated through rigorous field investigation can be used to educate and persuade, as needed, even in politically charged settings.

Examples of typical or common political issues for the field epidemiologist include territorial problems between large city and state health departments that can intensify when both health agencies will need to commit substantial resources to investigate an outbreak or other health event or when the timely sharing of information is integral. Generally, political considerations increase as the number of involved agencies and levels of government increases.

Naturally, there are varying views of the role of federal agencies by state and local level health officials, but efforts to generate positive partnerships are nearly always prudent and benefit the public's health. When federal resources are needed, the field epidemiologist may need to contend with pressure exerted by state or local policy makers who declare "We do not need any help from anyone." When there is a good track record of cooperation and benefit from such assistance, it is important to emphasize prudently, if not extol, the virtues of such assistance.

Conversely, when resources are limited, the pressure on the epidemiologist might be its corollary: "Why can't *you* do it? That's what the state is paying you to do!" Federal support in the form of assistance from federally assigned epidemiologists works best when there is continued participation and involvement by state or local field epidemiologists.

Whenever cooperation is needed, there are potential problems involving possession of data, authorship, responsibility, accountability, and other comparable issues. It is always valuable to discuss these issues early in an investigation or collaboration to obviate later concerns and to clarify roles that can ultimately enhance the conduct of the investigation.

## Media

Working cooperatively with the media is valuable and important at the state and local level. Within states the types and markets of the media vary, as do the catchment areas. Even so, the media are often instrumental in conveying important public health messages that can help you investigate successfully and implement control measures. The messages can be directive ("anyone who was sick, call this number" or "go to this location at such and such a time to get your immunization"), or instructive; that is, the media can also give to the public information they need during an investigation. During a pressing investigation, the media may seek increased access to you and your team. At that time, it is useful to create a specific time each day for the media to have access to the appropriate spokesperson of the team. In brief, you will need to keep the media informed. Patiently working with the media to assure the clearest of messages is key (see Chapter 13).

## ISSUES RELATED TO STATE AND LOCAL SURVEILLANCE

Public health surveillance, a critical activity for the field epidemiologist at all levels of government, is a core public health function, as defined by the Institute of Medicine in its 1988 report, *The Future of Public Health*.[7] Historically, surveillance efforts in the United States had their beginnings in the late 1700s and early 1800s and became more codified and universal in the late 1800s and early 1900s. These efforts took the form of requirements for investigating and reporting of specific diseases where public health measures like quarantine could be applied (e.g., smallpox, cholera). This direct link between surveillance and disease control activities currently an important feature of state and local public health practice.

The authority to conduct surveillance and require disease reporting is found in state laws and regulations. Some large cities also have health codes promulgated by boards of health that mandate surveillance activities. Ideally, these same laws and regulations specify the purposes for surveillance. State and local laws permit certain actions to manage disease threats and to specify the confidentiality protections for surveillance data. A model state statute on privacy of surveillance data has been developed[8] to aid states in ensuring that the confidentiality of surveillance data is adequately protected. Occasionally, distinctions must be made between public health practice and research pertaining to activities conducted by or under the authority of state or local health departments. Legal experts in partnership with a CSTE advisory committee prepared a practical report delineating these issues for public health practitioners.[9] A common misconception is that placing a disease or health event on a list of reportable conditions automatically means that it is under surveillance. True public health surveillance, as defined in Chapter 3, is not being practiced simply because a report is required from a health care provider. Resources must be available to set up surveillance systems, train staff and reporters, ensure timely analysis and dissemination of the data, and take appropriate action. Without each of these steps in place, a new reporting system will founder.

Physicians and other health care providers have historically not been effective disease reporters. Results of several statewide studies have demonstrated that a smaller proportion of communicable disease reports (only 6%–10%) originate from a physician's office compared to those (71%–77%) originating from clinical laboratories.[10, 11] Lack of knowledge about reporting and lack of incentives or time to report are common reasons given by physicians for not reporting diseases.[12, 13] Some studies have examined ways to improve physician reporting. Active surveillance, such as regular telephone calls to solicit reports, may result in increased reporting, but this approach is expensive and may not have a lasting effect if not continued.[10] For these reasons surveillance systems should try to harness data available in electronic form from laboratories, hospitals, and managed care plans wherever possible. However, you should not give up the traditional system of reporting by physicians, particularly for conditions that are not diagnosed by laboratory testing or may not result in hospitalization. The newer systems of reporting laboratory and health-care data can serve as an adjunct to the old system of reporting by individual physicians, but not as a replacement for it.

Maintaining the confidentiality of surveillance data is particularly important. While reporting is often a requirement of the system, surveillance and subsequent disease control efforts work best when those who report and the public cooperate. Breaches of confidentiality may damage the trust between these providers and the public health department. You should be aware that when analyzing data from small geographic or population areas, individuals may be identifiable by using small numbers in some table cells. This was a particular concern in the early phase of the AIDS epidemic. Most state health departments and the CDC have now developed data release policies that limit small cell sizes in tabulated data.

Funding for surveillance at the state and local level has been irregular and uncoordinated at best. For example, much of the specific funding support for infectious diseases surveillance comes from the federal government.[2] Many of these federal surveillance dollars are attached to categorical disease control programs (e.g., tuberculosis, AIDS/HIV, vaccine-preventable diseases) and public health preparedness activities. You should make every effort to coordinate and, if possible, integrate funding streams to develop core surveillance capacities in your health department. In the late 1990s and early 2000s, several federal grant programs acknowledged this need for integration and coordination; for example, bioterrorism and public health preparedness and the National Electronic Disease Surveillance System (NEDSS).

## ATTRIBUTES OF SUCCESSFUL STATE AND LOCAL FIELD EPIDEMIOLOGY PROGRAMS

At the risk of being prescriptive and encroaching on the definition of field epidemiologic capacity, we describe a variety of factors that can serve as goals and markers for a successful field epidemiology program.

### Goals

The field epidemiologist and field epidemiology programs:

- Foster a rich array of collaborative opportunities to benefit the public's health
- Have support from political leadership, the medical community, and the general public
- Have access to adequate training
- Promote good working relationships with laboratories and other partners
- Have the ability to analyze and disseminate findings in timely fashion
- Have adequate staffing, resources, and a team approach

### Markers for Success

The field epidemiologist:

- Has a considerable breadth of knowledge and is aware of cutting-edge issues
- Is mindful of traditional and emerging nontraditional partners
- Uses all opportunities to extend his or her ability to answer important public health questions

## EXAMPLES OF INVESTIGATIONS BY STATE AND
## LOCAL HEALTH DEPARTMENT FIELD EPIDEMIOLOGISTS

*1. State Responses to a Rapidly Emerging Disease: Wisconsin, Minnesota, and Iowa Responses to Toxic Shock Syndrome.* In December 1979, the Wisconsin Division of Health (DOH) received a call describing three hospitalized women from Madison, all of whom had rapid onset of fever, hypotension, erythroderma, and delayed desquamation of the palms and soles. The year before a similar syndrome in children had been described by Todd and was named toxic shock syndrome (TSS).[14] Apart from Madison residence, the only readily apparent common factor among these patients was being a woman. Because of the extreme rarity of this condition and the clustering of cases in women, an immediate field investigation began.

Record reviews rapidly generated four more cases in Madison hospitals; all had occurred within six months and were in females. Epidemiologic interviews revealed that six patients had been menstruating at onset of illness, and two had similar but milder illnesses during prior menstrual periods, suggesting the syndrome could recur. Because of the severity, rarity, and apparent newness of this syndrome, the DOH then informed all Wisconsin physicians of these patients, provided management recommendations, and established criteria for immediate statewide TSS surveillance.[15]

In Minnesota, also in December, five women with similar illnesses were hospitalized and subsequently were determined to have onsets during menstruation. These 12 cases from the two states and their apparent association of illness with menstruation was reported to the CDC in January by the state epidemiologists of Wisconsin and Minnesota. These reports served as the stimulus for the creation of a nationwide program of surveillance for TSS by CDC.[16]

Retrospective assessment of menstrual and other possible risk factors for TSS was now needed, and the Wisconsin DOH conducted a case control study in winter and early spring of 1980.[15] Thirty-five of 38 reported cases of TSS occurred during menstruation. Among menstruating women, 34 of 35 patients used tampons during every menstrual period compared to 80 of 105 controls ($p < .001$). TSS rates among women under 30 years old were 2.4- to 3.3-fold greater than among women 30 years old or older. Peak rates of nearly 15 cases per 100,000 menstruating women per year were noted among women 15–19 years old who were regular users of tampons. Lastly, analysis of tampon brand data in this study did not implicate a specific brand.[15]

By May 1980, 55 cases had been reported nationwide, including 31 from Wisconsin; 52 (95%) cases occurred in women; and 38 (95%) of 40 with known histories had onset during menses.[17] By June 1980, the use of tampons as a risk factor for TSS was corroborated in a national case control study conducted by the CDC. This study also showed no significant differences in brand use.[16] In September

1980, the CDC reported results of a second case control study that corroborated earlier findings regarding menses and tampon use as TSS risk factors. The results showed that, although cases occurred in association with multiple brands of tampons, significantly more cases compared to age-matched controls reported using Rely brand tampons; and that the relative risk of developing TSS was greater with use of Rely brand tampons when compared to other brands.[18] In mid-September the manufacturer of Rely brand tampons voluntarily withdrew the product from the market.

Meanwhile, during August 1980 epidemiologists from the Minnesota, Wisconsin, and Iowa state health departments with university colleagues in each of the states initiated a multistate collaborative comprehensive study of menses-associated TSS risk factors.[19] The Tri-State TSS Study included the use of proprietary tampon fluid capacity (as a measure of absorbency) and the chemical composition associated with all brand styles of tampons that had been used in the marketplace up to early September. Eighty women with TSS and 160 age- and sex-matched neighborhood controls were selected. The odds ratio for developing menstrual TSS with any tampon use compared to no tampon use was 18.0 ($p$ <.001). When individual tampon brand use was compared to no tampon use, the brand-specific odds ratios ranged from 5.9 to 27.2, and odds ratios for individual brand style use compared to no tampon use ranged from 2.6 to 34.5. In multivariate analysis, tampon fluid capacity (absorbency) and Rely brand tampon use were the only variables that significantly increased the relative risk of TSS; the risk associated with Rely brand tampon use was greater than that predicted by absorbency alone.[19]

Each of the studies used highly comparable TSS case definitions. Despite divergent methods, the association of menstrual TSS with tampon use was established in six different case control studies (four state-based studies conducted in five states and two CDC studies) by late 1980. The Tri-State TSS Study provides a superb example of an interstate–interagency collaborative field investigation that contributed seminal information for the prevention and control of TSS nationwide.

*2. State and Local Collaboration to Investigate and Analyze Disease Outbreaks: The New York State Department of Health–led Investigation of Widespread Shellfish-Associated Outbreaks.* A good example of state and local collaborative relationships occurred throughout New York State attendant to widespread outbreaks of gastroenteritis in 1982.

By way of background, the New York State Department of Health has a communicable disease epidemiology unit that oversees statewide surveillance and outbreak investigation activities. The 57 counties of New York State and the City of New York each have a public health officer who, under state law, acts as an agent of the state health commissioner. Each county has one or more communicable disease control specialists who are often public health nurses or sanitarians, particularly in rural areas of the state. Each county collects disease reports, conducts surveillance, performs outbreak investigations, and applies appropriate public health control measures. Only a few counties have public health laboratory services.

In the summer of 1982, this communicable disease surveillance and control system in New York was challenged by the occurrence of widespread outbreaks of gastroenteritis thought to be due to consumption of contaminated shellfish.[20] As the number of outbreaks reported to the county health departments increased in early summer of 1982, the state epidemiologists suspected a possible link between the outbreaks. However, it appeared that the source of the outbreaks would be difficult to determine because local health departments might not be conducting investigations in a standardized fashion. To ensure comparability, the state established a system to collect standard epidemiologic data, laboratory samples, and environmental information to trace the source of implicated shellfish. Standard epidemiologic case definitions, data collection tools, and analytic protocols for case-control studies were developed and disseminated to county health departments. Procedures for the proper collection, storage, and shipping of stool, blood, and food samples were developed; and special specimen containers were distributed. Standard procedures were designed to obtain shipping tags and other information to trace the origin of implicated lots of shellfish. Telephone and on-site technical assistance was provided by state staff to ensure proper application of the various protocols.

Using a standard protocol, 21 county health departments in New York investigated and reported 103 outbreaks of gastroenteritis that were definitely or probably associated with shellfish consumption. More than 1000 ill persons were interviewed statewide. In most cases the clinical and epidemiologic characteristics of these outbreaks were typical of Norwalk virus–like illness. Laboratory diagnosis of Norwalk virus was made in five of seven outbreaks when laboratory specimens were available. Norwalk virus was identified in shellfish specimens from two outbreaks. Northeastern U.S. coastal waters were the source of the shellfish when the source could be determined. Heavy spring rains with runoff into shellfish beds in 1982 may have been responsible for the widespread outbreaks.

The availability of high-quality epidemiologic and laboratory data from these outbreaks permitted the state health department to confidently warn consumers about the risks of raw or undercooked shellfish consumption, to strengthen record keeping procedures for selling shellfish, and to block the sale of shellfish from implicated beds.

*3. Mobilization of State/Local Field Epidemiologists to Investigate a Large-Scale Outbreak: Typhoid Fever among Conventioneers, New York 1989.* Large-scale communicable disease outbreaks constitute one of the true public health emergencies that a state or local health department may face. Epidemiologic forces must be marshaled quickly to get and analyze data from large numbers of persons at risk, to provide real-time information to release to the public, and to apply the correct control and prevention measures. Under conditions like these you may face some of the greatest challenges of your professional career.

An example of effective statewide mobilization occurred during the 1989 outbreak of typhoid fever among 10,000 conventioneers in New York.[21] This outbreak was detected when two persons with typhoid fever were reported to the state health department from different hospitals in Syracuse, New York, on the Friday evening after the Fourth of July. Typhoid fever is rarely reported in the United States in persons without a history of recent international travel, and neither of the patients had traveled out of the state recently. However, both had attended a convention of firefighters in the Catskill region of New York three weeks before the onsets of their illnesses. Initial information indicated that over 10,000 people had attended that convention, and additional case reports among attendees were being reported to the health department within a day or two of the initial reports. Because typhoid fever is an unusual and potentially fatal illness that physicians may not easily recognize and is often spread to others by a carrier; and because transmission had very possibly been ongoing for three weeks, potentially exposing tens of thousands of visitors to this resort area, a full-scale field investigation was immediately started.

During the weekend following receipt of the initial reports, the state health department mobilized multiple teams to start immediate investigation of the outbreak. All county health departments in the state and epidemiologists in neighboring states were contacted by one team to report possibly related cases to the New York State Department of Health. Standard data collection tools were disseminated, and stool specimens were requested for laboratory analysis. A second team began several cohort studies by telephone, using lists of firefighters who had attended the convention, as well as other convention groups that had met at the resort before or after the firefighters' group. The firefighters convention had occurred three weeks previously, and all attendees had returned to their homes throughout New York and the northeastern United States. The analysis sought to determine the duration, the time of exposure, and the origin of the epidemic, as well as possible vehicles of infection. A third field team began investigating the resort area, administering questionnaires, and collecting blood and stool specimens from staff at the suspect hotel where the first reported typhoid cases had stayed. This team also helped conduct an environmental investigation of the hotel kitchen and potable water supply.

A total of 44 culture-confirmed and 24 probable primary typhoid fever cases were reported in the outbreak from New York, several neighboring states, and Canada, making it the largest outbreak of typhoid fever in the United States in a decade. While complete reporting of the cases took several weeks, the initial telephone survey was completed and analyzed within 24 hours, implicating Hotel

A as the source of the outbreak. A second telephone survey of Hotel A guests identified a 48-hour time period as the likely period of transmission; no cases were found in persons staying at the hotel before or after this time period. The case-control study implicated orange juice as the likely vehicle (Odds Ratio = 5.6, 95% CI 1.1–54.7), and investigation of hotel employees revealed that the one and only ill employee had drunk orange juice. Another employee who prepared the orange juice had a positive stool culture for *Salmonella typhi*, the causative organism. This employee had no symptoms, was probably a typhoid carrier, and was presumed to have caused the outbreak.

Epidemiologists from the New York State Department of Health, several county health departments within New York, neighboring states, and CDC collaborated in the investigation of the outbreak, demonstrating that a large epidemiologic effort can be organized and conducted in a few days. The field studies provided critical information during the initial phase of the epidemic investigation: disease transmission was time limited, no other groups or time periods were implicated, the vehicle and source of the infection were identified quickly, and the culture-positive kitchen employee was removed from food preparation duties.

*4. Modern Social and Technological Advances in the Investigation of Disease Outbreaks: A Hepatitis A Outbreak in New York with a Distinctly Old-Fashioned Cause.* Computers are now a familiar and tremendously useful tool of the epidemiologist. The laptop computer has become as ubiquitous a symbol of the field epidemiologist as the worn-out shoe leather of old. Computers have become indispensable for tabulation of questionnaire responses and for analysis of outbreak data (see Chapter 7). However, as the computerization of all aspects of society increases and computer records are kept for even the most mundane commercial transactions, the potential for use of data already stored and available in the field also increases.

A good example of the value of technological advances occurred during a large hepatitis A outbreak in the Rochester, New York, area in 1994 among patrons of a retail buyers' club.[22] Retail buyers' clubs are large, members-only department stores and supermarkets. These clubs verify membership at the point of sale and can maintain detailed records of each member's purchases and often use them to market items to specific members based on their buying history. These data may also be useful to confirm potential exposure (at least purchase, if not consumption) to food items suspected in a food-borne outbreak. Such databases also establish a cohort that can be used for calculating rates of disease or serve as a sampling frame for epidemiologic studies.

In the spring of 1994, routine surveillance follow-up by the Monroe County Health Department staff of persons with reported hepatitis A revealed that a number of the persons either were co-workers at Buying Club A in Rochester or had purchased food from the club. The county health department then reviewed all recently reported hepatitis A cases in the Monroe County area where Rochester is located. Between April 9 and May 31, 79 cases of hepatitis A had been reported in Monroe and surrounding counties. Nine of the cases occurred in employees of Buying Club A, and 55 occurred in persons who ate food purchased at the club. To confirm the possible association of illness with the club, laboratory-confirmed hepatitis A cases were compared to controls matched by telephone prefix and interviewed by telephone. Eleven of 17 case households reported buying food at the club compared to 7 of 34 control households (matched Odds Ratio = 8.5, 95% CI 1.7–41.6). Cases by date of onset are shown in Figure 20–1—suggesting a common source of exposure.[22] To help identify food items as possible sources, a questionnaire was administered to the cohort of all employees. A history of eating any sugar-glazed item from the club bakery was associated with a relative risk of 4.4 (95% CI 1.2–15.9) for developing hepatitis A. No other food items were positively associated with illness.

Further investigation revealed that a food handler reported being ill with diarrhea, though jaundice was not noticed, approximately one month before the first club-associated cases began to occur (Figure 20–1). His duties during this time period included applying sugar glaze by hand to freshly baked items after cooking. Although the food worker claimed to wear plastic gloves for this task, other workers said that gloves were not always used. Furthermore, facilities for hand washing were not optimally designed and were reportedly used infrequently.

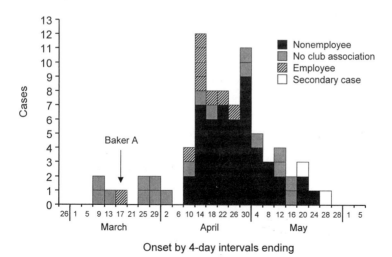

Onset by 4-day intervals ending

**Figure 20–1.** Cases of laboratory-confirmed acute hepatitis A by date of onset, greater Rochester area, New York, March 1–May 31, 1994 [*Source:* Weltman et al., 1996. Used with permission.]

Subsequently, the blood of the food handler was found to have antibodies to hepatitis A indicative of recent infection, leading to the conclusion that he was the source of the outbreak.

Although this investigation clearly implicated a logical source and mode of transmission of the hepatitis epidemic, the exact food item(s) and dates of purchase were not yet known. Since recall of food histories and other events fades with time—and because the incubation period of hepatitis A ranges from 15 to 50 days—it was decided not to administer a questionnaire to club members but, rather, to analyze computer purchasing records for this information. Record review showed that 42 club members with hepatitis had purchased sugar-glazed products from the bakery during the period in question. The dates of purchase were compared to the dates that the implicated employee worked in the bakery. All but three of the 42 members with hepatitis A purchased glazed bakery products during one or both time periods (March 10–12 and March 21–24) that the employee was working and presumably infectious.[22] This information strengthened the conclusion that the outbreak was due to glazed products from the bakery prepared by this employee.

As computerized records of commercial transactions become more common, you should be aware of the potential uses of these data in outbreak investigations. Large buying clubs and other "mega-stores," in particular, may have very detailed data available on purchases by their members. This is fortunate, since these stores serve large numbers of people with the potential for widespread transmission of food-borne agents, if strict hygienic standards are not maintained. An interesting sidelight of the Monroe County investigation was the mechanism of transmission of hepatitis A by hand contamination in preparing sugar-glazed baked products. A similar mechanism of transmission was found during the classic food-borne outbreak investigation in West Branch, Michigan in 1968.[23, 24] It seems that even though technology and computers are changing the world, some mechanisms of disease transmission never change.

*5. The Potential Pitfalls of Using Administrative Data for Public Health Surveillance: A Pseudo-Outbreak of Cholera in New York State, 1991.* The decade of the 1990s saw a dramatic increase in use of electronic systems to capture health-care system data. Administrative data, such as health insurance billing claims, is one source of computerized information available for analysis and for control of health-care costs. Field epidemiologists have been encouraged to look at electronic systems of health data as a potential way to conduct public health surveillance. Such systems have the advantage of containing data on large numbers of persons, if not population-wide data. These data may be more or less readily available to you (usually some red tape is involved in gaining access) and can be analyzed by computer. However, you must exercise great care in using such data for public health purposes, including surveillance, as the following example illustrates.

**Table 20–1.**   Health Insurance Billing Claims and Public Health Surveillance
Reports for Selected Reportable Communicable Diseases, New York, 1991

| ICD | | INSURANCE CLAIMS* | | SURVEILLANCE REPORTS[†] | |
|---|---|---|---|---|---|
| CODE | DIAGNOSIS | PATIENTS | RATE | PATIENTS | RATE |
| 001 | Cholera | 35 | 3.7 | 0 | 0.0 |
| 002 | Typhoid | 5 | 0.5 | 86 | 0.5 |
| 003 | Salmonella | 58 | 6.1 | 3474 | 19.3 |
| 004 | Shigella | 24 | 2.5 | 1058 | 5.9 |

*Health insurance billing claims for New York State and municipal employees, retirees, and their
dependents. Rate per 100,000 insured persons.
†Public health surveillance reports for New York State excluding New York City. Rate per 100,000
population. [*Source*: New York State Department of Health.]

In 1993, the communicable disease unit at the New York State Department of
Health examined electronic health data for possible use as a supplement to existing reportable disease surveillance systems. Data were obtained from the fiscal
intermediary for health insurance claims for 950,000 New York state and municipal employees, retirees, and their dependents for 1991. The analysis plan was to
examine ICD-9 diagnostic codes from the insurance data for reportable communicable diseases and to compare these data with communicable disease cases
reported to the state's communicable disease surveillance system. Table 20–1
shows the number of billing claims in the insurance database for 1991 for four
reportable communicable diseases: cholera, typhoid, salmonella, and shigella.
The rate per insured person for each disease was compared to the statewide disease rate calculated from the reportable disease surveillance data. Disease rates
were lower, but of the same order of magnitude, in the insurance data for salmonella and shigella, and were the same for typhoid. However, the insurance data
contained 35 patients with a diagnosis of cholera with an ICD-9 code of 001,
where none had been reported in the state that year through the traditional surveillance system.

    To check the validity of the billing codes further, the insurance records were
examined to see if a stool culture was done, which is needed to confirm a diagnosis of any of these conditions. This was determined by looking for billing codes
for stool cultures in the insurance data. Of salmonella insurance claims, only 29%
reported a stool culture. The proportion was less for the other diseases (cholera:
3%, typhoid: 0%, shigella: 13%). These findings seriously challenged the validity
of the diagnoses contained in the insurance database.

The cholera cases were of particular concern. No cases of cholera had been reported in New York that year, but it is possible that the diagnosis had been missed because physicians in the United States may not think of cholera in the differential diagnosis of watery diarrhea and may not order the appropriate laboratory tests. However, this number of missed cases would constitute a public health emergency and cast serious doubt on the traditional surveillance system. To gain further insight, detailed ICD-9 4-digit codes were examined. Of the 35 cholera patients, 25 (71%) were reported with an ICD-9 code of 001.1, indicating *V. cholerae*, el Tor strain, a particularly virulent strain of cholera of major worldwide importance. Particularly puzzling, moreover, was the fact that many of these records contained a medical procedure billing code for "destruction by any method including laser, of benign facial lesions or premalignant lesions"—a procedure clearly unrelated to cholera. The investigators then realized that, while ICD-9 001.1 coded for cholera, ICD-9 110.0 coded for "dermatophytosis including infection by trychophyton, etc."—a condition that might fit better with the procedure code for treatment of benign facial lesions. They surmised that a simple numerical transposition of the ICD-9 disease code, as might occur in manual data entry, might have been responsible for the apparent pseudo-outbreak of cholera.

Computers and computerized databases are a boon to the field epidemiologist. However, using these databases may have pitfalls. It is incumbent on you, the field epidemiologist, to learn as much about such databases as possible. Know where the data originate, how they are entered and handled, how they are checked and edited, and what coding systems are used before rushing to incorporate these data in surveillance or field investigation efforts. Such data must be completely characterized as to validity, sensitivity, specificity, and predictive value before pressed into use. In the case described here, a lot of unnecessary work by public health staff would have to be done to sort out the true diagnosis. Public health departments do not have the luxury of following up on too many blind alleys of this sort.

*6. Epidemiology and Laboratory Collaboration to Detect Outbreaks: The Minnesota Department of Health E. coli 0157:H7 subtyping system.* The public health laboratory is a key collaborator with the field epidemiologist in detecting and controlling communicable diseases at the state and local level. A good example of collaboration between epidemiologist and laboratory staff is the system established by the Minnesota Department of Health (MDH) to detect clusters of *Escherichia coli* 0157:H7 subtypes, each of which may have a common source of transmission.[25] *E. coli* 0157:H7 is a significant bacterial pathogen in the United States, causing outbreaks of severe, bloody diarrhea and, uncommonly, hemolytic uremic syndrome, a complication that can cause renal failure and death. *E. coli* 0157:H7 is found in the intestinal tracts of cows and other animals, and outbreaks can occur by consumption of contaminated uncooked meat, particularly ground

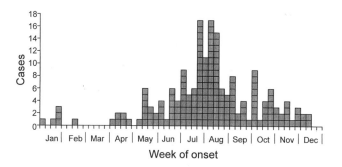

**Figure 20–2.**   Cases of *E. Coli* 0157:H7 by date of onset, Minnesota, 1995. [*Souce:* Bender et al., 1997.[25]]

beef, and potable or recreational water contaminated by animal feces. Prevention and control of these infections depend on surveillance for early detection of potential outbreaks and investigation of possible sources of the bacteria.

Historically, surveillance for *E. coli* 0157:H7 was based on clinical reports of clusters of patients with bloody diarrhea. However, *E. coli* are common in the human intestinal tract and may not be identified as pathogens in stool specimens. Now, since the emergence of the *E. coli* 0157:H7 strain as an important pathogen, clinical laboratories have been encouraged to type *E. coli* isolates or submit isolates to appropriate laboratories for typing. Over time and in many areas of Minnesota, this has provided a baseline number of *E. coli* 0157:H7 isolates for temporal, geographic, and demographic analysis. For example, Figure 20–2 shows the number of *E. coli* 0157:H7 reports by week for the state of Minnesota in 1995.[25]

This method of surveillance can detect large disease outbreaks, but it is limited in its ability to detect smaller clusters. For example, examination of Figure 20–2 does not suggest any clustering patterns except an increase in cases in the summer that is similar to many enteric diseases. Recognizing these limitations, epidemiologists and laboratory personnel at the MDH applied a new laboratory technique, pulsed-field gel electrophoresis (PFGE), to improve the identification procedure in hopes of uncovering disease clusters. As can be seen in Figure 20–3, this "molecular fingerprinting" technique applied to the same *E. coli* 0157:H7 isolates represented in Figure 20–2 shows multiple small clusters of subtypes that are probably related to a common source. Epidemiologists can then focus on each cluster as a discrete transmission event, determine the source, and implement control measures.

In Minnesota during 1994–1995, 10 outbreaks and 35 clusters of *E. coli* 0157:H7 disease were detected, in large part due to the application of PFGE subtyping of isolates. The public health benefits of this epidemiologic and public health laboratory collaboration included identification of a number of outbreaks

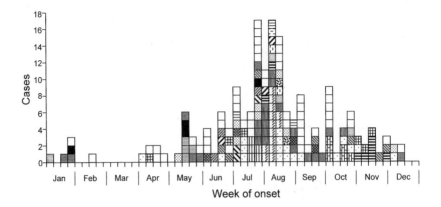

Note: Each white box represents a single, unrelated PFGE pattern, and each design represents multiple isolates of a unique PFGE pattern.

**Figure 20–3.** Cases of *E. Coli* 0157:H7 by date of onset, by pused-feild gel electrophoresis (PFGE) type, Minnesota, 1995. [*Souce:* Bender et al., 1997.[25]]

traced to consumption of contaminated meat and recreational water. Subsequently, with the benefit of enhancements of laboratory techniques and communications technology such as PulseNet, FoodNet and website postings, delineation of numerous local, statewide, multistate and international outbreaks of enteric diseases caused by bacterial pathogens has become increasingly rapid and accurate.[26, 27] Timely response to these data can result in rapid application of control measures and termination of serious outbreaks.

## SUMMARY

Beyond the disciplined application of epidemiologic methods, the conduct of field epidemiologic investigations and surveillance activities by state and local health department staff and their partners occurs within a framework that involves: understanding state and local laws and codes; awareness of personnel and resource constraints; effective collaboration, networking, and information sharing; maximizing information transfer and appropriate incorporation of technologic advances; sensitivity to local, state, and federal political issues that are germane to field epidemiologists; and cooperative and productive working relationships using print and electronic media. Successful field epidemiologists and field epidemiology programs foster collaboration and adequate training, have broad medical and political support and adequate staffing, generate and disseminate findings and important information in a timely fashion, and use investigative opportunities to expand important public health knowledge. The legacy of investigations conducted by state and local health department field epidemiologists is truly broad, deep, rich, and rapidly expanding. This legacy will continue to serve as a premier foundation for you and all current and future field epidemiologists.

## REFERENCES

1. Gostin, L.O. (2000). Public health law in a new century. Part II: public health powers and limits. *J Am Med Assoc* 283, 2979–84.
2. Osterholm, M.T., Birkhead, G.S., Meriwether, R.A. (1996). Impediments to public health surveillance in the 1990s: the lack of resources and the need for priorities. *J Public Health Manage Pract* 2, 11–5.
3. Dean, A.G., Arner, T.G., Sangam, S., et al. (2000). Epi Info 2000, a database and statistics program for public health professionals for use on Windows 95, 98, NT, and 2000 computers. Centers for Disease Control and Prevention, Atlanta.
4. Council of State and Territorial Epidemiologists. (2000). Support, development and implementation of the Epidemic Information Exchange (Epi-X). Position Statement EC-4. Available at http://www.cste.org/ps2000/2000-EC4.htm.
5. Ackman, D.M., Birkhead, G., Flynn, M. (1996). Assessment of surveillance for meningococcal disease in New York, 1991. *Am J Epidemiol* 144, 78–82.
6. Morse, D.L., Birkhead, G.S., Guzewich, J.J. (2000). Investigating foodborne disease. In Y.H. Hui, J.R. Gorham, K.D. Murrell, et al. (eds.), *Foodborne Disease Handbook: Diseases Caused by Bacteria*, 2nd ed., vol. 1, Marcel Dekker, New York. pp. 587–643.
7. Institute of Medicine (1988). *The Future of Public Health*. National Academy Press, Washington, D.C.
8. Gostin, L.O., Hodge Jr., J.G, Valdiserri, R.O. (2001). Informational privacy and the public's health: the Model State Public Health Privacy Act. *Am J Public Health* 91, 1388–92.
9. Hodge Jr., J.G., Gostin, L.O., CSTE Advisory Committee. (May 24, 2004). *Public Health Practice vs. Research: A Report for Public Health Practitioners Including Cases and Guidance for Making Distinctions*. Council of State and Territorial Epidemiologists. Available at: www.cste.org/pdffiles/newpdffiles/CSTEPHResRptHodgeFinal.5.24.04.pdf
10. Shramm, M., Vogt, R.L., Mamolen, J. (1991). Disease surveillance in Vermont: who reports? *Public Health Rep* 106, 95–7.
11. Harkess, J.R., Gildon, B.A., Archer, P.W., et al. (1988). Is passive surveillance always insensitive? An evaluation of shigellosis surveillance in Oklahoma. *Am J Public Health* 128, 878–81.
12. Konowitz, P.M., Petrossian, G.A., Rose, D.N. (1984). The underreporting of disease and physicians' knowledge of reporting requirement. *Public Health Rep* 99, 31–5.
13. Vogt, R.L., LaRue, D., Klaucke, D.N., et al. (1983). Comparison of an active and passive surveillance system of primary care providers for hepatitis, measles, rubella and salmonellosis in Vermont. *Am J Public Health* 73, 795–7.
14. Todd, J., Fishaut, M., Kapral, F., et al. (1978). Toxic-shock syndrome associated with phage-group-1 staphylococci. *Lancet* 2, 1116–8.
15. Davis, J.P., Chesney, P.J., Wand, P.J., et al. (1980). Toxic-shock syndrome: epidemiologic features, recurrence, risk factors, and prevention. *N Engl J Med* 303, 1429–35.

16. Shands, K.N., Schmid, G.P., Dan, B.D., et al. (1980). Toxic-shock syndrome in menstruating women: association with tampon use and *Staphylococcus aureus* and clinical features in 52 cases. *N Engl J Med* 303, 1436–42.
17. Centers for Disease Control (1980). Toxic-shock syndrome. *Morb Mortal Wkly Rep* 29, 229–30.
18. Schleck, W.F. III, Shands, K.N., Reingold, A.L., et al. (1982). Risk factors for development of toxic shock syndrome: association with a tampon brand. *J Am Med Assoc* 248, 835–9.
19. Osterholm, M.T., Davis, J.P., Gibson, R.W., et al. (1982). Tri-state Toxic-Shock Syndrome Study. I. Epidemiologic findings. *J Infect Dis* 145, 431–40.
20. Morse, D.L., Guzewich, J.J., Hanrahan, J.P., et al. (1986). Widespread outbreaks of clam- and oyster-associated gastroenteritis: role of Norwalk virus. *N Engl J Med* 314, 678–81.
21. Birkhead, G.S., Morse, D.L., Levine, W.C., et al. (1993). Typhoid fever at a resort hotel in New York: a large outbreak with an unusual vehicle. *J Infect Dis* 167, 1228–32.
22. Weltman, A.C., Bennett, N.M., Ackman, D.A., et al. (1996). An outbreak of hepatitis A associated with a bakery, New York, 1994: The 1968 "West Branch, Michigan" outbreak repeated. *Epidemiol Infect* 117, 333–41.
23. Schoenbaum, S.C., Baker, O., Jezek, Z. (1976). Common-source outbreak of hepatitis due to glazed and iced pastries. *Am J Epidemiol* 104, 74–80.
24. Roueche, B. (1982). The West Branch Study. In *The Medical Detectives*, pp. 233–52. Washington Square Press, New York.
25. Bender, J.B., Hedberg, C.W., Besser, J.M., et al. (1997). Surveillance for *Escherichia coli* 0157:H7 infections in Minnesota by molecular subtyping. *N Engl J Med* 337, 388–94.
26. National Center for Infectious Diseases, Centers for Disease Control. Update on multistate outbreak of *E. coli* 0157:H7 infections from fresh spinach, September 15, 2006. Available at: http://www.cdc.gov/ecoli/2006/september/updates/091506.htm
27. National Center for Infectious Diseases, Centers for Disease Control. Salmonellosis—outbreak investigation, February, 2007. Available at: http://www.cdc.gov/ncidod/dbmd/diseaseinfo/salmonellosis_2007/outbreak_notice.htm

# 21

## EPIDEMIOLOGIC PRACTICES IN LOW-INCOME COUNTRIES

Stanley O. Foster

This chapter covers three broad areas of consideration: (*1*) factors that are influencing the practice of epidemiology in low-income countries (*2*) examples of how some countries have used field epidemiology, and (*3*) practical tips and advice to help you prepare for and perform in this unique field setting.

### INFLUENCING FACTORS

In a world where 2.7 billion (41%) of the world's population live on less than $2 a day, and where 10 million children die each year before their fifth birthdays, epidemiology is an essential tool for identifying and eliminating health disparities.[1, 2]

For the epidemiologist, investigations in other geographic and cultural settings provide both opportunities and challenges. The settings in which epidemiology is practiced in low-income countries are changing. Five factors are contributing to these changes.

1. *International Health Regulations:* The 2005 revision of the International Health Regulations (IHR) became effective in 2007. The IHR states, "Parties … are required to develop, strengthen and maintain core

surveillance and response capacities to detect, assess, notify and report public health events to the World Health Organization (WHO), and respond to public health risks and public health emergencies."[3]

2. *SARS and Avian Influenza:* The emergence of global epidemics, SARS, and (potentially) avian influenza call for new global partnerships in surveillance, investigation, quarantine, and control. The emergence of SARS and the potential emergence of epidemic avian influenza exemplify the global connectedness of high case-fatality infectious diseases. The evolution of SARS in China and its subsequent spread to Hong Kong and Canada illustrate the need for coordinated action.[4, 5, 6] Accidental or purposeful release of highly pathogenic organisms, should it occur, will require the same epidemiologic skills.

3. *National and International Training Programs in Epidemiology:* Over the last two decades, countries have increasingly recognized the need for epidemiologic skills in assessing health needs, planning interventions, and monitoring and evaluating programs. While epidemiologic skills are being learned on the job and in academic settings, hands-on practical training has been particularly effective. Two programs, the Centers for Disease Control's (CDC's) Field Epidemiology Training Programs (FETP) and the Rockefeller Foundation's Public Health Schools without Walls, have used academic and field experiences to strengthen epidemiologic skills.[7]

4. *HIV/AIDS Epidemic:* HIV/AIDs has had both a positive and a negative effect on low-income country epidemiologic competence. The development of partnerships and the increase in resources for prevention, treatment, and research are providing more opportunities for collaborative and mentored skill development. On the negative side, the demands of HIV/AIDs programs and the morbidity, disability, and mortality from HIV/AIDS among health care workers are reducing epidemiologic capacity.

5. *Millennium Development Goals:* In the year 2000, the countries of the world, meeting under the auspices of the United Nations, established eight goals to be achieved by the year 2015.[8] Three of these goals are specifically health-related: Goal 4: Reduce child mortality; Goal 5: Improve maternal health; and Goal 6: Combat HIV/AIDS, malaria and other diseases. At the country level, epidemiologic skills are required for assessing current levels of morbidity, disability, and mortality; for identifying populations at risk; for assessing and improving program efficacy; and for program monitoring and evaluation.

## Examples of the Use of Epidemiology

Many low-income countries lack the established epidemiologic capacity of the high-income countries. In these countries, limited resources require the selection of epidemiologic methods that provide "data for action" or "data for decision making" at the lowest cost. The following are examples of how epidemiology is being used in low-income countries to address their health problems. Examples are provided under four categories: surveillance, epidemiologic investigations, population-based surveys, and prospective studies.

## SURVEILLANCE

### Routine Reporting

At the beginning of the 21st century, many surveillance systems in low-income countries relied on reported cases of disease through passive reporting systems. Sensitivity and specificity of outpatient data were low, and the data were of limited value and use. Peripheral health workers often spend two to four hours per month filling out forms. When queried by the author as to what happens to their forms, many workers replied that "the data go to district, region, and national levels where they are destroyed in a paper shredder." Hospital data, while of higher specificity, are seldom representative of the population at large and also are of limited use. A study from Uganda illustrates some of problems of data collection, analysis, and use at the field level (Table 21–1.)[9]

Improvements in surveillance, as being implemented by the Ugandan Ministry of Health, include the following actions:

1. Increasing health-worker understanding of the why and how of routine reporting
2. Confidence of these health workers that their reports are looked at in a timely manner and, when appropriate, acted upon
3. Capacity and commitment of district staff to review incoming reports in a timely and competent manner
4. Capacity of district staff to respond in a timely manner
5. Ongoing capacity-building through on-the-job training and "support-a-vision," in contrast to all-too-frequent critical and downgrading supervision.

### Unusual Event Reporting

Indonesia has developed an "unusual event" reporting system that identifies, investigates, and responds to unexpected rare events. Attention to the events may come from the media (press, radio, TV), through the civil administration, non-governmental organizations, a health facility seeing an unexpected increase in the number of cases of similar symptoms, or from an alert health care provider.

**Table 21-1.** Indicators of performance and support of infectious disease surveillance activities at health facilities* — Uganda, 2000

| INDICATOR | NO. | (%) |
|---|---|---|
| Case detection, registration, and reporting | | |
| Outpatient clinic register | 48 | (92) |
| Register correctly filled out | 29 | (56) |
| Official standardized case definitions | 18 | (35) |
| Adequate supply of reporting forms during preceding 6 months | 18 | (35) |
| Monthly report agreed with clinic register | 15 | (29) |
| Ability to confirm cases | | |
| Malaria | 27 | (51) |
| Tuberculosis | 23 | (44) |
| Meningococcal meningitis | 11 | (21) |
| Cholera | 0 | (0) |
| Shigellosis | 0 | (0) |
| Data analysis and use | | |
| Prepared line graphs or trend line of cases | 5 | (10) |
| Had a threshold for action for epidemic-prone diseases | 14 | (27) |
| Had conducted community prevention and control measures | 26 | (50) |
| Had a report of a communitywide public intervention | 8 | (15) |
| Feedback, supervision, and training | | |
| Received feedback at least once during preceding 6 months | 8 | (15) |
| Received performance review at least once during preceding 6 months | 11 | (32) |
| Received training on use of surveillance forms | 32 | (62) |
| Resources available | | |
| Stationery | 39 | (75) |
| Calculator | 40 | (77) |
| Telephone service | 14 | (27) |
| Radio-call | 7 | (14) |

*N=52 health facilities (e.g., dispensaries, health centers, and hospitals) surveyed.

Examples include common-source outbreaks of food-borne illness, outbreaks of infectious disease, or environmental toxic exposures. This system also increased the sensitivity of surveillance during the Aceh Tsunami and the current outbreak of "bird flu." At each level there is a time-specific target for action.

## Sentinel Surveillance

In most countries, HIV/AIDS programs have developed sentinel surveillance systems to estimate the burden of disease and to monitor trends over time. These systems utilize serologic surveillance of new attendees at selected prenatal clinics for HIV positivity. Figure 21–1 below demonstrates how Uganda has utilized prenatal surveillance to monitor trends in HIV/AIDS prevalence.[10] This figure, taken from the Uganda AIDS Bulletin, emphasizes the importance of providing regular feedback of surveillance data to the providers of data; to the policy makers; and to those planning, implementing, and monitoring prevention and control program.

## Epidemic Disease Surveillance

While routine surveillance systems are being strengthened, epidemic diseases that require rapid emergency response frequently require their own special surveillance. This is especially true for meningitis, yellow fever, cholera, and plague. In Africa, meningococcal meningitis is endemic in a belt across Africa—stretching from west to east. In this belt, known as the *meningitis belt*, epidemics occasionally emerge, creating medical emergencies. Based on work in Burkina Faso, WHO has developed guidelines enabling districts to identify their own action thresholds.[11, 12] For rural populations of more than 30,000, 5 cases/100,000 population in one week triggers: (*1*). an early warning, (*2*) an investigation, (*3*) an assessment of

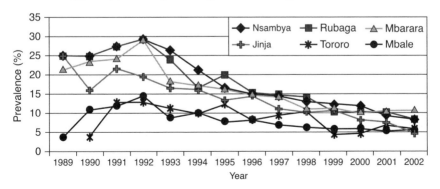

**Figure 21-1.** HIV infection prevalence rates among antenatal care antenatal clinic attendees (ANC) in major Ugandan towns from 1989–2002. [*Source:* Uganda Ministry of Health, STD/HIV/AIDS Surveillance Report, June 2003.]

epidemic preparedness, and (4) a vaccination campaign, provided disease is present in adjoining districts.

## Active Surveillance

Disease-eradication programs such as smallpox in the 1960s and 1970s and polio-myelitis today require intense surveillance aimed at detecting every case. The polio program has the goal of identifying every case of Acute Flaccid Paralysis (AFP).[13] This involves an active search of caretakers (traditional healers, practitioners, and health facilities) for cases of AFP. Each identified case is investigated, a stool specimen is collected for laboratory diagnosis, and cases are followed up at 60 days. Since there is a baseline rate of non-polio AFP of 2 cases of AFP per 100,000 children ages 0–15, the sensitivity of AFP surveillance can be monitored by the non-polio AFP rate. Polio surveillance is continually monitored at country, region, and global levels using the following criteria: AFP Cases, Non-Polio AFP rate (target 2 AFP cases per 100,000 <15), % AFP with 2 stool specimens collected within 14 days, and wild virus isolations (Table 21–2).

## EPIDEMIOLOGIC INVESTIGATIONS

A major epidemiologic priority is the investigation of health problems identified through surveillance. Four examples illustrate the range of issues and methods.

**Table 21-2.**   Performance of AFP surveillance and reported wild poliovirus cases, 2004 and 2005, by WHO Region

| WHD REGION | NO. OF REPORTED AFP CASES* | | NON-POLIO AFP RATE | | PRESENT AFP WITH ADEQUATE STOOL SPECIMENS | | WILD VINUS CONFORMED POLIO CASES | |
|---|---|---|---|---|---|---|---|---|
| | 2004 | 2005 | 2004 | 2006 | 2004 | 2006 | 2004 | 2006 |
| AFR | 9719 | 11685 | 2.90 | 3.30 | 89% | 85% | 934 | 851 |
| AMR | 2309 | 2202 | 1.38 | 1.33 | 79% | 80% | 0 | 0 |
| EMR | 6176 | 8345 | 2.70 | 3.69 | 89% | 88% | 187 | 727 |
| EUR | 1516 | 1473 | 1.14 | 1.10 | 81% | 82% | 0 | 0 |
| SEAR | 16270 | 31519 | 2.70 | 5.21 | 83% | 82% | 134 | 373 |
| WPR | 6521 | 6898 | 1.61 | 1.65 | 88% | 88% | 0 | 0 |
| GLOBAL | 42511 | 62422 | 2.29 | 3.34 | 86% | 84% | 1255 | 1951 |

*Data in WHD as of 02 May 2006

*Source:* WHO: Global Polio Eradication Initiative Annual Report. 2005.

## Renal Failure

In 1990, the trainers of an epidemiology course in Jos, Nigeria, solicited the assistance of the Ministry of Health in identifying a health problem to serve as a class field exercise. A cluster of pediatric renal failure cases was identified. Using a case-control methodology, the class identified intake of paracetamol syrup as highly associated with renal failure. Use of paracetamol syrup was stopped. Eighty-five of 102 cases died, for a case fatality rate of 83%.[14] When a subsequent outbreak occurred at Oluyoro Catholic Hospital, Oke-Ola, Ilorin, Oyo State, further investigation identified a common source of a renal toxin, ethylene glycol, instead of the required propylene glycol. The Minister of Health stopped all distribution of paracetamol syrup until the source of the toxin was identified and removed from the market.[15] Manufacturers were required to pass raw-material inspection before restarting production.

## Injuries

Until recently, mortality from injuries, suicide, and violence has been under-recognized. Table 21–3 summarizes the estimated number of deaths from these three causes for 2005 and (projected) 2030.[16]

Given that nine percent of deaths, one in every 11, are attributed to these four causes, studies need to be carried out to identify risk factors and develop and test risk-reduction strategies. One such example is described below.

Razzak and Luby studied traffic deaths and injuries in Karachi, Pakistan. Using a two-sample capture-recapture method, they estimated 972 deaths and 18,936 injuries over a 10-month period.[17] The police system had identified only

**Table 21-3.** Estimated Deaths Due to Injuries, Sucide, Violence & War World Wide, 2005-2030

|  | 2005 | | 2003 | |
|---|---|---|---|---|
|  | NUMBER | PERCENT | NUMBER | PERCENT |
| Unintentional Injuries | 3,700,00 | 6.3 | 4,763,000 | 6.4 |
| Self Inflicted | 912,00 | 1.6 | 1,138,000 | 1.5 |
| Violence | 593,000 | 1.0 | 805,000 | 1.1 |
| War | 184,000 | 0.3 | 318,000 | 0.4 |
| Sub-Total | 5,389,000 | 9.2 | 7,024,000 | 9.4 |
| Total | 58,26,000 | 100.0 | 74,273,000 | 100.0 |

Source: World Bank.Burden of Disease Project http://www.who.int/healthinfo/statistics/bodpro jectionspaper.pdf

56% of cases and 4% of severe injuries. The annual traffic death and injury rates for 1994 were 11.2 deaths and 185 injuries per 100,000 population.

## Ebola Fever

In the Gulu District of Uganda, a remote area near the Sudanese border, cases of hemorrhagic fever were recognized and reported in 2002. Ebola virus was isolated at the National Virology Laboratory in South Africa. Widespread active surveillance and community education were initiated to inform and educate the public. Identified cases were hospitalized; isolation and barrier nursing were instituted to prevent nosocomial spread. By the time transmission had been interrupted, 425 cases and 224 deaths had been identified.[18]

## Toxic Exposures

Environmental hazards are increasingly being recognized as contributors to the burden of disease. Examples include the 1984 Bhopal Union Carbide industrial accident, which released methyl isocynate into the air and caused an estimated 6000 deaths and significant morbidity in India.[19] In neighboring Bangladesh, contamination of ground water with arsenic has been identified as a major health risk.[20] In both outbreaks, prospective follow-up studies were instituted to look at the long-term health consequences of acute exposure in Bhopal and the long-term exposure to arsenic in Bangladesh.[21, 22]

## POPULATION SURVEYS

### Censuses and National Surveys

For national planning, policy making, and revenue allocation, national surveys are needed. Such surveys range from national censuses carried out every 10 years, to the Demographic and Health Surveys (DHS) carried out primarily in low-income countries every four years.[23] The DHS surveys are multiple-indicator surveys that measure demographic and fertility data at the sub-national and national levels. Surveys have a large sample size, 5000 to 30,000 households, and have been carried out in 75 countries. Data are available on-line and can be summarized by simple on-line statistical packages. The data can also be downloaded by responsible investigators.

### Natural Disasters

In 1970, Sommer and Mosley reported on the use of a rapid helicopter survey in the assessment of a cyclone that killed somewhere between 225,000 and 500,000 people in Bangladesh.[24] While the medical response teams were being mobilized around the world, the assessment showed that injuries were not the priority, and that the greatest needs were for draft animals and farm tools. As Bangladeshi disaster-preparedness, including the building of cyclone shelters, improved, investigation of a later cyclone in 1991 documented the effectiveness of the shelters, and three mortality risks: children under 10, women over 40, and individuals not getting to shelters.[25] Following the tsunami of December 26, 2004, the Thai Ministry instituted their emergency response plan and provided important data to document the impact of the tsunami and the mobilization of resources.[26]

## War-Related Noncombatant Casualties

Warring parties often consider noncombatant deaths as an expected collateral of fighting. The aggressor seldom allows or facilitates the measurement of noncombatant deaths. Surveys are, however, important to alert global policy-makers of the human-rights injustices of war, the mortality cost to noncombatants, the needs of the affected population, and to provide a framework for disaster response. Two studies document war-related noncombatant mortality: in the Democratic Republic of Congo in 2004, and in Iraq in 2005. In the Democratic Republic of Congo, a survey by an International Rescue Committee team estimated 3.9 million deaths, most of whom were noncombatants.[27] In Iraq, a similar survey documented a 58-fold increase in violent deaths and an estimated 98,000 excess deaths.[28]

## PROSPECTIVE POPULATION STUDIES

Prospective studies of populations are used to provide important epidemiologic data on at-risk populations including:

1. Documentation of changes in health status; for example, the emergence of obesity, diabetes, and cardiovascular disease as populations experience an epidemiologic transition and a shift from rural to urban lifestyles
2. Assessment of the contribution of a risk factor to disease emergence; for example, tobacco smoking and cancer
3. Long-term follow-up of toxic exposures as occurred in Bhopal, India and Bangladesh as described above.[21, 22]
4. Assessing the effectiveness of health promotion, prevention, and treatment on disease morbidity, disability, and mortality.

Listed below are four studies that have documented improved strategies in disease control.

## Presumptive Treatment of Pregnant Women for Malaria[29]

Working in a highly endemic malaria area in Malawi, Steketee and colleagues compared the effectiveness of presumptive treatment of malaria in pregnant women. Comparing the Chloroquine and Mefloquine groups, the women in the chloroquine group had significantly increased risk of parasitemia: persistent (OR=30.9), breakthrough (OR=11.1), and at delivery: peripheral (OR=8.7), placental (OR=7.4), and cord blood (OR=4.1) parasitemia. This study was key to the development of the current policy of presumptively treating pregnant women with an effective antimalarial drug.

## Reduction of Neonatal Mortality

In Ghadchiroli, India, Bang and colleagues identified neonatal mortality as responsible for 75% of infant mortality. Further investigations demonstrated that traditional birth attendants (TBAs) were only attentive to mothers; the lack of attention to newborns and traditional practices contributed to respiratory distress, airway obstruction, hypothermia, hypoglycemia, and sepsis. In a study of intervention and non-intervention communities, training village women ("barefoot neonatologists") in clearing the airway, warming, immediate breastfeeding, and recognition and treatment of sepsis led to a reduction in neonatal mortality from 62 to 25 and infant mortality from 75 to 39.[30]

## Pneumonia in Nepal

Pandev and colleagues carried out a controlled intervention trial among 13,404 children in the highlands of Nepal. In the intervention group, community health workers were trained to diagnose and treat pneumonia. Compared to the non-intervention group, overall under-five mortality was reduced by 28% in the intervention group.[31] This study was important in showing the feasibility and effectiveness of developing a community program of malaria diagnosis and treatment.

## Handwashing in Pakistan

In urban Karachi, Luby and colleagues randomly assigned neighborhoods into three groups: (1) handwashing with antibacterial soap, (2) handwashing with plain soap, and (3) controls. The intervention group with handwashing and soap (both types) had a 50% lower incidence of pneumonia, 53% lower incidence of diarrhea, and 34% lower incidence of impetigo.[32] Clearly the challenge of this research is to find ways for handwashing promotion and support at the community level.

## Practical Advice

Envision yourself assigned to investigate an epidemic of an unknown disease in an unfamiliar area of the world and in a country where both the language and the culture are different from anything you have previously experienced. Such an assignment encapsulates the challenge of field epidemiology in the international setting. Although the approach to international field investigations is similar to that described in Chapter 5, carrying out an investigation in unfamiliar settings has unique aspects.

## Be Prepared

If you have an interest in global health or are in a position that provides opportunities for global epidemiologic assistance, it is essential to be prepared, even though you never know what is coming. Twice in my career, Alexander D. Langmuir, the founder of the Epidemic Intelligence Service at CDC, called me and said, "If you are not on the plane by sundown, you are not going."

Being prepared to accept an international assignment often requires weeks (passport) or months (immunization). Those who are prepared get to go; those not prepared do not go. Preparation includes:

- an up-to-date valid passport, two photocopies of the identification page (in case the passport is stolen), and at least four extra pictures for visas;
- up-to-date immunizations for hepatitis A, hepatitis B, diphtheria, tetanus, poliomyelitis, and yellow fever (for tropical areas of Africa and South America). Rabies vaccine is recommended for veterinarians collecting specimens from animals and for joggers, and an international certificate verifying yellow fever immunization is required by international sanitary regulations;[*]
- a box of key items that you can easily forget in the last moment, such as: a first-aid kit, flashlight with extra batteries, insect repellent, canteen, water purification tablets, and a solar-operated calculator.

## Getting Ready

Because many countries in the developing world have rudimentary disease-reporting systems at best, most requests for epidemiologic assistance arise from adverse health events brought to the government's attention through the press or the political system. Outbreaks are generally of two types: (*1*) large outbreaks of a major

* A list of recommended vaccinations for adults can be found on the CDC website: http://www.cdc.gov/nip/recs/adult-schedule.pdf.

epidemic disease (yellow fever, cholera, meningococcal meningitis), or (2) acute episodes of unexplained mortality, such as those caused by adulterated drugs or foods, toxic exposures, or rare hemorrhagic fevers. Detection is frequently delayed because of inadequate surveillance, poor communications, or the tendency of officials to overlook potential problems in the hope that the problems will eventually disappear. When the outbreaks do become public, there is often a sense of panic. For the public health official pressured to act, the arrival of technical assistance provides a visible sign of government response to the emergency. The request frequently carries with it the expectation of external resources to control the problem.

When a request for assistance is received, it is important to acknowledge receipt and provide a time frame in which a response will be forthcoming. Contact should be made with WHO, international and bilateral agencies working in the country, and the diplomatic mission to which you will be attached. These early contacts are useful in verifying the need for epidemiologic assistance; providing additional information on the outbreak; identifying other ongoing requests for assistance; and, most important, opening the channels of communication for in-country collaboration and support.

The typically short lead time between receipt of a request and departure (hours to days) requires that you prepare carefully. Place a high priority on arranging travel (some countries have only one flight in and out per week) and obtaining a visa or visas. The latter will require a current passport, passport-sized photos, and contact with the diplomatic mission accredited to grant visas. Clearances on the provision of technical assistance, preferably in writing, should be obtained from the requesting country, the funding agency, and your own supervisor. Advance information on the flight number and the arrival time should be communicated to an in-country contact with a request for airport assistance. Airport assistance will frequently reduce the hassle of immigration and customs and is especially important when the investigation requires carrying a computer (restricted in some countries); specimen collection materials such as needles, syringes; or laboratory equipment.

Your personal health merits attention. Written health guidelines for international travel are available from WHO and from many public health agencies. Sites relating to travelers' health available on the Internet can identify health hazards for individual countries. Experts on travelers' health can be found in larger health departments, major hospitals, and quarantine facilities. Travelers to malarious areas need to initiate appropriate chemoprophylaxis. If travel is to an area where *Plasmodium falciparum* is endemic and drug-resistant strains have been identified, a malaria expert should be contacted about current recommendations for chemoprophylaxis and back-up disease treatment. As medical facilities may be limited or of questionable quality in-country, you should assemble a basic medical kit for personal use that includes: a thermometer, antipyretics, antihistamines, antibiotic eye ointment, chapstick, oral rehydration salts (ORS) for treatment of dehydrating diarrheas, water purification tablets, antibiotics for severe diarrheal illness, and simple bandages. Pack lightly. Men should include a jacket, and for women, native dress or a simple dress (long with long sleeves if custom expects it) for official visits. Take two sets of hand-washable comfortable clothes, good walking shoes, and sneakers. A small daypack and a carry-on roll-on bag are often sufficient and enable the traveler to avoid the hassle of waiting for baggage. Other important items to pack include a canteen, a flashlight with extra batteries, a Swiss Army–type knife (in checked baggage), hat, soap, towel, and plastic gloves (in case you are required to provide first aid), and an extra pair of glasses. While sunglasses are useful during travel, they are, in many cultures, a barrier to effective communication. Clear, not tinted, glasses are recommended during conversations.

As checked luggage may be delayed or lost en route, carry all essential items such as prescription medicines, one change of washable clothes, and toiletries *in your hand baggage*. If your luggage is lost, airlines will frequently provide money for an extra set of clothes. Replacements can often be obtained in the local market in a few hours.

Consider your money carefully. As credit cards and travelers' checks are not always accepted, cash may be needed. If it is possible that you will need to fund in-country travel, gasoline, or field staff, establish a mechanism for transfer of funds. For personal safety reasons, carrying large amounts of cash is not recommended. Wear a money belt. As investigations scheduled for a few weeks may on occasion last for several months, set aside one evening before departure for family or close friends.

As international investigations frequently involve unknown or unfamiliar conditions, use the few available hours to read up on possible disease etiologies; collect a few key references; identify potential back-up technical expertise that will be available to respond if needed (e.g., epidemiologic, statistical, laboratory); and talk to individuals who have worked in the country. Depending on the nature of the request, consider the need for clerical supplies, a portable computer, and specimen collection and shipping materials. Keep a diary of events, persons met, and data in a bound notebook (loose pieces of paper can be a disaster). Be sure that any electrical equipment is compatible in voltage and plug type to what is available at your destination. Plugging a 110-volt computer into a 220-volt line will destroy the computer. It is important to back up your data on disks or flash drive frequently; keep backup disks at a separate place. Computer crashes, theft, or accidents have compromised the results of many investigations. Solar calculators are an excellent investment, both for work in remote villages without electricity and as a token of appreciation for collaborating field staff.

Perhaps the most important part of your preparation is to collect one or two books on the country and culture for reading in transit. Cultural differences are significant and important.[2, 3] In certain societies, it is inappropriate to shake hands with members of the opposite sex. In others, showing the sole of your shoe is a major breach of etiquette. Mistakes will be made, but a few small steps demonstrating good faith and affirming your recognition and appreciation of the new culture will facilitate the development of effective working relationships. Knowledge of a country's history, geography, and greetings in the local language is a good place to start. Many cultures require that women's arms and legs be covered. While Western dress is acceptable for women, wearing clothes similar to those of the women that you are working with is preferable and often more comfortable. Care should be taken not to wear the clothes of the elite.

E-mail and long-distance telephones are both a blessing and a curse to the field epidemiologist. Both provide an opportunity to solicit information and advice that you and your national colleagues see as important. On the curse side is the tendency of some supervisors to micromanage the investigation from afar, frequently disrupting and paralyzing the collegiality of a field investigation. It is therefore important to establish ground rules with your supervisor in advance.

## The First Day

The first day is important both in terms of whom you meet and the order in which you meet them. Critical to success is your attitude. Are you the knight in shining armor coming to solve an important problem, or a colleague coming to work with national authorities to help them solve their problem?[4] The latter approach is the only appropriate one. In many cultures, it is necessary to establish rapport before proceeding with substantive discussions. Finding areas of common interest is an art that bears preparation and practice. During the protocol visits, a dependable national should be identified as responsible for the investigation. If you are not fluent in the language of the country, you will need an interpreter. Frequently, they are provided by the government. If you are responsible for recruiting an interpreter, be specific as to what you want—an individual willing to travel under difficult circumstances and to work long hours. Be sure to identify the source of funding and finalize the terms of employment in writing before departure to the field.

Before heading to the field, obtain maps, collect information on what is already known about the affected area, the health hazard, and the basic epidemiologic questions of who, what, when, and where. It is useful to determine how the outbreak came to public attention, the nature and timing of the response, and the reasons for the request. Be sure that you understand what is expected of you, and allocate top priorities to those tasks.

Logistics is a major challenge for the field epidemiologist. Request a vehicle with seat belts. Reliable transport, a driver, maps, gasoline, spare tire(s), a jack, and a lug wrench often require ingenuity and time to acquire. Do not take the driver's word that the vehicle is field-ready; check out the transport yourself. Take the time to discuss with the driver your expectations regarding his driving, such as obeying the speed limit and not passing on hills. Ensuring compliance, especially during the first hour of travel, is good prevention. If the driver starts driving dangerously, ask the driver to stop. Calmly discuss again the rules of the road. The possibility of an accident in areas where blood supplies are not safe justifies expecting and enforcing safe driving practices. A reliable driver is worth his weight in gold. In most countries, it is dangerous to drive at night; so don't. If safe water and food are not available in the affected area, these, too, need to be procured in advance.

## The Investigation

Naturally, after days of preparation you will want to get on with the investigation and examine cases. However, the prelude to any field investigation is the introduction to the local authorities. These visits should be viewed not as protocol but as team recruitment. Local authorities will serve as guides, provide introductions at the community and household level, and facilitate community and family participation in the investigation. In addition, local authorities may have access to the only comfortable places to sleep and eat.

Once the existence of a health problem has been established, the next step in the investigation is the establishment of a case definition. This will require collecting a clinical history and a physical examination on several, preferably recently, affected individuals. It is important to know that diseases often have a local name. For example, a search for yellow fever survivors for serologic tests in Ghana was totally unsuccessful until the investigators learned the local name— "horse-piss eye disease"*. With that local definition, over 100 cases were found in an area where the descriptions "yellow skin," "jaundice," or "dark urine" had failed to identify a single case. If timely laboratory support is not available, cases will usually be defined on clinical grounds. Where possible, use simple and workable definitions, such as those established by WHO. For example, the WHO case definition of poliomyelitis is "acute onset of asymmetric flaccid paralysis without sensory change"; that for neonatal tetanus includes "breast-fed, cried normally during the first few days of life, stopped sucking, developed spasms, and died between days 3 and 21"; and that for shigellosis is simply "diarrhea with blood."

---

* Newberry, D., personal communication.

Once a case definition has been established, the next task is finding cases. Determining when and where cases occurred will frequently require the ingenuity and assistance of local political, religious, and traditional authorities. With a lay-adapted case definition and a list of geographic subunits (e.g., districts and villages), the challenge is to find the most efficient way to identify cases. This may utilize telephone contact among local authorities, police radio contact, or sending out traditional messengers on foot. On some occasions, it may be necessary to organize an active community-to-community search. Such surveys need to be well planned and involve several key steps: (1) recruitment and selection of personnel; (2) development and testing of the data collection instrument; (3) on-the-job training of the staff in field survey techniques; (4) utilization of field training to refine the survey instrument; and (5) mobilization of logistic support (see Chapter 6).

The conduct of the investigation will require an understanding of cultural norms and practices. For example, in some Muslim cultures, where men are not allowed to enter a house or talk to women, enumerators will have to be female. In developing the survey instrument and in carrying out interviews, knowledge of the local health belief model is useful. For individuals who traditionally attribute illness to a curse or to the supernatural, biological causality does not make sense. You may often encounter events worthy of in-depth investigation and eventual publication. It is, however, important to give priority to the reasons for which your assistance was requested: the identification of etiology, the route of exposure, risk factors, and potential control strategies. Once an etiology is identified and control measures are agreed upon, control activities should become the primary focus of attention. Monitoring the quality and effectiveness of these control actions often requires new and creative approaches.

Fieldwork, even under ideal conditions, can be stressful. Absence from home, long hours, unfamiliar food, difficult climates, especially if accompanied by illness, often pose a health risk to the visiting epidemiologist. Consider your physical and mental well-being. A short half-day break may lead to a renewed sense of purpose and perspective. It is important to drink adequate "safe" fluids (kidney stones are an occupational hazard in dry climates). At times it will be difficult to stay calm when "things fall apart." Ability to laugh at yourself and a good sense of humor are essential..

## Communicating and Reporting

An important aspect of the investigation is keeping those responsible informed. This includes the officials who requested the investigation, local health officials, political or traditional leaders cooperating in the investigation, and technical experts at the investigator's home institution. In areas where telephones do not exist or do not function, alternative means of communication need to be identified (e.g., police or short-wave radio). If communication is difficult, it is useful to set up a schedule for contact. Radio messages need to be discreetly worded to avoid misinterpretation by others with radio access. In some remote areas, couriers may be needed to transport messages via local transport or on foot.

Before leaving the country, the investigative team has the responsibility to report the investigative findings and the recommended actions; first, to those responsible and, additionally, to others involved in the request or follow-up actions. It is important that your national counterpart have a prominent role in these debriefings. While hand-prepared audiovisuals such as transparencies are often useful in making the presentation, handouts or flip charts provide backup in case of power failure. Separate debriefings for those with different interests are often useful. This allows the debriefing messages to be targeted to meet special needs. Results of the investigation need to be clearly presented in a language understandable to the intended audience. Acknowledgments should be given to the individuals assisting in the investigation. Prepare and distribute a written draft report prior to departure. Promises of a report "next week" are seldom met, as one returns to family and long lists of urgent messages and e-mails. Delay in the availability of a report, frequently two to three months, compromises the implementation of recommendations.

As indicated in several chapters of this book, there is one key rule regarding the role of the visiting epidemiologist and the press: requests for information should be referred to the appropriate national authority. On rare occasions, when national authorities request a briefing with the media, the interviews should be carried out jointly.

## Publication

When publication is appropriate, it needs to be sensibly handled. Authorship, including local collaborators, should be agreed to in advance. In large outbreaks, acknowledgment of the team with all contributors listed alphabetically merits consideration. In some field investigations the laboratory component deserves separate treatment in a companion article. All articles need clearance in writing from both the host country and the visiting epidemiologist's institution prior to publication.

## Maintaining a Perspective

As a visiting epidemiologist, your salary may be 50 to 100 times that of your national colleagues. Living and working in such a situation require both wisdom and tact. Acceptance of hospitality from an impoverished village leader is difficult but necessary. As the leader's youngest children may go hungry when visitors are fed, a modest appetite is suggested. Maintaining team rapport often requires accepting accommodations that national team members can afford, rather than "fancy hotels." Small tokens of appreciation such as picture books of your city or country, commemorative stamps, postcards, or solar calculators are appropriate gifts. Except for drivers, monetary gifts are not recommended. Always carry a few family pictures both to keep in touch and to share.

On your return home, thank-you notes, technical publications, and copies of photographs, provide appreciation and continuity to friendships that have developed.

## CONCLUSION

In low-income countries where epidemiologic capacity is being strengthened, obtaining needed data requires a selection of most appropriate methods based on:

1. Need for data
2. Population at risk
3. Choice of methodology that is epidemiologically appropriate, logistically feasible, and affordable
4. Presentation of data in a format that promotes appropriate action

In this era of globalization, sharing your talents with individuals working in a low-resource setting is a challenge, an opportunity, and a privilege. It is essential to act as a guest in your international colleague's home. Working with national colleagues provides an opportunity to learn about the epidemiology of a new disease in a different culture. It also provides an opportunity to develop the capacity of your colleagues as you work to describe health problems and initiate control activities. If you do it right, you will gain much more than you give.

## REFERENCES

1. Chen S., Ravallion M. How have the world's poorest fared since the early 1980s? World Bank 2004. http://www.worldbank.org/research/povmonitor/MartinPapers/How_have_the_poorest_fared_since_the_early_1980s.pdf
2. Black R, Norris S., Bryce J. (2003). Where and why are 10 million children dying each year? *Lancet* 361, 2226–34.
3. WHO. International Health Regulations-2005. http://www.who.int/csr/ihr/en/index.html
4. Zhong, N., Zeng, G. (2006). What we have learnt from SARS epidemics in China. *BMJ* 333, 389–391.

5. Leung G., Hedley A., Lai-Ming, H. et al. (2004). The epidemiology of severe acute respiratory syndrome in the 2003 Hong Kong epidemic: an analysis of all 1755 patients. *Ann Intern Med* 141, 662–73.

6. Poutanem S., Low, D., Henry, B., et al. (2003). Identification of severe acute respiratory syndrome in Canada. *N Engl J Med* 348, 1995–2005.

7. White M., McDonnell S., Werker, D., et al. (2001). Partnerships in international applied epidemiology training and service, 1975–2001. *Am J Epidemiol* 154, 993–9.

8. United Nations. The Millenium Goals Report—2006.

9. CDC (2000). Assessment of Infectious Disease Surveillance—Uganda, 2000. *Morb Mortal Wkly Rep*, 49, 687–91.

10. Uganda Ministry of Health (2003). STD/HIV/AIDS Surveillance Report. June.

11. Moore, P., Plikaytis, B., Bolan, G., et al. (1992). Detection of meningitis epidemics in Africa: a population-based analysis. *Int J Epidemiol* 21, 155–62.

12. WHO (2000). Detecting meningococcal meningitis epidemics in highly endemic African countries. *WER* 38, 306–9.

13. WHO (2005). Global Polio Eradication Initiative Annual Report.

14. Okuonghae, H., Ighogboja, I., Lawson, J., et al. (1992). Diethylene glycol poisoning in Nigerian children. *Ann Trop Paediatr* 12, 235–8.

15. Alubo, S. (1994). Death for sale: a study of drug poisoning and deaths in Nigeria. *Soc Sci Med* 38, 97–103.

16. World Bank (2005). Burden of Disease Project. http://www.who.int/healthinfo/statistics/bodprojectionspaper.pdf

17. Razzak J., Luby, S. (1998). Estimating deaths and injuries due to road traffic accidents in Karachi, Pakistan, through the capture-recapture method. *Int J Epidemiol* 27, 866–70.

18. Okware, S., Omaswa, F., Zaramba, S. et al. (2002). An outbreak of Ebola in Uganda. *Trop Med Int Health* 7, 1068–75.

19. Mehta, P., Mehta, A., Mehta, S. (1990). Bhopal's tragedy's health effects; review of methyl isocyanate toxicity. *JAMA* 264, 2781–7.

20. Rahman, M., Chowdhury U., Mondal, K., et al. (2001). Chronic arsenic toxicity in Bangladesh and West Bengal, India, a review and commentary. *J Toxicol Clin Toxicol* 39, 683–700.

21. Dhara, R. (2002). The Union Carbide disaster in Bhopal: a review of health effects. *Arch Environ Health* 57, 391–404.

22. Ahsan, A. Chen, Y. Parvez, F., et al. (2006). Arsenic exposure from drinking water and risk of premalignant skin lesions in Bangladesh: baseline results from the health effects of arsenic longitudinal study. *Am J Epidemiol* 163, 1138–48.

23. Measure DHS (2008). Demographic and Health Surveys. http://www.measuredhs.com/

24. Sommer, A., Mosley, W. (1972). East Bengal cyclone of November 1971: epidemiologic approach to disaster assessment. *Lancet* 1029–36.

25. Bern C., Sniezek, J., Mathbor, G. et al. (1993). Risk factors for mortality in the Bangladesh cyclone of 1991. *Bull WHO* 71, 73–8.

26. Thailand Ministry of Health (2005). Rapid health response, assessment, and surveillance after a tsunami, Thailand, 2004–2005. *WHO WER* 55–60.

27. Coghlan, B., Brennan, R., Ngoy, P. et al. (2006). Mortality in the Democratic Republic of Congo: a nationwide survey. *Lancet* 367, 44–51.

28. Roberts, L., Lafta, R., Garfield, R. et al. (2004). Mortality before and after the 2003 invasion of Iraq: cluster sample survey. *Lancet* 364, 1857–64.

29. Steketee, R., Wirima, J., Slutsker, L. (1996). Malaria parasite infection curing pregnancy and delivery in mother, placenta, and newborn: efficacy of chloroquine and mefloquine in rural Malawi. *Am J Trop Med Hyg* 55, 24–32.
30. Bang, A., Reddy, H., Deshmukh, M. et al. (2005). Neonatal and infant mortality in the 10 years (1993–2003) of the Ghadchiroli field trial: effect of home-based neonatal care. *J Perinatol* 25, S92–S107.
31. Pandey, M., Daulaire, N. (1991). Reduction in total under-five mortality in western Nepal through community based antimicrobial treatment of pneumonia. *Lancet* 338, 993–7.
32. Luby, S., Agboatwalla, M., Feikin, D. et al. (2005). Effect of handwashing on child health: a randomized controlled trial. *Lancet* 366, 225–33.

# 22

## TERRORISM PREPAREDNESS AND EMERGENCY RESPONSE FOR THE FIELD EPIDEMIOLOGIST

Daniel M. Sosin
Richard E. Besser

Rarely will you fulfill a public health role more challenging or compelling than in *terrorism preparedness* and the associated activities of *emergency response*, abbreviated here as TPER. This chapter will attempt to prepare you for your role in such a multi-disciplinary response.* We will cover an *all-hazards* approach to preparedness and not strictly a focus on bioterrorism. While many decision makers have focused on bioterrorism because of its potential to create a large-scale event, persistent exposure, and social destabilization, the breadth of possible threat scenarios demands that our planning be directed to common response functions across these threat scenarios. Therefore, rather than committing our preparedness efforts to accurately predicting the next terrorist incident (e.g., chemical, radiological, or biological; indoor or outdoor; food, water or air; mass exposure or mass fear and limited exposure; etc.), "all-hazards" means that multi-use strategies take precedence. A thorough understanding of and experience with principles of *surveillance, epidemiologic investigation, joint law-enforcement investigation, incident management, transportation and delivery of mass countermeasures, professional* and *public communications*, and *evaluation* will serve well for

---

* A more comprehensive perspective on the TPER enterprise can be found in documents such as the National Response Framework, which addresses the full range of emergency support functions that must work together for effective response (http://www.fema.gov.emergency/nrf/).

most emergency response scenarios, even though the particulars will vary among incidents.

This chapter takes an American perspective in describing a preparedness and response system, though its concepts could be extrapolated for use in other countries. The role and relevant skills of the field epidemiologist in TPER are grounded in the application of conventional epidemiologic methods to public health emergencies (see chapters 2 and 3). With an emphasis on surveillance and supplemental data collection to support detection, investigation, and evaluation, your contributions would be made throughout a temporal cycle of planning and response. You are likely to be involved in planning and exercising for the public health requirements of a health catastrophe, assessing a threat, and/or investigating the health effects of terrorist incidents or health events of national significance. A broad knowledge of the action-oriented principles of field epidemiology is vital to your effectiveness. The special considerations highlighted in this book, such as legal considerations (see Chapter 14), environmental problems (Chapter 18), occupational hazards (Chapter 19), operating at a state and local public health level (Chapter 20), natural disasters (Chapter 23), and laboratory support (Chapter 24) are also important for your work in TPER. You will support all of these functions, yet you are uniquely qualified to lead in public health surveillance and the epidemiologic investigation.

A recurring theme in this chapter is that the roles and tools of the field epidemiologist in TPER are similar to those seen in other public health activities, only driven to be faster, bigger, and better: *faster* in that effective mitigation of a disaster, manmade or natural, is premised on how quickly an event can be identified, the exposed population can be recognized and treated, and the exposure contained; *bigger* because the potential for incidents of catastrophic scale drives planning and preparedness efforts toward the worst-case scenarios, with the expectation being that lesser requirements will be met if we are prepared for the most demanding ones; and *better* because leveraging resources and expertise across organizations and disciplines will be needed to effect the greatest impact, recognizing that resources always will be inadequate to prepare for all the possible threats we face.

## BACKGROUND

Terrorism preparedness became an explicit interest for field epidemiology after World War II when, in 1951, the United States Public Health Service created an on-the-job training program for physicians and allied health professionals called the Epidemic Intelligence Service (EIS).[1] The mission of this program was to promote the application of epidemiology to disease control, whether naturally occurring or a result of bioterrorism or warfare. Headquartered at the Communicable Disease Center (now the Centers for Disease Control and Prevention [CDC]) in Atlanta, Georgia, this two-year program continues to teach the trainees how to perform disease surveillance and investigate epidemics in real-life situations to improve disease control nationwide. With the support and cooperation of the state and local health departments, more than 2500 epidemiologists were trained in the first 50 years and many remain in active public health practice.[2]

The anthrax letters of 2001 and the rising global threat of terrorism have elevated the relevance of robust public health preparedness for deliberate events. Similarly, the unmet demands on the public health system in response to large humanitarian disasters, such as Hurricane Katrina on the U.S. Gulf Coast in 2005, have increased attention on the need for public health preparedness for catastrophic events from all hazards. The U.S. federal government's investment of $5 billion to upgrade public health systems across the country in order to respond to large-scale emergencies from 2002–2005 is a reflection of the elevated role of public health in national security.[3]

## BASIC AREAS FOR ACTION

### Planning

Given the infrequency of terrorism and disasters in any particular location, planning and exercising to improve readiness is the predominant phase in the TPER cycle. Preparedness covers actions necessary to build, sustain, and improve the capability to prevent, control, respond to, and recover from public health emergencies. Preparedness is ongoing and cross-cutting, involving all levels of government and a diversity of disciplines and nongovernmental organizations. Lessons discovered in previous responses, exercises, and drills can be addressed during the planning phase to mitigate the effects of future emergencies.

One of the primary objectives during the planning phase should be the integration of response sectors. Resources are always constrained. Integrated response supports resource efficiency and better decisions. The purpose of response planning is to appropriately define roles and relationships to other responders under different scenarios, and to assure that the skills and resources are in place to meet the expectations.

Public health response plans (e.g., to an anthrax aerosol release or a nuclear explosion) are designed to identify and control public health threats and maintain health services. Response plans are a vital part of preparedness because they provide context for envisioning specific response requirements and the roles and relationships of responders. Each response sector (e.g. public health) develops response plans to meet its responsibilities and to align with the National Response Framework (NRF) (see below) so that the sector response integrates smoothly with other sectors.

You should be familiar with public health response plans in your jurisdiction. As a field epidemiologist, you may be looked to for scientific leadership in planning the response to health emergencies. You will likely be an "agent expert" or be expected to have ways to reach national experts in order to plan control and prevention measures. You will be expected to be familiar with the application of disease control measures such as quarantine, isolation, and personal protective equipment. Emergency response modeling tools may assist policy-makers and planners in choosing between preparedness options.[4, 5, 6] Improved simulation to produce realistic scenarios may aid in exercising and drills. These tools, however, are only as good as the quality of information they are built on and require your careful review to assure proper inputs and realism.

Response plans should address the delivery of medical measures needed to counter an act of terrorism, including procedures when local resources are overwhelmed. Local, state, and federal public health have established mechanisms of stockpiling and managing inventories of countermeasures that might be needed for various priority threat scenarios and you may have a role in establishing the policies for appropriate use of these resources. The Strategic National Stockpile (SNS), executed through the CDC, is a system which manages procurement, storage, and delivery of medical countermeasures and equipment and supports local and state public health agencies to receive and distribute the countermeasures. The mission of the SNS is to augment state and local public health response capabilities by delivering critical medical supplies when needed. Experience with civil unrest during the dire circumstances of search and rescue during Hurricane Katrina demonstrated that response plans must also consider security and continuity of operations.

Due to the infrequent and unique nature of emergency responses, it is difficult to rely on experience to fully inform preparedness needs and measure readiness. Exercises allow for quality improvement of response systems by measuring the effectiveness of preparedness activities outside of real emergencies. Exercises have become a vital tool to ready and test the response system, from table-top activities designed to strengthen relationships and familiarize officials with common response issues to full-scale exercises framed around priority scenarios and intended to test operational details of the response. Full-scale exercises are a rapidly evolving, elaborate, and highly integrated method of quality improvement for complex responses. It is important for you, the field epidemiologist involved in TPER, to be familiar with the terminology and exercise products under development so that you can provide input to (1) define the roles and relationships of field epidemiology relative to the other disciplines and governmental entities,

(*2*) support the development and interpretation of performance assessments, and (*3*) contribute to the solutions that will be effected through corrective actions.

A National Preparedness Goal (NPG) was developed under leadership of the U.S. Dept. of Homeland Security (NPG; http://www.ojp.usdoj.gov/odp/assessments/hspd8.htm). The NPG defines the capabilities that must be in place to prevent and respond to current and future threats and hazards and establishes measurable targets and priorities to guide national planning. The following represent the capabilities-based planning tools and products under the NPG:

- *National Planning Scenarios* provide parameters for 15 terrorist attacks and natural disasters and provide the basis to define prevention, protection, response and recovery tasks, as well as the capabilities required to perform them.
- The *Universal Task List* provides a comprehensive menu of tasks to be performed by different disciplines at all levels of government to address major events.
- The *Target Capabilities List (TCL)* describes the capabilities (e.g., epidemiological surveillance and investigation) needed to perform critical homeland security tasks found in the Universal Task List. The TCL is designed to assist local, state, and federal entities understand and define their respective roles in a major event; the capabilities required to perform a specified set of tasks; the people, equipment, and supplies needed; and where to obtain additional resources if needed.
- *Exercise Evaluation Guides (EEG)* define the relationship between work activities and desired outcomes for the target capability. Key activities in the successful realization of a target capability are subject to standard performance measurement and observation by exercise evaluators. Figure 22–1 provides an example EEG framework for epidemiology and surveillance. Performance measurement focuses on markers of quality between the epidemiology and surveillance functions and the desired outcomes.

Field epidemiologists often have a breadth of knowledge to serve in a unique leadership role that bridges many disciplines and organizational boundaries, builds consensus around common goals, and empowers multi-disciplinary teams to optimal effectiveness. A type of integrating leadership coined "*meta-leadership*" (overarching leadership that provides guidance across organizational lines to produce a shared course of action and commonality of purpose) captures the principles of effective leadership that will enable you to accomplish your mission effectively.[7] The integrated operations necessary for public health responses to be "better" begin with leadership that embraces all components of the response system and builds connections among them to leverage their strengths in support of public health.

**Epidemiology &
Surveillance Functions**

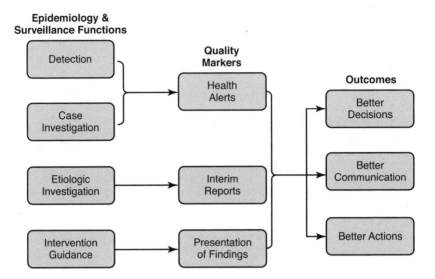

**Figure 22-1.** Exercise Evaluation Guide (EEG) framework: From a depiction of the workflow and key functions for a given Target Capability, work products for performance measurement are identified where variation in quality is influential on performance outcomes. The hand-off of information between Capabilities and responders is exceptionally vulnerable to failure. Measurement is focused on the quality markers. If the work that comprises the quality markers does not get handed off in a timely manner, is of poor quality, or does not get handed to the correct Capability or responder, the emergency response system becomes disorganized and performance outcomes suffer.

## Detection

The principles of public health surveillance for the field epidemiologist described in Chapter 3 are intrinsic to TPER. The driving purposes of surveillance with TPER are early detection of incidents of interest and provision of standard information during an event to feed awareness of needs (i.e., situational awareness). A number of advances in disease surveillance have followed the terrorist incidents of 2001 triggered by increased availability of electronic data and increased interest in timely detection. The surveillance system attributes of elevated importance for detection in TPER are extreme timeliness, sensitivity, the accuracy of positive and negative results, and the integration of information across response organizations and disciplines.

Time is of the essence when detecting and appropriately responding to deliberate disease outbreaks and those from new etiologic agents. The timeliness of outbreak detection can be improved through 1) more rapid and complete reporting and follow-up on notifiable diseases, 2) routine application of statistical methods and modeling that draws the attention of public health investigators at an earlier stage (e.g., fewer cases), and 3) analysis of new types of data that can signify an outbreak before it would otherwise be apparent.[8]

The foundation of disease and outbreak detection is *the reporting relation-ship between clinical medicine (including laboratories) and the local public health system*. For example, recent concerns about terrorism and emerging infectious diseases (e.g., SARS, West Nile Virus, avian influenza) have increased the appreciation among clinical communities and the public for the role of public health surveillance. With improved awareness of the interdependent roles of public health and clinical medicine, and improved technology to communicate between the two, the linkage between medicine and public health is strengthened, and the stronger linkage has created opportunities for improved timeliness and completeness of disease reporting.

Statistical tools enhanced through software applications facilitate the regular, automated analysis and early identification of nascent disease clusters. Since 2001, these tools have become more sophisticated, expanding from process control algorithms to detect temporal clusters to include other regression models, time-series methods, and scan statistics to add a geographic axis to aberration detection.[9]

Expanding data types for surveillance can also be considered to support earlier detection of disease outbreaks, although this often comes with less specificity and more false-positive findings. The implementation of electronic health records holds great promise for expanding the data for surveillance and improving their timeliness, completeness, and accuracy. While awaiting the robust implementation of electronic health records, alternative electronic data sources for outbreak detection and population health status monitoring are being explored. New data types for public health action include *environmental monitoring* to detect threat agents at the time of exposure; *health-related behaviors* such as product purchases, absenteeism, and health queries to capture disease manifestations in communities before individuals present to the health care system; and *early clinical indicators* such as diagnostic test orders and results, and presenting complaints and preliminary diagnoses (Figure 22—2). Additionally, *exposure surveillance* and *registries* may be implemented to track long-term health effects following potentially toxic exposures.

A relatively new term in the lexicon of surveillance is *syndromic surveillance*: the ongoing, systematic collection, analysis, interpretation, and application of timely indicators for disease and outbreaks. This kind of surveillance is being pursued for detection of outbreaks before public health authorities would otherwise note them.[10] Syndromic surveillance for terrorism detection applies automated analysis and visualization tools to screen nonspecific indicator data in electronic form for unexpected patterns that warrant investigation. It will not necessarily

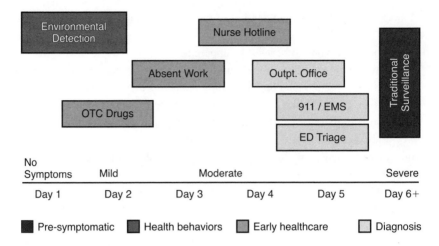

**Figure 22-2.** Stylized depiction of a detection timeline by data type: New data types for public health action include environmental monitoring for exposure to threat agents; health-related behaviors such as product purchases, absenteeism, and health queries; and early clinical indicators such as diagnostic test orders and results, and presenting complaints and preliminary diagnoses.

result in earlier diagnosis of a specific disease, but it may provide lead time for public health to mobilize outbreak investigations and response capabilities sooner. Syndromic surveillance and volume surveillance (measuring the frequency of types of presentations without individual-level data) may be implemented manually or electronically in order to discern outbreaks at an earlier stage, although manual surveillance systems that require volition on the part of reporters are difficult to sustain. In the presence of a credible threat, either from evidence of disease in another jurisdiction or during a high-profile event that might be vulnerable to a large-scale attack, such as gatherings for sports championships or political conventions,[11] enhanced surveillance efforts including syndromic surveillance may be implemented in a time-limited manner.

Limited evidence has been published to establish the effectiveness of syndromic surveillance for prospective identification of all but the largest seasonal outbreaks (e.g., influenza and viral gastroenteritis).[12] The role of syndromic surveillance in providing situational awareness during events also remains undocumented as of the writing of this chapter. These gaps in our knowledge reinforce the importance of systematic evaluation of these emergency preparedness surveillance systems and the need to share results through the referenced biomedical literature.[13] System coverage needs to be evaluated because the more completely the surveillance data represent the community, the more quickly and completely outbreaks will be detected and tracked. Cost and impact need to be assessed to determine the potential for syndromic surveillance to complement traditional surveillance systems. The implications of emphasis placed on timeliness and sensitivity need to be weighed against reduced specificity and an increase in falsely labeled events leading to misapplication of busy epidemiology staff and resources.

The laboratory plays a pivotal role in detection. The need for rapid laboratory assays with coordinated testing and information exchange is particularly important for TPER and uncommon but potentially catastrophic conditions.[14] The capability to conduct analyses in a manner consistent with the protection of legal evidence (e.g., chain-of-custody) is important for incidents precipitated by deliberate action. Additionally, accelerated operations to identify unknown agents and characterize their susceptibility to medical countermeasures are a special need for mitigation of terrorism and emerging infectious diseases. Since 1999, the Laboratory Response Network (LRN) has served as the integrating focus for rapid laboratory response to biological and chemical threats. With CDC, the Federal Bureau of Investigation, and the Association of Public Health Laboratories as founding partners, the LRN is comprised of more than 140 laboratories that are affiliated with local/state public health departments, federal agencies, military installations, and international partners. LRN bioterrorism preparedness and response activities emphasize local laboratory response by helping to increase the number of trained laboratory workers in local and state public health facilities; distributing standardized test methods and reagents to local labs; promoting the acquisition of advanced technologies; providing secure communications and consultation; and supporting proficiency testing and facility improvements.

The chemical side of the LRN employs a more centralized structure. This approach is necessary because the analytical expertise and technology resources required to respond to a chemical event are great. As a result, initial clinical testing in a suspected chemical event will usually occur at CDC. Using sophisticated analytical techniques, including mass spectrometry, CDC laboratories perform comprehensive testing to identify and characterize human exposure and target further testing requirements. Results of these tests are reported to affected jurisdictions, and if needed, appropriate LRN members may be asked to test additional samples for specific agents. Laboratory capabilities are stratified and member labs are classified accordingly to National, Reference, or Sentinel status. National laboratories have the capability to perform forensic analyses, handle highly infectious or lethal agents, and look for modifications in agents that would make them harder to detect or treat with standard measures. Reference laboratories are responsible for confirmatory identification of threat agents using advanced technology and assays of the network. These laboratories are strategically located and include local and state public health laboratories and military, veterinary, agricultural, food, and environmental laboratories. Sentinel laboratories provide initial testing for threat agents using commercial tests and follow referral proto-cols for further testing as appropriate to the situation. Technical guidance regard-ing public health laboratory support for emergency field operations can be found in Chapter 24.

As a direct component of the national terrorism surveillance infrastructure, the LRN also conducts laboratory analyses with the environmental monitoring BioWatch program. BioWatch monitors population-dense urban environments for an aerosol release of select biological threat agents.[15] BioWatch leverages the strengths of research and development in the Department of Homeland Security, the air-monitor-ing expertise of the Environmental Protection Agency, and the laboratory and applied public health expertise of local, state, and federal public health agencies associated with the LRN, to analyze and interpret samples for public health action. As the tech-nology for environmental monitoring evolves to provide more rapid results and expands to cover additional agents, the greatest challenge for the field epidemiologist will be the rapid evaluation of positive environmental test results, possibly in concert with other data streams, to establish exposure probabilities and direct decision-making for further investigation and delivery of countermeasures.

True to the priority for timeliness, you should review surveillance data and reports daily, keeping in mind the possibility of early detection of all types of significant public health events.[16] Your level of suspicion for an outbreak should be elevated when:

- A *large number* of people have a similar illness, particularly a group with common features (e.g., time of onset, personal characteristics, similar geography, work setting, common event, etc.).
- A *cluster* of unexplained deaths or severe illnesses with common expo-sures occurs.
- *Animal populations* have the same disease concurrently.
- A *commercial product* that should be free of pathogens is suspected, e.g., medication, pasteurized milk, or peanut butter.

Suspicion of a *deliberate* event is further increased when:

- Individual *cases of a rare and serious disease* occur, particularly those caused by an agent seen as a terrorism threat (e.g., anthrax).
- *Unusual severity* or manifestation of a specific disease occurs.
- Seasonal or geographic *patterns are unusual.*
- An *unusual strain* or treatment resistance is discovered.
- *Transmission* occurs through an *unusual* mode.
- Law enforcement or the intelligence community provides *evidence of a credible threat.*

## Response

Public health response includes immediate actions to save lives and meet basic needs to maintain health. Interdisciplinary coordination for complex responses large and small is supported through the Incident Command System (ICS). ICS has evolved through years of experience in emergency response disciplines, such as wildland fire management. Although the overall responsibility for leading an emergency response will rest on other shoulders, you may be asked to fill specific roles in the public health response which must be integrated in the larger incident response.

### Incident management

As relative newcomers to the large and complex field of emergency preparedness and response, you will need to learn and conform to the principles, terminology, and processes of emergency management and you should be familiar with the National Response Framework (NRF) (http://www.fema.gov/emergency/nrf/), where the principles of effective incident management are exemplified. The NRF is an all-hazards plan for integrating and applying federal resources before, during, and after an incident. It incorporates best practices from a wide variety of incident management disciplines, including fire, rescue, emergency management, law enforcement, public works, and emergency medical services.

A National Incident Management System (NIMS) provides a cascading framework for coordination among local, state, federal, tribal, nongovernmental, and private-sector organizations, regardless of the cause, size, or complexity of the incident. A guiding principle of NIMS is that the organizational structure is scalable and flexible, and thus to be used in all responses. Core concepts of incident management include:

- Common terminology
- Modular organization scalable to the size and complexity of the incident
- Chain of command (orderly line of authority) and unity of command (every individual has 1 supervisor at the scene)
- Manageable span of control limiting supervision to 3—7 subordinates
- Resource typing to standardize the application of human and materiel resources
- Integrated communications and information management
- Training standards

An extensive library of resources on the NRF, NIMS, and incident management is available from the Federal Emergency Management Agency (http://www.training.fema.gov/) and other sources.[17, 18, 19]

Depending on the magnitude and nature of the public health emergency, you might be assigned to support one of many emergency operations functions. The CDC incident management system, for example, includes upwards of 100 "desks" that serve as a single contact point at CDC for specific and non-redundant public health response functions. The CDC role is to assure that the functions are being served, whereas the field sites are responsible to execute these functions. If called for, any of the science desks might expand to a team to meet the requirements of responding to an incident. Some of the functions that field epidemiologists might serve include:

- Epidemiology: to determine the epidemiological characteristics of the event (time, place, person), the risk factors for disease and severity, potential methods of prevention and control, and evaluation of intervention impact
- Surveillance: to meet routine, ongoing information requirements to direct public health actions
- Laboratory: for guidance on sampling, collection, and analysis of specimens
- Clinical Care/Infection Control: to provide guidance on the diagnosis, treatment, and prevention of disease in clinical settings
- Environmental and Occupational Health: to assess environmental hazards and provide guidance for protection of workers and indigenous populations
- Quarantine and Displaced Populations: to address the vulnerabilities and special health needs of populations displaced from their homes
- Communications: to translate public health situational awareness into messages for external constituencies and stakeholders and assure proper sharing with those who need to know
- Various event-specific teams: such as immunizations, food and water safety, mental health, veterinary, chemical, radiological, injury/trauma, chronic diseases and vulnerable populations.

## Primary epidemiology response functions

It is important that you plan for and then *implement standardized response surveillance*. Response surveillance includes enhancements to existing public health surveillance that are implemented to monitor for disease and injury outbreaks anticipated to be of higher than usual risk. As with routine surveillance, standard case definitions, data collection templates, and reporting mechanisms are developed in advance and must be adhered to over the course of the event to assure that case counts are accurate. When multiple sources of data contribute to case counts and other epidemiological data requirements, differences must be reconciled through a systematic process. It is important to quickly establish which data source will represent ground truth for event reporting and to set a routine frequency of reporting (usually once daily) to minimize confusion regarding changing information.

Once a response is initiated, you will be called to apply the fundamental principles of epidemiology and laboratory practice described elsewhere in this book, particularly *rapid surveys* to assess population health needs and investigate the epidemiological parameters of the event. These surveys establish health risks unique to the event and help determine the geographic extent, size and characteristics of the affected population, and mechanism of agent dissemination and disease transmission in the population. Whereas the investigation principles are similar, they must be applied under increased pressures of time, scale, and interdisciplinary coordination. Statistical and mathematical methods are increasingly being applied to surveillance and investigation data to forecast the progression of events and the impact of interventions and to facilitate decision-making under intense time pressures. These decision-support tools need to be informed and validated by the experienced field epidemiologist.

## Additional response considerations

Epidemiologists must work closely with other disciplines in complex investigations. For example, epidemiologists and *industrial hygienists* need to be closely aligned with *laboratory practice* in the field investigation. The study of threat agents in the environment is critical to understanding the introduction, spread, and control of diseases in human populations. Recent investigations of outbreaks caused by emerging or newly recognized pathogens such as the SARS coronavirus or avian influenza, or terrorism-associated events, such as the anthrax-contaminated letters, have hinged on being able to detect and characterize these agents in environmental samples (e.g., air, water, surfaces, soil, and non-animal bulk substances such as powders) rapidly and accurately. *Environmental investigations* are also critical for drawing conclusions about virulence, transmission, and persistence of threat agents and to provide guidance on decontamination and personal protective measures to prevent and control exposures. The industrial hygienist develops the sampling strategy, understands the limitations of the sampling (e.g., limits of detection, bias, range, recovery, how the sample was collected, etc.), and can provide interpretation to maximize the value of the information from environmental sampling. As a field epidemiologist you also play an important role in interpreting laboratory data to guide public health actions.

Field investigations will need to be coordinated with the *law enforcement investigation* when terrorism or criminal intent is suspected. Law enforcement assumes the lead for these investigations and it is vital that strong working relationships are in place between you and law enforcement officials in advance of such events. Training in forensic epidemiology has been implemented to bridge differences in terminology and align epidemiologic investigation methods between public health and law enforcement (http://www.publichealthlaw.info/forensicepi-more.htm). Legal authorities for public health investigation and intervention are further considered in Chapter 14.

One of the more challenging facets of terrorism preparedness is that fundamental principles of public health and medicine under natural conditions may not apply with deliberate acts. *Occam's razor*, or the law of parsimony, for example, would have us apply the simplest explanation for a scenario when more than one theory would explain it, yet deliberate acts aim to confound us and keep us off balance. A single point source might explain a pattern of disease, yet in a deliberate act there actually may be multiple simultaneous exposures in different locations. A deliberate act may precipitate exposure to multiple agents, whereas concurrent exposure to multiple threat agents might be virtually impossible under natural conditions. One deliberate act with a biological agent, salmonella, was investigated by local and state health departments with CDC assistance in The Dalles, Oregon in 1984.[20] Seven hundred and fifty-one cases of salmonellosis occurred among residents who ate in local restaurants. Intensive investigation failed to implicate a single food item as the source of salmonella consistent with establish patterns for foodborne outbreaks. Later, with assistance from the public health laboratory, law enforcement officials were able to confirm a report that a religious commune had purposely contaminated the salad bars at the affected restaurants—an unnatural presentation of an all-to-common occurrence, a foodborne outbreak. The uncommon concentration of an agent in a deliberate act may alter the time course and presentation of illness in ways that distract us from looking for alternative explanations. With terrorism preparedness, the epidemiologist, who is trained to see patterns and decipher the most common explanation, must carefully anticipate the unexpected.

## Information Management and Communication

Sophisticated *information management tools* are needed to leverage the wealth of existing public health science; support evidence-based planning decisions; analyze and apply electronic health surveillance data, including pattern recognition for early detection; support response decisions during an incident, and improve exercise simulations. If you are to be a leader in the application of science into preparedness, you need to be attentive to information management and to foster tools to better leverage existing knowledge. Public health preparedness needs are similar to the knowledge management and decision support requirements of the clinical environment and decision-support tools available in the clinical environment can serve as a foundation for public health. The end-point of effective management of information is the timely sharing of information for decision-making across the response community and with the public.

As with the principles of surveillance and epidemiologic investigation, the principles of communication by the field epidemiologist during an emergency response build on the lessons of other chapters in this book (see Chapters 12 and 13), yet are distinguished by the needs for timeliness and credibility of the message. Five keys to successful communication by public health authorities during a crisis are:[21]

- Execute a robust communication plan that describes roles, responsibilities, and resources for your organization.
- Be first with relevant information.
- Have and express empathy early.
- Show competence and expertise.
- Remain honest and open with what you know and don't know.

Communications research has shown that the first message received by a person seeking information about a subject with which he is unfamiliar will carry more weight than subsequent messages. Additionally, the first messenger can establish credibility for being prepared by being timely. Timeliness will always be in tension with the accuracy of the message, especially for the scientist, and must be balanced with clear and careful explanation of what is known, what is not known, and what is being done to answer the unknown questions. This candor can build credibility and lessen the predictable human emotions of anxiety, helplessness, and uncertainty during a crisis. Credibility also is enhanced by the consistency of messages from government officials. The damage that ensues from inconsistent messages from officials and experts reinforces the importance of coordinated communications among health agencies and across the response infrastructure. (see Appendix for examples of epidemiologic information exchange systems).

## After-Action Review

The quality improvement cycle for emergency response culminates in the systematic review of response actions and outcomes to identify lessons for improvement. Performance is observed and measured during the response and reviewed upon its termination or transition to the recovery phase. This process is known as the after-action review. The review can be as simple as a short debriefing, or "hotwash," or as complex as a full study with additional data collection and analysis. The after-action report then drives corrective actions to improve inadequacies or extend successful practices of the response, and these are assigned to the appropriate organizational entities to execute. This assessment is expected to influence funding decisions and may result in policy changes or re-assignment of authorities. You will play an important part of this review and improvement cycle by reflecting on the epidemiological functions that were needed and performed and how they could be strengthened. For example, many after-action reviews and lessons-learned were captured following the response to Hurricane Katrina in 2005. This table is a high level depiction of the types of findings and actions taken by CDC in its after-action quality improvement cycle (http://www.cdc.gov/about/news/2006_11/katrina.htm).

It behooves you to stay abreast of these evaluation concepts and templates because of the significant implications for ongoing resources and institutionalization of response roles.

**Table 22-1.** Examples of Hurricane Katrina Lessons Learned that Led to Corrective Actions

| KATRINA LESSON LEARNED | CORRECTIVE ACTION |
| --- | --- |
| Missing mission statement and clear objectives | Incident Action Plan and Mission Statement standardized |
| Lines of authority confused | Standard Operating Procedures written and exercised; Incident Management System staffing standardized in the DEOC |
| Inadequate support staff to support experts | Support staff integrated into deployed teams |
| Procurement and Grants Office overtaxed | PGO developing surge-capacity plan |
| Financial Management Office overtaxed | FMO developing surge-capacity plan |
| Partner/stakeholder communication spotty | CDC developed partner database and protocol and identified a "partner desk" in the DEOC |
| HQ Briefing documents cumbersome | Briefing template standardized |
| CDC staff lacked understanding of the nature and demands of emergency deployments | Deployment training for staff institutionalized based on U.S. Forest Service "Red Card" training |
| Collaboration with federal partners spotty | Now play books, checklists in place |
| SNS role too restrictive for Katrina disaster | CDC is assessing expansion of SNS formulary |
| Responder resilience not fully addressed | CDC expanded existing responder resilience program |
| Cross-cutting agency roles unclear | All agency elements defining roles for natural disaster response |

## SUMMARY

Principles highlighted in this chapter differentiate TPER from standard field epidemiology practice in the following ways:

1. Public health practice is a relative newcomer as a full partner in the highly integrated, multi-disciplinary emergency response infrastructure. The field epidemiologist brings many skills and talents, yet must conform to the language and operating procedures of the enterprise.
2. "All-hazards" refers to a common platform for responding to natural and deliberate disasters of large scale. An all-hazards strategy focuses preparedness efforts on common issues and optimizes the use of resources in a threat environment that is changing and unpredictable.
3. A new form of cross-cutting or meta-leadership is needed for the highly integrated environment of TPER. Successful response depends on making the most of what every participant and organization brings to the effort and minimizing cross-jurisdictional differences and tensions.
4. Speed, scalability, and connectivity (faster, bigger, better) are core values in the TPER environment.
5. Integrated management of surveillance and epidemiologic investigation is a critical requirement of effective response and is the foundation of what the field epidemiologist brings to TPER.
6. Crisis communication is a special field that can define success or failure of a response effort. Communications must be timely, accurate, and credible.
7. Exercises and proxy responses are the essence of the preparedness quality improvement cycle and field epidemiologists should contribute to defining their role in response, establishing measures of performance, interpreting results, and devising corrective solutions to gaps and vulnerabilities.
8. Deliberate events can be counter-intuitive. You should remain skeptical and open-minded to unusual explanations for health events.
9. Deliberate acts have legal implications for investigation methods and data sharing, and you need to work effectively with law enforcement when crime or terrorism might be involved.

You are an essential member of the team responsible for preparedness and response to terrorism. The activities that you perform are similar to those undertaken during other public health emergencies. By understanding the changes that occur in roles and responsibilities during deliberate events, you will effectively contribute to health security through what must be a cross-disciplinary response.

## APPENDIX: INFORMATION EXCHANGE SYSTEMS

Coordinated communications is a central tenet of incident management and is supported through structural features of the incident management system. Vehicles for epidemiologic information exchange within the response community can support the discipline of applied epidemiology (e.g., the Epidemic Information Exchange [Epi-X; http://www.cdc.gov/epix/]) as well as a national response infrastructure (e.g., the National Biosurveillance Integration System [NBIS]). Established to share outbreak and related information at the earliest stages among public health practitioners and to initiate appropriate detection and control efforts as soon as possible, Epi-X is a secure, moderated, bi-directional web-based communications and alerting system. Using advanced encryption and verification technologies, the system can rapidly establish secure channels of communication between its users, giving public health officials a safe way to send and receive preliminary information. The system is designed to provide early warning of developing situations and response efforts. As significant health threats develop, local and state officials use Epi-X to communicate with each other and the command centers at the national level. Less secure communications and alerting systems (e.g., the Health Alert Network; HAN http://www2a.cdc.gov/han/Index.asp) have been developed for sharing early notifications to a broader range of health professionals at, local, state, and national levels. Being able to link these cascading technologies and information assets holds promise for improved cross-jurisdictional response.

Just as local and state public health departments serve as hubs to manage and apply surveillance and investigation data from the reporting sources within their jurisdictions and share a subset with CDC for regional and national awareness, CDC serves as a node for public health surveillance in a larger preparedness and response enterprise and shares analyzed information with higher levels of the national response hierarchy. NBIS is an example of culling public health surveillance information in support of a broader preparedness and response mission. NBIS is a system under development through the leadership of the U.S. Department of Homeland Security that intends to provide situational awareness through the exchange of information about human disease, food, agriculture, water, meteorology, and the environment in a single locus. Standardized routines for early interagency notification of potential threats and actions being taken (e.g., situation reports, or sitreps) facilitate timely and coordinated multi-disciplinary response.

## REFERENCES

1. Langmuir, A.D., Andrews, J.M. (1952). Biological warfare defense—2: The Epidemic Intelligence Service of the Communicable Disease Center. *Am J Public Health* 42, 235–8.

2. Thacker, S.B., Dannenberg, A.L., Hamilton, D.H. (2001). The Epidemic Intelligence Service of the Centers for Disease Control and Prevention: 50 years of training and service in applied epidemiology. *Am J Epidemiol* 154, 985–92.

3. Lurie, N., Wasserman, J., Nelson, C.D. (2006). Public health preparedness: Evolution or revolution? *Health Affairs* 25(4), 935–45.

4. Ferguson, N.M., Keeling, M.J., Edmunds, W.J., et al. (2003). Planning for smallpox outbreaks. *Nature* (Oct. 16) 425(6959), 681–5.

5. Georgopoulos, P.G., Fedele, P., Shade, P., et al. (2004). Hospital response to chemical terrorism: personal protective equipment, training, and operations planning. *Am J Ind Med* (Nov.) 46(5), 432–45.

6. Koopman, J.S. Infection transmission science and models. (2005). *Jpn J Infect Dis* (Dec.) 58(6), S3–8. [cited 10/30/2006]. Available from: http://www.nih.go.jp/JJID/58/S3.pdf.

7. Marcus, L.J., Dorn, B.C., Henderson, J.M. (2006). Meta-leadership and national emergency preparedness: A model to build government connectivity. *Biosecurity and Bioterrorism: Biodefense Strategy, Practice, and Science* 4(2), 128–34.

8. Wagner, M.M., Tsui, F.C., Espino, J.U., et al. (2001). The emerging science of very early detection of disease outbreaks. *J Public Health Mgmt Pract* 7(6), 51–9.

9. Farrington, P., Andrews, N. (2004). Outbreak detection: application to infectious disease surveillance. In: R. Brookmeyer, D.F. Stroup (eds.), *Monitoring the Health of Populations*, Oxford University Press, New York. pp. 203–31.

10. Sosin, D.M. (2003). Syndromic surveillance: the case for skillful investment. *Biosecurity and Bioterrorism: Biodefense Strategy, Practice, and Science* 1(4), 1–7.

11. Gesteland, P.H., Gardner, R.M., Tsui, F.C., et al. (2003). Automated syndromic surveillance for the 2002 Winter Olympics. *J Am Med Inform Assoc* (Nov.-Dec.), 10(6), 547–54.

12. Beuhler, J.W., Sosin, D.M., Platt, R. Evaluation of surveillance systems for early epidemic detection. In N.M. M'ikantha, R. Lynfield, C.A. Van Beneden, and H. de Valk (eds.), *Infectious Disease Surveillance*, Blackwell Publishing, Oxford UK: 432–42.

13. Centers for Disease Control and Prevention (2004). Framework for evaluating public health surveillance systems for early detection of outbreaks). recommendations from the CDC Working Group. *Morb Mortal Wkly Rep* 53(No. RR-5), 1–13.

14. Pien, B.C., Saah, J.R., Miller, S.E., et al. (2006).Use of sentinel laboratories by clinicians to evaluate potential bioterrorism and emerging infections. *Clin Infect Dis* 42(9), 1311–24.

15. Shea, D.A., Lister, S.A. (2003). The BioWatch Program: Detection of Bioterrorism. Congressional Research Service Report No. RL 32152. November 19, [cited 10/30/2006]. Available from: http://www.fas.org/sgp/crs/terror/RL32152.html#_1_19.

16. Treadwell, T.A., Koo, D., Kuker, K., et al. (2003). Epidemiologic clues to bioterrorism. *Public Health Rep* (Mar.–Apr.), 118(2), 92–8.

17. Couig, M.P., Martinelli, A., Lavin, R.P. (2005). The National Response Plan: Health and Human Services: the lead for Emergency Support Function #8. *Disaster Management & Response* 3(2), 34–40.

18. Qureshi, K., Gebbie, K.M., Gebbie, E.N. (2005). Public Health Incident Command System: A Guide for Management of Emergencies or Other Unusual Incidents with Public Health Agencies, Volume I. October 24, (http://www.ualbanycphp.org/pinata/phics/guide/default.cfm).

19. Walsh, D.W., Christen, H.T., Miller, G.T., et al. (2005). *National Incident Management System: Principles and Practice*, Jones and Bartlett Publishers, Sudbury, Mass.

20. Torok, T.J., Tauxe, R.V., Wise, R.P., et. al. (1997). A large community outbreak of salmonellosis caused by intentional contamination of restaurant salad bars. *JAMA* 278, 389–95.

21. Reynolds, B. (2004). *Crisis and Emergency Risk Communication: By Leaders for Leaders*, Centers for Disease Control and Prevention, Atlanta.

# 23

# FIELD INVESTIGATIONS OF NATURAL DISASTERS AND COMPLEX EMERGENCIES

Ron Waldman
Eric K.Noji

No matter where you live and no matter what your "day job" might be, as a practicing epidemiologist you may be called upon to respond to the needs of people in your own community who are affected by a natural disaster, or, in some cases, you might volunteer to lend your skills and expertise to organizations that provide humanitarian assistance to victims of war, drought, famine, or other catastrophes that regularly occur in the poorer countries of the world. In 2006, 427 natural disasters were reported around the world, more than one per day. These affected more than 143 million people, killing more than 23,000 of them, and taking an economic toll of more than \$34.5 billion.[1]

The future may bring even more calamities. Increasing populations in floodplains and in earthquake- and hurricane-prone areas around the world suggest that individual disasters may take a higher toll. Global climate change is no longer a controversial topic and, with it, may come an increased number of natural disasters of increased intensity. In addition, although there has been evidence of a decline in their numbers,[2] war and civil strife continue to plague many parts of the world, from Côte d'Ivoire to the Middle East, from Afghanistan to Burma, and the lives of people who have been forcibly displaced or otherwise affected by disasters that are fundamentally political in nature also depend, to a large extent, on the ability of trained professionals to objectively assess their needs and to respond appropriately.

Both kinds of disasters, natural and man-made, frequently occur in remote, hard-to-reach areas, far from tertiary-care centers. Roads are frequently impassable, bridges destroyed, air transport disrupted or dangerous. Even in this age of almost instant communications, the remoter the area, the longer it takes for the world, and the first-response community, to learn of the magnitude of a disaster with any degree of accuracy, and the longer it takes to get desperately needed help to those in need.

## THE HISTORICAL DEVELOPMENT OF FIELD EPIDEMIOLOGY IN DISASTERS AND EMERGENCIES

The application of epidemiological principles to disaster response is generally thought to have begun during the massive international relief effort that was mounted in response to the civil war in Nigeria in the late 1960s. When the region of Biafra, the traditional home of the Ibo ethnic group, sought to secede from the central authority of Nigeria, dominated by the Yoruba, the latter responded by instituting a blockade that resulted in widespread starvation, mass internal displacement, and high mortality. Epidemiologists developed survey tools, measurement devices, and other epidemiological methods that helped to determine the health status of large populations so that appropriate assistance could be delivered to the most vulnerable. Nutritional surveillance was further developed over the subsequent years and, by the late 1970s, internationally approved guidelines for measuring nutritional status had been developed.[3]

Toward the end of that decade, the genocidal practices of Pol Pot's Khmer Rouge regime in Cambodia resulted in a massive exodus of those who survived to Thailand, where they were gathered, by relief authorities, in large refugee camps. Outbreaks of disease transformed the camps of Sa Keo and Khao-i-Dang into so-called death camps, but it was not until epidemiologists from the Centers for Disease Control and Prevention, building on lessons learned from the Guatemala earthquake of 1976, instituted a formal surveillance system and conducted methodologically sound surveys that the extent of morbidity and mortality was measured in quantifiable terms.[4, 5]

Prior to these efforts, disaster relief was guided mostly by the best intentions of relatively inexperienced medical and surgical teams with inappropriate skills and inadequate logistic support. Clinicians frequently worked from makeshift clinics, providing services for only a small proportion of the population, those fortunate enough to be able to access those facilities. In most cases, the services provided did not match the public health needs of the populations. Program planners and managers with little or no public health expertise were put into the untenable position of having to direct major relief efforts with little information to guide their efforts. However, as sound epidemiological practices began to generate more accurate information as to how disasters unfolded, a more disciplined approach to the delivery of humanitarian assistance in the health sector slowly evolved.

Unfortunately, during the 1980s and 1990s, there was no lack of opportunity to further hone the epidemiological approach to disaster relief. Refugee relief efforts in Somalia, Sudan, and Ethiopia became increasingly guided by a more formal approach to assessment, surveillance, monitoring, and evaluation. Floods in Bangladesh, earthquakes in Central America, and wars in Iraq, the Balkans, and Central Africa all required distinctive responses, but eventually patterns of morbidity and mortality emerged and training programs were established as disaster epidemiology became a minor sub-specialty.[6–9]

However, the dissemination of epidemiological findings proved to be inadequate and the relief community was shown to be tragically unprepared when, in July 1994, in the wake of the genocide in Rwanda, more than 45,000 refugees from that war-torn country died of cholera in a three-week period, despite the presence of literally hundreds of non-governmental organizations, United Nations agencies, medical contingents of at least nine Western armed forces, and other public health officials. The terrible failure of the humanitarian response, other aspects of which will be discussed later in this chapter, did have at least one positive outcome, though: recognizing the need to develop indicators of what might constitute a successful humanitarian intervention in response to disasters of any kind, the international community came together to develop the Sphere Project, a set of minimum standards that all actors in disaster relief should strive to achieve.[10] In addition to establishing standards in the areas of shelter, food security, food aid and nutrition, water and sanitation, shelter, and health services, the Sphere Project provided an opportunity for epidemiologists and other public health experts to agree on a relatively standardized approach to disaster relief.

Since the first edition of this book appeared, a number of serious natural and man-made disasters have tested the ability of the global response community to effectively provide needed assistance to those affected. Specifically, the south Asian tsunami of December 1994 and the devastation wreaked by Hurricane Katrina in the United States provide contrasting disaster-response experiences from which much can be learned. On the man-made side, the continuing agony of the people the Democratic Republic of Congo and those of Darfur in the Sudan is clear evidence of the difficulty faced by the humanitarian community in providing effective relief to those oppressed or ignored by their governments. Practicing epidemiologists should become as familiar as possible with the mistakes made and the lessons learned from past disaster-response efforts, both domestic and international. As the philosopher George Santayana put it, "those who cannot remember the past are condemned to repeat it."

## THE ROLE OF THE EPIDEMIOLOGIST IN DISASTER RESPONSE

The objectives of post-disaster epidemiologic activities are to establish the magnitude of the public health consequences of the disaster, assess the needs of disaster-affected populations, promote epidemiologically derived data as a principal source of resource allocation, guide the implementation of public health programs to prevent additional morbidity and mortality, monitor the progress of the relief effort, and evaluate the effectives of the response. In the immediate post-disaster period, as those responsible for mounting a first response are getting organized, you may be called upon to provide advice regarding the probable health effects of the specific disaster and to suggest, on the basis of past experiences, likely priorities for intervention. Be aware, though, that most lay people, and many health professionals, will be more aware of the clinical needs of individuals than of the public health needs of the population. You will frequently have to argue about the importance of conducting methodologically sound data-collection activities in order to contribute to intelligent decision-making. Be prepared, though, to encounter skepticism and scorn: "Why don't you stop asking questions and do something?" is a frequent complaint heard by epidemiologists in disaster settings. Still, you will make a maximum contribution by not ceding ground to the "act first, think later" proponents.

Specifically, you should consider tasking yourself and your team with the following, while remaining flexible and understanding that there is no cookbook approach to disaster response:

- determine the impact of the disaster on the public's health (see Table 23–1).
- initiate disease surveillance as quickly as possible (see Chapter 3).
- identify risk factors for morbidity and mortality (see Chapter 5).
- strongly advocate the early initiation of appropriate public health interventions and disease-control programs
- insist that health actions of lesser priority be deferred until the situation has stabilized
- work with first responders and others to design an evaluation of the relief effort

The contribution of epidemiologists working in disaster response will be measured by (1) the ability to provide timely and accurate data on important issues in a way that can be easily understood and acted on by decision makers; and (2) the effective implementation of appropriate public health measures, as determined by those data, by those decision makers. The collection and provision of potentially useful information that is not acted upon by those responsible for its use in the decision-making process is a failure for field epidemiology. The successful epidemiologist coordinates closely with decision makers, prepares them

**Table 23–1.** Characteristics of data collection methods in disaster settings

| ASSESSMENT METHOD | REQUIREMENTS | | DATA-GATHERING TECHNIQUES | |
|---|---|---|---|---|
| | TIME | RESOURCES | INDICATORS | ADVANTAGES |
| 1. Pre-disaster "background" data | Ongoing | Trained staff | Reporting from, health facilities and *practitioners.* Disease patterns and seasonality | Provides baseline data for detecting problems and assessing trends |
| 2. Remote: airplanes, helicopter, satellite | Minutes/ hours | Hardware | Direct observation, cameras. Destroyed buildings, roads, dams, flooding. | Quick; useful when ground transport out; useful to identify area affected |
| 3. On-site "walkthrough" (ride through) | Hours/ days | Transportation, maps | Direct observation, talks with local *leaders and health workers.* Deaths, homeless persons, numbers and types of diseases | Quick; visible; does not require technical (health) background |
| 4. "Quick and dirty" Surveys | 2–3 days | Few trained staff | Rapid surveys. Deaths, no. hospitalized, nutritional status, (see also 3) | Rapid quantitative data; may prevent mismanagement; can provide data for surveillance |
| 5. Rapid health screening system | Ongoing (as needed) | Health workers; equipment that depends on the data that are collected | Collect data from fraction of persons being *screened.* Nutritional status, demography, hematocrit, parasitemia. | Can be established quickly; collects data and provide* services (vaccines, vit A, triage) in migrating populations |
| 6. Surveillance systems | Ongoing | Some trained staff; standard diagnoses; method of communicating data | Routine data collection *in standardized manner.* Mortality/ morbidity by diagnosis and age | Timely; expandable; can detect trends |

*Continued*

**Table 23–1.** Characteristics of data collection methods in disaster settings—Continued

| ASSESSMENT METHOD | REQUIREMENTS | | DATA-GATHERING TECHNIQUES | |
| --- | --- | --- | --- | --- |
| | TIME | RESOURCES | INDICATORS | ADVANTAGES |
| 7. Survey | Variable: hours/ days | Experienced field epidemiologist statistician; reliable field staff | Random or representative *sample selection.* Varies according to purpose of survey | Large amount of specific data obtained in brief time |

Source: Adapted from Nieburg's model for data collection methods in disaster situations, in *Health Aspects and Relief Management After Natural Disasters.* Center for Research on the Epidemiology of Disasters. Bruxelles, Belgium, 1980.

for using the data that will be collected and analyzed, suggests appropriate interpretations of those data, and successfully advocates the initiation of data-based interventions. In other words, you must use not only your epidemiological skills, but also management, communications, and advocacy skills in order to succeed (see chapters 4 and 13).

## PROBLEMS YOU WILL FACE IN THE FIELD

### Logistics

The post-disaster environment is always chaotic. Every responder will have the same needs—transportation, communication, labor, food, water, and a place to sleep. As a first priority after arriving on the scene, you should make sure you have arranged for your own needs to be met before throwing yourself into your work—don't forget that if others have to respond to your needs they will be diverted from the more important task at hand.

In the wake of a natural disaster, telecommunications systems can be destroyed and slow to rebuild; in other settings, they might never have existed, and those responsible for establishing communications might have difficulty doing so, as was the case after the 1994 tsunami in Indonesia. Destroyed or blockaded roads can impede transportation. Health facilities may be destroyed, either by the forces of nature or, increasingly, because they are specific targets of armed militia seeking to destabilize societies. For these reasons, and others, it may be difficult to recruit qualified staff, and you may have to press lay workers into service. Often, interpreters are needed, and important information can be lost in translation.

If possible, one or more members of the epidemiological team should speak the local language and be familiar with the customs and culture of the affected population (see Chapter 21). Finally, transportation, communications, and hiring may be expensive—always be sure to have sufficient cash available to be able to work productively.

## Establishing Rates

In most cases, in the period immediately following a disaster, accurate figures concerning the size of the population and its health status will be missing and very difficult to re-establish. Still, for an epidemiologist, the determination of a reasonably precise denominator on which to base the calculation of crude, age-specific, and disease-specific mortality rates, the prevalence of malnutrition in the affected community, incidence rates of high-priority diseases, health service utilization rates, and so on, is crucial. The inability to establish a reliable denominator in the Goma disaster mentioned above, for example, despite the use of aerial and satellite photography, and the application of a number of relatively new (at the time) epidemiological methods, posed a considerable obstacle to determining the magnitude of the catastrophe and, more important, to the ability to determine the needs for food and other relief commodities.

Determining rates is crucial for making comparisons between population groups and for prioritizing public health programs. Because the impact of a disaster within a specific geographic area is frequently not uniform, these comparisons are important for guiding the response. For example, the Sphere Project has established one death per 10,000 people per day or, if baseline data are available, a doubling of the baseline rate, as thresholds for determining whether or not an emergency exists.* Determining the numerator—meaning, for a crude mortality rate, the number of people who have died—can be quite difficult, as the experience of relief teams after the Pakistan earthquake of 2005 and Hurricane Katrina discovered; and even controversial, as recently published estimates of the number of civilians killed in Iraq during since the 1993 invasion has demonstrated.[12] Innovative methods, such as counting fresh graves in northern Iraq after the Kurdish population fled, fearful of reprisals after the defeat of Saddam Hussein's government in 1991, or the distribution of burial shrouds to religious leaders when disasters occur in Moslem societies where bodies are traditionally covered prior to burial, have helped, when the situation has been relatively calm.

---

* This figure represents a doubling to tripling of baseline mortality rates in developing countries. It is extremely high, yet mortality rates higher than this persist for years in some parts of the world.

## RAPID ASSESSMENT

The critical component of disaster response is, of course, the speed with which appropriate relief goods and services can be provided to the affected population. A rapid quantitative needs assessment can be of life-saving importance. Nevertheless, a practical combination of timeliness and accuracy is more important at the outset of a relief effort than the use of more sophisticated, more scientifically sound methods of data collection and analysis to establish the most precise data possible. One shies away from the term "quick and dirty" epidemiology, but it does convey a sense of what is needed. The field epidemiologist responding to a disaster should also be familiar with simple qualitative methods that can shed considerable light on a situation. A lot can be learned just from educated observation during a walk-through of the affected area. For example, if commodities are being sold, their price can be a good indication of their availability or, conversely, their scarcity. Black markets spring up quickly in post-disaster settings, and the willingness of people to pay exorbitant prices for everyday commodities can indication of desperate need. In slow-onset natural disasters such as famine and drought, indicators such as the amount of jewelry worn by women can be important—the absence of adornment in a society in which it is customary can be an important sign of impending starvation, a signal that everything of value has already been sold. Interviews with community leaders, transect walks through the affected areas, and the constellation of methods that fall under the umbrella of "participatory rapid appraisals" can also be quite informative. The important thing is to get out to the field as quickly as possible after a disaster has occurred and visit all affected areas and population groups.

## SURVEYS

Because of the disruption of routine systems mentioned above, data collection, especially in the early phases of disaster response, is usually by survey (see Chapter 6). Again, you might not be able to establish a precise sampling frame, and you may have to exercise considerable judgment in order to be able to draw a representative sample. Talking to people to ensure that vulnerable population groups are not omitted from the sample is important. In every case, a nearly representative sample is better than a convenience sample if relief is to be apportioned equitably.

The most commonly used survey method is *two-stage cluster sampling*, first developed by the World Health Organization to measure vaccination coverage rates in children.[7] The huge advantage of this method compared to either simple random sampling or systematic random sampling is that the logistical demands are far less—relatively few clusters, usually around thirty, need to be visited in order to obtain statistically valid results with a reasonable degree of precision. The sample size may be considerably larger, and a design effect can be calculated, but in disaster areas it is usually easier to work in a relatively confined area. One major disadvantage of cluster sampling is that it is not well suited for measuring characteristics that are not homogeneously distributed through the population—when mortality, or malnutrition, to cite two examples, are "clumped," then cluster sampling may miss them or, on the other hand, over-sample them, giving skewed, non-representative estimates. Another disadvantage, not to be sneered at, is that the method is difficult to explain those who will be using the data to make decisions. When using this method, your ability to communicate what you have done and what the results mean will be challenged.

Finally, for any survey, whatever method is used, non-sampling error is likely to far outweigh sampling error. Surveyors need to be trained carefully, albeit quickly, to understand the objectives of the survey and to ask questions and make measurements in a way that minimizes the introduction of bias. When individuals and their families desperately need assistance, as is the case in the immediate post-disaster period, they always aim to please. Both surveyors and those they are interviewing will give you the answers they think you want, and you may get a very sincere, but not necessarily accurate, picture of what is happening. You should always be aware of the reasons why people may be providing misleading information—for example, people will not report deaths in their household if they feel that it will result in a smaller food ration—and take steps to ensure that none of your activities are contributing, or are believed to be contributing, to a further deterioration of living standards.

## Organizing Priority Interventions

Médecins Sans Frontières (Doctors Without Borders) in their book *Refugee Health*, cited above, lists what they, on the basis of their experiences through the mid-1990s, feel to be the "ten top priorities" in mounting a relief effort in the health sector (see Table 23–2). You, as a field epidemiologist, should be aware of this list and take it into account when organizing your work. It is quite important to note that, of the first five priorities in disaster relief, only one, measles immunization, is a health-specific intervention. We have already discussed some aspects of rapid assessment and the identification of risk factors. It should be intuitive, but is not always the case, that the most attention should be paid to ensuring that all those affected by disaster have access, as quickly as possible, to adequate amounts of culturally appropriate food of reasonable nutritional value. As difficult as it may seem to believe, epidemiologists working in disaster response over the past twenty years have been called upon to diagnose and react to large outbreaks of exceptionally rare diseases such as scurvy, pellagra, and beriberi, in addition to staggeringly high levels of acute malnutrition.

**Table 23–2.**   The Ten Top Priorities in Disaster Response as Determined by Doctors without Borders)[9]

- initial assessment
- measles immunization
- water and sanitation
- food and nutrition
- shelter and site planning
- health care in the immediate post-disaster phase
- control of communicable diseases and epidemics
- public health surveillance
- human resources and training
- coordination

The quantity, in addition to the quality, of water supplies is also of major concern, crucial to the health of a population, although usually addressed by non–health professionals. The Sphere Project, mentioned above, establishes a level of 15 liters of water per person per day (for all purposes) as the minimum required in a relief effort. As has been seen countless times, from the desert of East Africa to the Superdome of New Orleans in the wake of Hurricane Katrina, achieving even this bare minimum has been quite challenging.

Public health surveillance is, of course, a critical element of disaster response and falls squarely in the realm of the epidemiologist. Earlier chapters of this book have been devoted to this topic (see chapters 3 and 20). The important aspect of surveillance in disaster settings is the need to use it to establish and re-establish priorities on an ongoing basis. When resources, whether financial or human, are constrained, as they always are in the post-disaster period, a clear sense of priorities must be maintained. Assessment and reassessment should be conducted on a continuous basis and, each time a problem is managed, the next most important one should be addressed until the situation comes under control.

In disaster settings, you will encounter a number of major obstacles to establishing good surveillance. These include: (*1*) the need to collect data rapidly *and* accurately in adverse conditions; (*2*) the need to integrate multiple sources of sometimes conflicting data, distinguishing between those that are objective and those that are not; (*3*) persuading others to participate in an effective surveillance system when they may not believe that it is the most important thing to do; (*4*) getting decision makers and those charged with intervening to act on the basis of your surveillance data. Beyond a shadow of a doubt, the successful response to the December 2004 tsunami in Indonesia, successful because it minimized excess morbidity and mortality after the cataclysmic event had occurred, was due to the very rapid establishment of an effective surveillance system. The job was greatly facilitated by the presence, on the scene, of the most experienced disaster epidemiologists from a wide array of international, governmental, and private organizations. Individual cases of diarrhea, measles, and other diseases with epidemic potential were identified shortly after they occurred, and interventions were rapidly mounted.

Sensitivity—the ability to detect cases or events of interest—is an essential feature of surveillance systems in disaster settings. Reporting of untoward events should occur by any means necessary. Cell phones are a very useful tool, but web-based surveillance can also be mounted if computer systems can be maintained. In all cases, a clear message regarding the reporting system must be disseminated as rapidly as possible, and the individual or organization receiving reports must be able to ensure that a rapid and appropriate response will ensue.

In regard to the diseases of interest to be included in any surveillance effort, all depends on the setting. In most developing countries, a simple surveillance form calling for the reporting of cases of acute respiratory illnesses (a proxy for pneumonia), acute watery and acute bloody diarrhea (cholera, bacillary dysentery), measles,[*] fever (malaria), and suspected meningitis can be developed and widely disseminated. In other settings, such as during the Balkan wars of the 1980s and following Hurricane Katrina and other natural disasters in the industrialized world, addressing the needs of the chronically ill who might be cut off from their medications or procedures; of those with diabetes, hypertension, and other cardiovascular conditions; and of the disabled is usually of higher priority than the common communicable diseases that are the leading causes of morbidity and mortality in poorer countries. In all instances, surveillance should focus on those who might be most vulnerable, in order to ensure an equitable distribution of health services. Children, the elderly, women, and, as was seen graphically following Hurricane Katrina, those of lower socio-economic groups, should get special attention, and epidemiologists should ensure that data are always disaggregated in a way that would allow the problems of those high-risk groups to be analyzed separately.

A few words are in order regarding the importance of coordination. Disaster response always takes place in an emotionally charged environment. Both those needing assistance and those there to provide it tend to be quite anxious and short-tempered. Everyone realizes that there is a need for highly coordinated action— one expert has even suggested that "poor coordination" should be considered a valid entry as the cause of death on death certificates—but, because everyone feels that what they are doing is the most important thing to do, no one wants to

---

\* Although it is no longer the case, during the 1980s measles was the leading cause of death in many refugee settings, despite the existence of a safe and effective vaccine, which accounts for its prominent position on the Doctors without Borders priority list. Through the efforts of epidemiologists who documented a number of major outbreaks, mass vaccination against measles is now fairly routine in disaster-response efforts in developing countries.

"be coordinated." You—the epidemiologist who has organized the collection of appropriate data, analyzed it, and recommended the prioritization of certain interventions on the basis of that analysis (and the relegation of others to a place of secondary importance)—will frequently find yourself on the proverbial hot seat. Relatively few of those on the scene will be as familiar with the published literature as you. Relatively few will have the ability to view the chaos through the objective lens of unbiased data. Whether you have asked for it or not, you are likely to be thrust into a position of responsibility and authority, and the respect which you are accorded may be unfamiliar and even uncomfortable. Responding to a disaster will tax your ability to make life-or-death decisions in a calm, confident manner. If you think of your job as the public health equivalent of running an emergency room during a mass casualty event, you can understand why people will look to you guidance, for leadership, for direction. You will have to rise to the occasion.

## SPECIAL CONSIDERATIONS

### Dead Bodies

Natural disasters are frequently characterized by the large numbers of deaths they cause in the acute phase. Whether it is an earthquake, a tsunami, or, rarely, a virulent epidemic such as the cholera epidemic that afflicted the Rwandan refugees in Goma in 1994, both relief workers and the survivors will have to cope with the presence of many dead bodies requiring disposal. Inordinate attention is sometimes paid to this problem, at the expense of dealing with other pressing health concerns that should be aimed at ensuring that no further preventable deaths occur. A common myth that accompanies disaster relief is that dead bodies can be the cause of epidemics of communicable disease—this has been shown many times to not be the case. On the other hand, the presence of cadavers in the midst of a community seriously retards recovery efforts and is a profoundly depressing psychological burden on all involved. When a society is rocked by a serious disaster, it tends to do what it can to maintain itself through its customs, rituals, and traditions: one of the most powerful of which is the funeral and burial ceremony. Ironically, relief authorities frequently insist that even this pillar of social activity be abandoned, and arrangements for the collection and mass burial of corpses, without identification or attempts at family notification, is the norm. You, an epidemiologist interested in the enumeration of the dead in order to establish mortality rates, need to be particularly sensitive to the emotional needs of the community and take all measures to not contribute further to the psychological trauma that has affected it.[15]

## The Laboratory

In many cases, usually in developing countries, communicable diseases have caused substantial morbidity and mortality after both natural and man-made disasters. As mentioned above, surveillance systems generally use syndromic proxies for common disease conditions, but interventions must be guided by confirmation of the exact cause. A field laboratory, with essential diagnostic capabilities, can be a very useful tool in directing both prevention and case-management efforts.

Nevertheless, it is important not to rely too heavily on field laboratories. It is certainly unnecessary to try to diagnose each case of a particular illness. Once a confirmed diagnosis is made, the proper public health approach is to assume that patients who present with similar symptoms have the same illness. Action to contain the spread of any communicable disease should always be instituted on the grounds of clinical suspicion. The laboratory's role is one of confirmation—you should act on the basis of clinical and epidemiological judgment.

## SUMMARY

Disaster response settings are the emergency rooms of public health. Life-saving, irreversible decisions are frequently made in the early phases of the relief effort. The fundamental task of the field epidemiologist responding to either a natural or man-made disaster is to collect and circulate to the appropriate authorities essential data regarding the health and nutrition status of the affected population as accurately as possible in the shortest possible time. The purpose of these data is to be able to direct the first responders to prioritize the interventions that are most likely to limit excess preventable mortality to the greatest extent possible. Given that the environment in which you will be working is one characterized by chaotic coordination, marked logistical and resource constraints, a lack of appreciation for the power and value of the epidemiological approach, and (frequently) blurry lines of authority, you will have to be calm, assertive, and somewhat authoritative in your approach. Communications skills and the ability to convince decision makers that you can help guide their relief efforts are essential. In the end, a successful epidemiological contribution to a disaster response will be measured, not on the basis of the elegance of your epidemiologic investigations, but rather as a function of how many lives are saved.

## REFERENCES

1. Centre for Research on the Epidemiology of Disasters (CRED) (2007).. Annual Disaster Statistical Review: Numbers and Trends, 2006. Université Catholique de Louvain, Brussels, May.

 2. Human Security Centre (2005). Human Security Report—2005. University of British Columbia, Vancouver.
 3. de Ville de Goyet, C., Seaman, J., Geijer, U. (1978). *The Management of Nutritional Emergencies in Large Populations.* World Health Organization, Geneva..
 4. Spencer, H.C., Campbell, C.C., Romero, A., et al. (1977). Disease-surveillance and decision-making after the 1976 Guatemala earthquake. *Lancet* (Jul. 23) 2(8030), 181–4.
 5. Glass, R.I., Cates, W. Jr, Nieburg, P., et al. (1980). Rapid assessment of health status and preventive-medicine needs of newly arrived Kampuchean refugees, Sa Kaeo, Thailand. *Lancet* (Apr. 19) 1(8173), 868–72.
 6. Toole, M.J., Waldman, R.J. (1990). Prevention of excess mortality in refugee and displaced populations in developing countries. *JAMA* (Jun. 27) 263(24), 3296–302.
 7. Toole, M.J., Waldman, R.J. (1997). The public health aspects of complex emergencies and refugee situations. *American Review of Public Health* 18, 283–312.
 8. Centers for Disease Control and Prevention (1992). Famine-affected, refugee, and displaced populations: recommendations for public health issues. *Morb Mortal Wkly Rep* (Jul. 24) 41, RR-13.
 9. Médecins sans Frontières (1997). Refugee health—an approach to emergency situations. Macmillan, London.
10. The Sphere Project (2004). *Humanitarian Charter and Minimum Standards in Disaster Response*, 2nd ed., Oxfam Publishing, Oxford, U.K.
11. Cliff, J., Noormohamed, A.R. (1988). Health as a target: South Africa's destabilization of Mozambique. *Soc Sci Med* 27(7), 717–22.
12. Burnham, G., Lafta, R., Doocy, S., et al. (2006). Mortality after the 2003 invasion of Iraq: a cross-sectional cluster sample survey. *Lancet* (Oct. 21) 368(9545), 1421–8.
13. Henderson, R.H., Sundaresan, T. (1982). Cluster sampling to assess immunization coverage: a review of experience with a simplified sampling method. *Bull World Health Organ* 60(2), 253–60.
14. Waldman, R.J. (2001). Prioritizing health care in complex emergencies. *Lancet* (May 5) 357(9266), 1427–9.
15. Pan American Health Organization (2006). *Management of Dead Bodies after Disasters: A Field Manual for First Responders.* Washington, D.C.

## APPENDIX 23–1

## SUMMARY OF THE MEDICAL AND PUBLIC HEALTH EFFECTS OF MAJOR NATURAL DISASTERS

### Floods

Floods are the most common natural disaster. They affect more people worldwide and cause greater mortality than any other type of natural disaster. They occur in almost every country, but 70% of all flood deaths occur in India and Bangladesh. In the United States, floods cause more deaths than any other natural disaster, with most fatalities resulting from flash floods. Fast-flowing water carrying debris such as boulders and fallen trees accounts for most flood-related injuries and deaths— the main cause of death being drowning, followed by various combinations of trauma, drowning, and hypothermia. Although the health impact of many floods has not been studied at all or only rudimentarily, the few that have been well studied suggest that among flood survivors, the proportion requiring emergency medical care is reported to vary between 0.2% and 2%. Most injuries requiring medical attention are minor and include lacerations, skin rashes, and ulcers, although in the 2004 Asian tsunami, these led to a substantial number of cases of tetanus, a condition not previously documented as a consequence of natural disasters. For some floods, substantial numbers of casualties caused by fire have been documented, because fast-flowing water can break oil or gasoline storage tanks.

Floods may disrupt water purification and sewage disposal systems, cause toxic waste sites to overflow, or dislodge chemicals stored above ground. There may be the potential for water-borne disease transmission of such agents as *Escherichia coli*, *Shigella*, *Salmonella*, and hepatitis A virus. In endemic areas, the risk of transmission of mosquito-borne diseases such as malaria, yellow fever, and the encephalitides may be increased because of enhanced vector-breeding conditions. Upper-respiratory-tract diseases can increase and be rapidly spread in overcrowded temporary shelters for flood victims. Despite the potential for communicable diseases to follow floods, mass immunization programs are almost always counterproductive: they divert limited personnel and resources from other critical relief tasks, and they may create a false sense of security. Unfortunately, after floods, the public often demands typhoid vaccine and tetanus toxoid, although no epidemics of typhoid after floods have ever been documented in the United States. The vaccine can produce mild to moderate systemic reactions, takes several weeks to develop immunity, and even then produces only limited protection. Likewise, mass tetanus vaccination programs are not indicated. Management of flood-associated wounds—like any wounds—requires a tetanus immunization history and immunization only if indicated. As with all disasters, the proper approach to communicable disease prevention and control is to set up a public health surveillance system to monitor disease occurrence.

## Tropical Cyclones (Hurricanes or Typhoons)

The greatest natural disaster in U.S. history occurred on September 8, 1900, when a hurricane struck Galveston, Texas, and killed more than 6000 people. Cyclones, hurricanes, and typhoons have killed hundreds of thousands and injured millions of people during the last 20 years. In 1970, deaths resulting from a single tropical cyclone striking Bangladesh were estimated to exceed 250,000. As population growth continues along vulnerable coastal areas, deaths and injuries resulting from tropical cyclones will increase. Although hurricane winds do great damage, wind is not the biggest killer in a hurricane. Hurricanes are classic examples of disasters that trigger secondary effects such as tornadoes and flooding that, together with storm surges, can cause extraordinarily high rates of morbidity and mortality. This was seen following the 1991 cyclone and sea surge in Bangladesh in which 140,000 people drowned, and during Hurricane Mitch in Central America in 1998 with thousands of drowning deaths. The most graphic recent example was Hurricane Katrina, when most morbidity and mortality was incurred as a result of the rupture of the levees that resulted in the severe flooding of New Orleans.

Nine of 10 hurricane fatalities are drownings associated with storm surges. The major rescue problem is locating people stranded by rising waters and evacuating them to higher ground. Other causes of deaths and injuries include burial beneath houses collapsed by wind or water, penetrating trauma from broken glass or wood, blunt trauma from floating objects or debris, or entrapment by mud slides that may accompany hurricane-associated floods. Many of the severest injuries occur to persons who are in mobile homes during the storm or who are injured or electrocuted during the post-disaster cleanup. Most persons who seek medical care after hurricanes do not require sophisticated surgical or intensive care services and can be treated as outpatients by primary care physicians. The great majority suffer from lacerations caused by flying glass or other debris; a few have closed fractures; and others, mostly penetrating injuries. As with flood-related wounds, emergency medical care providers should be aware that such wounds may contain highly contaminated material such as soil or fecal matter.

People are often severely crowded in storm shelters. As with flood disasters, this crowding increases the probability of disease transmission via aerosol or fecal–oral routes, particularly when sanitary facilities are insufficient. Trauma after a cyclone is not usually a major public health problem when compared with the need for water, food, clothing, sanitation, and other hygienic measures. Sending fully equipped mobile hospitals and specialized surgical teams that usually arrive much too late at the disaster site is an ineffective response to a cyclone disaster. Nonmedical relief (such as epidemiologists, sanitary engineers, shelter, food, and agricultural supplies) is probably more effective in reducing mortality and morbidity. However, field hospitals and emergency medical teams from outside the disaster-affected area may, indeed, be useful to provide ongoing primary health-care services to the community when all other health-care facilities have been destroyed or severely damaged.

## Tornadoes

Tornadoes are among the most violent of all natural atmospheric phenomena. Although almost 700 tornadoes occur in the United States each year, only about 3% result in severe injuries requiring hospitalization. Of 14,600 tornadoes between 1952 and 1973 for which data exist, only 497 caused fatalities, and 26 of these events accounted for almost half of the fatalities. The destruction caused by tornadoes results from the combined action of their strong rotary winds and the partial vacuum in the center of the vortex. For example, when a tornado passes over a building, the winds twist and rip at the outside. Simultaneously, the abrupt pressure reduction in the tornado's eye causes explosive pressures inside the building. Walls collapse or topple outward, windows explode, and the debris from this destruction can be driven as high-velocity missiles through the air. Buildings of nonreinforced masonry, wood-frame buildings, and those with large window areas are likely to suffer the most. The leading cause of death is craniocerebral trauma, followed by crushing wounds of the chest and trunk. Lacerations and fractures are the most frequent nonfatal injuries. Also frequent are penetrating trauma with retained foreign bodies and other soft-tissue injuries. A high percentage of wounds among tornado casualties are heavily contaminated. In many instances foreign materials, such as glass, wood splinters, tar, dirt, grass, and manure, are deeply embedded in areas of soft-tissue injury. Sepsis is common in both minor and major injuries; sepsis affects one-half to two-thirds of patients with minor wounds.

## Volcanic Eruptions

The U.S. Geological Survey has identified approximately 35 volcanoes in the western United States and Alaska that are likely to erupt in the future. Most of these are in remote rural areas and are not likely to result in human disaster. A few, like Mt. Hood, Mt. Shasta, Mt. Rainier, and the volcano underlying Mammoth Lakes in California, are located near population centers. Most volcanic deaths are caused by immediate suffocation and, to a lesser extent, by burns or blunt trauma. Eruptions have immediate life-threatening health effects through suffocation from inhaling massive quantities of airborne ash, scalding from blasts of superheated steam, and surges of lethal gas. Pyroclastic flows and surges are particularly lethal. These are currents of extremely hot gases and particles that flow down the slopes of a volcano at tens to hundreds of meters per second and cover hundreds of square kilometers. Because of their suddenness and speed, pyroclastic flows and surges are difficult to escape. Sudden release of these gases can be catastrophic: carbon dioxide released from Lake Monoun and Lake Nyos in Cameroon in 1984 and 1986, respectively, claimed 1800 lives. Other toxic effects of these gas releases include pulmonary edema, irritant conjunctivitis, joint pain, muscle weakness, and cutaneous bullae. Mud flows, or lahars, account for at least 10% of volcano-related deaths. These are flowing masses of volcanic debris mixed with water. The mud is sometimes scalding hot, causing severe burns. A volcanic eruption may also generate tremendous quantities of ash-fall. Buildings have been reported to collapse from the weight of ash accumulating on roofs, resulting in severe trauma to the occupants. The ash can also be irritating to the eyes (causing corneal abrasions), mucous membranes, and the respiratory system. Upper airway irritation, cough, and bronchospasm, as well as exacerbation of chronic lung diseases, are common findings in symptomatic patients. With extremely high concentrations, volcanic ash may cause severe tracheal injury, pulmonary edema, and bronchial obstruction leading to death from acute pulmonary injury or from suffocation.

After the eruption of Mount St. Helens in 1980, 23 immediate deaths were reported. Post-mortem examinations revealed that 18 of these deaths resulted from asphyxia. Finally, a delayed onset of ash-induced mucus hypersecretion or obstructive airway disease may occur. Hospitals in the vicinity of both active and dormant volcanoes should be prepared to deal with a sudden influx of victims with severe burns and lung damage from inhalation of hot ash, as well as multiple varieties of trauma.

## Earthquakes

An earthquake of great magnitude is one of the most destructive events in nature. During the past 20 years, earthquakes have caused more than a million deaths and injuries worldwide. Hospitals and other health-care facilities are particularly vulnerable to the damaging effects of an earthquake. The primary cause of death and injury from earthquakes is the collapse of buildings. Deaths may come from severe crushing injuries to the head or chest, external or internal hemorrhage, or drowning from earthquake-induced tidal waves (tsunamis). Rapid death occurs within minutes or hours and may come from asphyxia from dust inhalation or chest compression, hypovolemic shock, or exposure. Heavy dust, produced by crumbling buildings immediately following an earthquake, may cause asphyxiation or upper airway obstruction. Asbestos and other particulate matter in the dust are both sub-acute and chronic respiratory hazards for trapped victims, as well as for rescue and cleanup personnel. Burns and smoke inhalation from fires are also major hazards after an earthquake.

Paralleling the speed required for effective search and extrication is the speed needed for emergency medical services—for speed is of the essence. The greatest demand occurs within the first 24 hours. Injured people usually seek medical attention at emergency departments only during the first three to five days; afterwards, the case mix patterns return almost to normal. Moreover, a surprisingly large number of patients require acute care for nonsurgical problems such as acute heart attacks, exacerbation of chronic diseases such as diabetes or hypertension, anxiety and other mental health problems, and near-drowning because of flooding from broken dams.

Finally, an earthquake may precipitate a major technological disaster by damaging or destroying nuclear power stations, hospitals with dangerous biological products, hydrocarbon storage areas, and hazardous chemical plants. As with most natural disasters, the risk of secondary epidemics is minimal, and only mass immunization campaigns based on results of public health surveillance are appropriate following earthquakes.

## Drought and Famine

Although frequently considered natural disasters, drought, which sometimes leads to localized or widespread famine, is often the result of long-term socio-political factors, including the oppression of minority ethnic groups in some areas. Those most vulnerable to these slow-onset disasters are most often those who were the poorest and most down-trodden elements of society prior to their occurrence. For this reason, the humanitarian crises engendered by them have come to be referred to as "complex emergencies." The combination of political oppression and deteriorating environmental conditions frequently leads to the forced migration of large populations, and many of the disasters that have stimulated an international response over the past two decades have been those in which the provision of relief to refugees and/or internally displaced persons has been the paramount concern.

The principal causes of morbidity and mortality associated with slow-onset disasters generally reflect the same pattern as that which existed prior to the disaster, although the magnitude may be much greater, and high levels of acute malnutrition make an important contribution.

## War and Civil Strife

Although the number of wars has been declining since the end of the Cold War in the early 1990s, the nature of war and its consequences have changed. It is estimated that 90% or more of the current victims of war are civilians, and that the indirect consequences of armed conflict, with some notable exceptions including the continuing conflict in Iraq and the Balkan wars of the last decade, far outweigh the death and injury caused by combat itself.

The indirect consequences of war include food scarcity, and the contribution of armed conflict to famine has been alluded to above. In addition to the disruption of the marketplace, irrigation systems may be destroyed, sowing and reaping cycles impossible to maintain, and normal distribution channels interrupted. The plight of those fleeing intense conflict or the threat of conflict can further compromise their nutritional status. For example, in Darfur, Sudan, in 2004, it was found that only 7% of those displaced had access to sufficient food, compared to 50% of those who had remained in their villages. One aspect of war that is all too often ignored by epidemiologists and other public health officials is the gross violations of human rights that can result, through torture, sexual violence, and other illegal acts resulting in elevated morbidity and mortality.

As might be imagined, it is difficult, if not impossible, to practice public health during times of violent conflict, and the ability of the epidemiologist to collect, analyze, and use data is often severely compromised. Whatever data can be generated can and perhaps should be used for advocacy purposes, to inform the public and appropriate political authorities of the serious toll that wars, sanctioned or ignored, take on the health of the public. Public health officials can usually only try to limit the consequences of war—preventing it is the job of politicians and diplomats—but accurate documentation of the damage that armed conflict inflicts on the health of civilian populations and its effective communication to those who can intervene might be a major contribution.

# 24

# LABORATORY SUPPPORT FOR THE EPIDEMIOLOGIST IN THE FIELD

Elaine W. Gunter
Joan S. Knapp
Janet K. A. Nicholson

This chapter provides general guidelines on what specimens are appropriate to collect when investigating an infectious disease problem or when studying a potentially toxic chemical or radionuclide exposure, and what types of tests should be done to confirm an exposure or infection. The lists we have provided of specimens to collect and tests to perform may not be exhaustive and may not include all the newer investigative or research tools. The microbial agents included are only the more common ones that you are likely to encounter; no effort was made to include all possible agents. Because most field investigations will involve specimen collection, *it is absolutely essential to contact the appropriate laboratory personnel prior to entering the field to determine the appropriate specimens to collect and the precise methods for preserving and shipping them to the laboratory* (see Chapter 5). Although these guidelines are intended for epidemiologists doing field investigations, they also apply to specimens collected in other settings, as indicated in the sections below. Many local support laboratories can perform the tests described below—particularly those relating to infectious diseases. However, the laboratory services of the Centers for Disease Control and Prevention (CDC) will always serve as a necessary backup. Remember, make early contact with your support laboratory, and seek out the local, state, or provincial laboratory as appropriate. This chapter is divided into four parts: the first deals with specimen collection for the detection of toxic chemicals; the second covers the identification of infectious pathogens; the third provides information about the Laboratory Response Network (LRN); and the last addresses general issues.

## COLLECTION OF SPECIMENS FOR POTENTIAL CHEMICAL TOXICANTS

### General Instructions

In cases of suspected chemical toxicant exposure, it is extremely important to work in conjunction with your analytic support laboratory or, if needed, with the Division of Laboratory Sciences (DLS) in the Coordinating Center for Environmental Health and Injury Prevention (CCEHIP) of CDC. DLS will provide laboratory support for environmental health studies and emergency response in these situations, and, as with other epidemiologic investigations, these studies must be planned and submitted for all appropriate processing as early as possible. For all analyses to be performed by DLS, it is imperative to contact the laboratory personnel prior to specimen collection, because a detailed specimen collection protocol must be prepared and included as an appendix to any study protocol. The section below describes only general instructions on how to collect specimens. An example of the necessary detail and care required to collect certain kinds of specimens is also given to emphasize the critical nature of the methods used (see Appendix 24–1). *In the rare event that you might be part of a team responding to chemical or biological terrorism events, see Appendix 24–2*, which outlines simplified instructions for first responders who will be collecting specimens for identification of suspected chemical terrorism agents. All such specimens will be sent to the DLS/CCEHIP Sample Logistics group/lab. A subset of the samples will be sent to CDC's Rapid Response and Advanced Technology Laboratory (RRAT Lab), where they will be initially triaged for detection of selected infectious agents. If, on the other hand, you are contemplating collection and transport of specimens for chemical toxicant examination at CDC, it is imperative that you make contact with the CCEHIP DLS laboratory prior to collection. This is absolutely essential because of the highly specialized collection and analysis required for these toxicants. In some cases DLS is the only place where certain assays are performed. DLS has or will create detailed protocols for you. If there is an emergency, DLS is on call and will send materials and instructions as soon as possible—and, if necessary, provide personnel to assist in field specimen collection. In chemical exposures, many toxicants or their metabolites may be rapidly cleared from easily accessible specimens, such as blood, either through excretion or sequestration in tissues. One must know the proper specimen matrix to collect to reflect either recent acute exposure, or body burden through chronic exposure.

To meet this need, DLS maintains dedicated specimen collection supplies that have been pre-tested for any background contamination, and abbreviated collection instructions (by specimen type) that can be rapidly shipped by air or prepared to accompany the investigator. The information that follows and the urine collection procedure in Appendix 24–1 are examples of these instructions. A good rule of thumb in the case of an emergency where acute exposure(s) may have occurred is to obtain biological specimens (blood, serum, and urine) as soon as possible, even if it means using materials not pre-tested by the support laboratory or CDC. In these cases, follow the basic guidelines to control extraneous contamination, and try to cryo-cool (dry-ice) the urine and cool the blood specimens as soon as possible. To allow evaluation of possible extraneous contamination from the collection materials, randomly select at least three of each item used (e.g., three randomly selected, empty test tubes), seal them in a clean container, and store and ship them with the specimens. However, it is still important to obtain the state support laboratory or CDC-supplied collection materials as soon as possible for all subsequent sampling. For both regularly scheduled studies and emergency response, laboratory results are only as good as the specimens collected, regardless of how sophisticated the analytic method may be. The small amounts of clinical specimens that are often collected and the low toxicant concentrations in the specimens require methods with sensitivities as low as parts per quintillion ($10^{-18}$). Extraneous substances from the ambient air or a person's skin or clothing, or interfering substances in collection supplies, will be concentrated and measured along with the specimens. Specimens must be kept at low temperatures to prevent degradation. For these reasons, detailed specimen collection protocols are found below.

## Materials Required

### Materials available locally

The following materials must be supplied or available locally by prior arrangement with a support laboratory:

- Centrifuge capable of spinning tubes as large as 16 mm in diameter by 100 mm long for separation of serum. After the blood in the red-topped Vacutainer™ (no anticoagulant) tubes has been allowed to clot at room temperature for at least 30 and no more than 60 minutes, centrifuge the tubes for 15 minutes at 2400–2800 RPM (i.e., RPMs necessary to attain a force of 1000 x G)
- Refrigerator (4 °C –8 °C) and freezer (< –20 °C, *not* frost-free)
- Dry ice, 20 lb–30 lb on hand (10 lb–12 lb per shipping container)

## Materials supplied from DLS

- Materials: All other materials needed are contained in the supplies provided by DLS. A collection protocol will be provided, since specimen collection requirements may vary for each study. All of these materials (collection tubes, pipettes, aluminum foil, etc.) will have been pre-screened or specially washed to minimize extraneous contamination. Use only the materials supplied for specimens if they are to be sent to CDC, and do not open the supplies until they need to be used. Return any unused intact and nonexpendable supplies to CDC. *Instructions*: Detailed instructions for collecting each specimen type should be included, as well as the protocol for packing and shipping specimens. These instructions have been abbreviated to the extent possible to accommodate emergency situations.

## Four general considerations

*These considerations must be kept in mind at all times:*

- Specimen collection and processing conditions should be aimed at minimizing contamination from extraneous sources, such as hands, body parts, clothes, and ambient air.
- Specimens should be refrigerated or frozen, as instructed, as rapidly as possible after collection. If the field situation prevents access to specimen processing for six to eight hours, the laboratory staff will provide stability information about the specimens. A cooler and reusable cold-packs will be provided for this purpose during specimen collection and transport for processing.
- Bar-coded labels with CDC's unique specimen identifiers required for "cradle-to-grave" specimen tracking will be provided by the laboratory to label all tubes collected, vials processed, and related paperwork. A specimen transmittal list must be prepared to accompany the specimens. If time permits in advance of leaving for field collection, epidemiologists may contact CDC receiving laboratories that use electronic Laboratory Information Management System (LIMS) software. These labs may be able to provide an Excel™ template file that will allow the importation of specimen identifiers and epidemiologic information directly into their LIMS module when the specimens and data are received at CDC.
- Specimen collection teams should be given copies of these instructions and trained in their use prior to the time of anticipated need.

## Guidelines for Collection of Clinical Specimens

Table 24–1 is provided to help collection teams determine which specimens should be collected by priority in various situations based on the type of toxicant exposure.

**Table 24–1.** Blood or Urine to Collect for Suspected Environmental Toxicant Exposures

| SUSPECTED TOXICANT | SPECIMEN PREFERRED (IN DECREASING ORDER OF PRIORITY) | ADULTS AND CHILDREN (10 YEARS OLD AND OLDER) | BABIES AND CHILDREN (LESS THAN 10 YEARS OLD) |
|---|---|---|---|
| Organic | Serum | Two 10-mL tubes, no anticoagulant | One 5-mL tube, no anticoagulant |
| | Urine† | 30 mL | 10–20 mL† |
| | Whole blood (heparin) | One 7-mL tube (if available), three 4-mL tubes, or four 3-mL tubes | Two 3-mL tubes‡ |
| Inorganic | Urineᵈ | 30 mL | 10–20 mL |
| | Whole blood (EDTA) | One 3-mL tube | One 3-mL tube |
| | Serum¶ | One 7-mL trace metals-free tube | One 7-mL trace metals-free tube |
| Unknown | Serum | Two 10-mL tubes, no anticoagulant | One 5.0-mL tube, no anticoagulant |
| | Urine* | 30 mL | 10–20 mL |
| | Whole blood (EDTA) | One 2-mL tube | One 2-mL tube |
| | Whole blood (heparin) | One 7-mL tube (if available), three 4-mL tubes, or four 3-mL tubes | Two 3-mL tubes‡ |

*Urine is the preferred specimen to be collected if a cholinesterase inhibitor is suspected, such as organophosphate pesticide.

†For babies and children too young to be toilet trained, disposable urine bags or special collection tampons placed in the diaper may be used.

‡Preferred specimen if toxicant is a suspected volatile organic compound. If time permits, the preferred tube here is a 7- or 10-mL gray-top tube (sodium oxalate/sodium fluoride anticoagulant) prepared and provided by DLS.

ᵈSpecimen pretreatment is required only for a separate aliquot for urine mercury if toxic mercury exposure is suspected. DLS will provide specimen collection containers with a small amount of sulfamic acid and Triton X-100™ (a surfactant) to stabilize this specimen. Urine specimens for all other metals (e.g., As, Ni, Sn, Sb, Pb, Cd, Cr) or heavy radionuclides (e.g., U, Th, or Pu) will be stabilized with Ultrex™ nitric acid upon receipt at DLS.

¶For essential trace metals such as Se, Fe, Zn, Cu, Mg, Mn only, in case of overload.

For example, if problems are encountered while collecting specimens from a six-year-old boy by venipuncture for a suspected inorganic toxicant such as lead, cadmium, or mercury, the EDTA-anticoagulated whole-blood tube should be obtained before collection of additional blood for serum yield is attempted.

Contact the support laboratory or the DLS, CCEHIP (770–488–4305 or 770–488–7950) and establish the date and time to ship the specimens. Examples of possible environmental toxicants are:

- *Organic:* dioxins, furans, coplanar and non-coplanar polychlorinated bis-phenol compounds (PCBs), volatile organic compounds (VOCs), perfluorinated compounds, cotinine and other markers of tobacco exposure, persistent pesticides, non-persistent pesticides, pyrethroid pesticides, organophosphate pesticides, polyaromatic hydrocarbons (PAHs), phthalates, paranitrophenol, brominated flame retardants (BFRs)
- *Inorganic:* heavy metals such as lead, arsenic, nickel, mercury, chromium, beryllium, or tin (including Speciated forms of mercury and arsenic); essential trace metals such as selenium, iron, zinc, copper, calcium, magnesium, manganese (in overload cases); perchlorates; radionuclides such as uranium (including U isotope ratios), thorium, plutonium, and radioactive iodine.

For autopsy material such as liver, adipose, kidney, and lung tissues, and for fluids such as whole blood, urine, and stomach contents, place freshly cut tissues or fluids in sterile plastic screw-capped containers provided by DLS. Do *not* submit formalinized tissues.

ACKNOWLEDGMENT    The authors wish to thank the following persons who contributed to the preparation of this chapter.

From the Coordinating Center for Infectious Diseases:

Matthew J. Arduino. M.S., Dr.P.H., Division of Healthcare Quality Promotion National Center for Preparedness, Detection and Control of Infectious Diseases (NCPDCID); Amanda Balish, B.S., Influenza Division, National Center for Immunization and Respiratory Diseases (NCIRD); Ronald C. Ballard, Ph.D., Division of Sexually Transmitted Disease Prevention, National Center for HIV/AIDS, Viral Hepatitis, STDs, and TB Prevention (NCHHSTP): Bernard Beall, Ph.D., Division of Bacterial Diseases (DBD), NCIRD; C. Ben Beard, Ph.D., Division of Vector-Borne Infectious Diseases (DVID), National Center for Zoonotic, Vector-Borne, and Enteric Diseases (NCZVED); Cheryl Bopp, M.S., Division of Foodborne, Bacterial, and Mycotic Diseases (DFBMD), NCZVED; Maria da Glória S. Carvalho, Ph.D., DBD, NCIRD; Mark L. Eberhard, Ph.D., Division of Parasitic Diseases, NCZVED; Barry S. Fields, Ph.D., DBD, NCIRD; Barbara W. Johnson, Ph.D., DVID, NCZVED; Thomas G. Ksiazek, DVM, PhD., Division of Viral and Rickettsial Diseases (DVRD), NCZVED; Susan Maslanka, PhD, DFBMD, NCZVED; J. Steven McDougal, M.D., Division of HIV/AIDS

Prevention, NCHHSTP; Paul Mead, MD, MPH., DVID, NCZVED; M. Steven Oberste, Ph.D., DVD, NCIRD; Pierre Rollin, M.D., Division of Viral and Rickettsial Diseases, NCZVED; David Turgeon, M.S., M.M.S., Ph.D., Division of Scientific Resources, NCPDCID; Mary Brandt, Ph.D., DFBMD, NCZVED; Wendi Kuhnert, Ph.D., Division of Viral Hepatitis, NCHHSTP.

From the Coordinating Center for Environmental Health and Injury Prevention:

Robert L. Jones, Ph.D., Division of Laboratory Sciences, CCEHIP; John Osterloh, M.D.,M.S., CCEHIP; David L. Ashley, Ph.D., DLS, CCEHIP; J. Jerry Thomas, M.D., DLS, CCEHIP; Dorothy Sussman, R.N., B.A., M.F.A. CCEHIP; Charles Dodson, M.T.(ASCP), DLS, CCEHIP; Charles Buxton, M.P.H., M.T.(ASCP)SBB, DLS, CCEHIP; Jacob Wamsley, M.P.H., E.M.T., DLS, CCEHIP.

## APPENDIX 24–1. URINE COLLECTION PROCEDURE FOR SPECIMENS FOR METALS AND PESTICIDES ANALYSIS

### URINE COLLECTION (FIRST MORNING VOID SPECIMEN IF POSSIBLE)

Urine collection cups will be provided for each participant. Instruct each person to do the following for urine collection to obtain a "clean catch" sample:

- Wash hands with soap and water.
- Do not remove the cap from cup until ready to void. Exposure to air should be minimized.
- Collect at least 30 mL urine in the cup as a midstream collection.
- Do not touch the inside of the cup or the cap at any time.
- Recap the specimen and deliver to investigator.
- Place a label for URINE CONTAINER on cup.
- For a child younger than three years of age, pediatric urine collection bags may need to be used. Follow the directions accompanying the bags for use.

A total of 3 aliquots is needed. Prepare them in the order given below. If the sample is insufficient for all aliquots, do as many as possible with the amounts required for each test.

1. *Urine Pesticides:* Gently swirl the capped container to re-suspend any dissolved solids. Pour 20–30 mL urine into the provided 2- or 4-oz plastic specimen container. (At DLS, one 1.0-mL aliquot of this specimen will be used for a urine creatinine measurement to correct the concentration of the metals or pesticides for specimen volume differences.) If a pediatric

collection bag was used, tilt the bag slightly so the corner of the bag can be clipped with clean stainless steel scissors. Carefully pour the urine into the containers through this small hole.

2. *Urine Metals:* Transfer 4 mL urine to a 5-mL plastic cryotube.

3. *Urine Mercury:* Add urine to 4.5-mL line on tube with red dot. This tube contains a small amount of a sulfamic acid (a mild acid) and Triton X-100™ (a surfactant) to preserve the mercury, and must be mixed well by inversion after being securely capped to dissolve this preservative mixture.

All aliquot tubes should be labeled with the appropriate barcoded label with the participant ID number and aliquot type. Ship specimens on dry ice to DLS.

## SHIPPING LIST

A transmittal log is provided to record samples that are collected. Mark the appropriate spaces indicating which aliquots were collected, the date collected, and any problems that were encountered in collection, storage, or shipping.

## SHIPPING PROCEDURE

1. Pack the shipping box with the boxes of urine samples. Place each box in the resealable plastic bags before packing. Fill the shipper with dry ice, cover with the Styrofoam™ lid, and tape down the cardboard outer flaps. Place a dry ice label on the outside of the container, and write in the amount of dry ice in the shipper.

2. Ship to the following address: Specimen Receipt Coordinator, Division of Laboratory Sciences, Centers for Disease Control and Prevention, Building 110 Loading Dock, 4770 Buford Highway NE, Atlanta, GA 30341–3724.

3. Call (770) 488–4305 on the day the shipment is made, or if any questions arise.

## COLLECTION OF SPECIMENS FOR MICROBIAL IDENTIFICATION

### General Instructions

It is essential that the field epidemiologist contact the specific support laboratory prior to collecting specimens, because each testing laboratory has its own protocols. If you plan to send your specimens to CDC, you should know that specimens sent to the Coordinating Center for Infectious Diseases (CCID) may be tested in one of many laboratories. To ensure that specimens are received in the Data and Specimen Handling section and distributed to the appropriate laboratory for testing, packages should be shipped to:

CENTERS FOR DISEASE CONTROL AND PREVENTION

STAT Laboratory
Attn: (Unit #/disease agent)
1600 Clifton Road, N.E.
Atlanta, GA 30333
(404) 639–3931

CCID provides laboratory services to state health departments under special, clearly defined circumstances. CCID does not normally accept specimens submitted to it from county health departments, hospitals, or private physicians, as these specimens should initially be sent to the state health department laboratory. If the state laboratory subsequently deems it necessary to call upon the laboratories of CCID for support and if the specimens satisfy the CDC requirements, then the CCID laboratories will accept the specimens. Under some circumstances, individual CCID laboratories will accept specimens directly; however, these are special circumstances, and these arrangements must be made in advance with the specific laboratory that will perform the testing. Reports from testing will be sent to the corresponding state health department. Laboratories wishing to submit specimens directly to CCID laboratories should contact their state health department to obtain permission to ship specimens directly to a CCID laboratory and obtain a state health department patient/specimen number with which to identify the specimens; a completed copy of the CDC specimen submission form (Form 50.34) should accompany individual specimens. Specimen test reports will be sent to the state health department for distribution to the submitting laboratory. When an epidemiologist encounters an illness likely to be of infectious etiology, there is no substitute for good clinical judgment. Inappropriate, insufficient, or inappropriately collected specimens may result in misidentification or in the ability to identify the causative agent. In this regard, many of the suggested laboratory tests provide information to support a clinical diagnosis, not make it.

*Universal precautions statement*

Since medical history and examination cannot reliably identify all persons infected with HIV or other blood-borne pathogens, "universal blood and body fluid precautions" should be used when obtaining and handling specimens of blood and certain other body fluids from *all persons* (*Morbidity and Mortality Weekly Report* 37:377, 1988; http://www.cdc.gov/hiv/resources/reports/mmwr/1988.htm). Other body fluids include amniotic, pericardial, peritoneal, pleural, synovial, and cerebrospinal fluids (CSF), and semen and vaginal secretions. In addition, any body fluid containing visible blood and body tissues should be handled as though it may be infectious.

Gloves should be worn whenever handling blood or the specified body fluids and when performing phlebotomy. Barrier precautions should be used whenever appropriate to prevent skin and mucous membrane exposure during specimen acquisition and handling. Gowns should be worn if splashing or spattering of fluids is likely. If splashing of the mouth and face are possible, masks and protective eyewear are indicated. Specimens are to be transported in leakproof containers.

Take care to prevent injuries when using needles, scalpels, and other sharp instruments or devices and when disposing of used sharp instruments. Do not recap or remove needles from disposable syringes by hand; and do not bend, break, or otherwise manipulate used needles by hand. Dispose of needles and sharp equipment in puncture-resistant containers designed for this purpose.

## Specimen Collection

Tables 24–2 to 24–9 provide information on the type of specimen needed and the assays used for identification of the microbial agent. Some considerations for collection and shipment of specimens are found below. In addition, one should contact the nearest LRN laboratory, the CDC Bioterrorism Rapid Response and Advanced Technologies (BRRAT) laboratory, or other CCID laboratory for precise instructions on the selection, collection, and transport of specimens for testing. Investigators of outbreaks may contact the Division of Scientific Resources (DSR) Emergency Supply Coordinator to obtain supplies:

Business hours (8:00 AM–4:30 PM EST/EDT, Mon–Fri): call 404–639–2402 and ask for the DSR Emergency Supply Coordinator.

After hours: call Director's Emergency Operations Center (DEOC) (404–639–2436) or contact Physical Security (404–639–2888) and ask for DEOC.

### Serum

Serum specimens for serology should be separated from whole blood using aseptic technique. Contaminated serum specimens are unsuited for almost all testing purposes. Paired serum specimens are preferred and in many cases required. The first specimen should be obtained as soon after the onset of illness as possible and refrigerated. The second specimen should be collected two to four weeks later. The optimal interval for collecting the serum specimens will vary with different infectious diseases. Paired serum specimens, though desirable, are difficult to obtain and are not required for serologic tests of mycotic or parasitic diseases. Serologic tests for neurosyphilis require both serum and CSF specimens.

**Table 24–2.** Bacterial Diseases—General*

| AGENT OR DISEASE | SPECIMEN(S) TO COLLECT | METHOD OF CONFIRMATION OR IDENTIFICATION | COMMENTS |
|---|---|---|---|
| Brucellosis | Blood, bone, marrow, or site of localization<br>Sera | Culture<br>Tube agglutination or EIA | Prolonged incubation (4–5 days) may be necessary<br>2-mercaptoethanol agglutination test distinguishes IgG from IgM antibodies and may be diagnostic for chronic brucellosis. *B. canis* infection requires specific serologic test |
| Cat scratch disease | Skin biopsy<br>Lymph node<br>Blood Pus | Culture, FA | |
| *Chlamydia pneumonia* | Nasopharyngeal swab<br>OP swab<br>Serum | Culture, PCR<br><br>MIF | Maintain cultures at 4 °C, or −70 °C if transport time >24 hr |
| Diphtheria | Throat swab | Culture, PCR | Put swab directly into Pai or Loeffler slants. Silica gel package can also be used for transport. |
| *H. influenzae* | Blood | Culture<br>CSF<br>Sterile site specimen | Antigen tests sensitive but culture strongly preferable |
| Legionellosis | Sera<br>Lung tissue<br>Resp. secretions<br>Urine<br>Sera | IFA<br>DFA, culture<br>PCR<br>Antigen detection (ICT or EIA)<br>MAT | Positive IFA not conclusive, culture strongly preferable |
| Leptospirosis | Blood<br>Urine<br>Sera | Culture<br><br>MAT | Leptospiremia occurs during first week of illness.<br>Leptospiruria occurs after the second week of illness.<br>Growth occurs after several days to several weeks |

*See Appendix 24–3 for definitions of acronyms.

*Continued*

**Table 24-2.** Bacterial Diseases—General*—Continued

| AGENT OR DISEASE | SPECIMEN(S) TO COLLECT | METHOD OF CONFIRMATION OR IDENTIFICATION | COMMENTS |
|---|---|---|---|
| Listeriosis | CSF | Culture, PCR | Serology neither sensitive nor specific |
| | Blood | | Serotyping and subtyping indicated for epidemiologic investigation; not for confirmation or identification |
| | Site of infection | | |
| | Placenta | | |
| | Food | | |
| Lyme disease and other borrellioses | Sera | EIA (or FA), WB | Clinical case definition necessary |
| | Blood | Culture, PCR | For tick-borne relapsing fever |
| | CSF | EIA (or FA), WB | May be indicated for patients with neurologic disease |
| | Plasma or Skin Biopsy | Culture, PCR of cultures | For early Lyme disease (research) |
| | Synovial fluid | PCR; rarely EIA, WB | For Lyme arthritis |
| | Sera | CF, EIA, indirect hemagglutination, IIF | |
| *Mycoplasma pneumoniae* | NP swab, Throat swab, sputum | PCR, Culture | |
| | Sera | CF, EIA, indirect hemagglutination, IIF | |
| *Neisseria meningitidis* | CSF | Culture, serotype, latex agglutination | Serotyping and molecular subtyping indicated for epidemiologic investigation; not for confirmation or identification |
| | Blood | | |
| | Throat | | |
| | Sera | | |
| Plague | | | |
| All clinical forms | Blood | Culture, PCR | Cultures can be recovered on general lab media such as sheep blood agar (SBA). |
| Bubonic | Aspirate of lymph node | Culture, DFA, PCR | |
| Pneumonic | Respiratory secretions | Culture, PCR | |
| Septicemic | Blood | Culture, DFA, PCR | |

| Disease/Form | Specimen | Test | Comments |
|---|---|---|---|
| All clinical forms | Serum | Passive hemagglutination/Passive hemagglutination inhibition | |
| Trachoma (C. trachomatis) | Conjunctival swab | NAAT | Maintain at −70 °C in sucrose phosphate transport medium without penicillin |
| Tularemia All clinical forms | Blood | Culture, PCR | Culture requires cysteine enhancement; cysteine heart agar with 9% chocolatized blood (CHAB) recommended; All work with cultures should be done at Biosafety Level 3. |
| Pneumonic tularemia | Respiratory Secretions | Culture, PCR | |
| Ulceroglandular or oculoglandular | Swabs of visible lesions or affected areas | Culture, DFA, PCR | |
| Ulceroglandular, glandular or oropharyngeal | Aspirates from lymph node or lesions | Culture, PCR, DFA | |
| All clinical forms | Serum | Microagglutination, tube agglutination | |
| Group A streptococcus | Throat swab, skin lesions, blood, any tissue, | Culture, serogroup carbohydrate, subtyping | |
| Group B streptococcus | Placenta, blood, CSF, vaginal swab, anorectum swab, lesional material, soft tissue | Culture, serogroup carbohydrate, subtyping | |
| Streptococcus pneumoniae | blood, CSF, sputum, ear fluid, eye secretion | Culture, PCR, optochin, bile solubility | |
| Psittacosis (C. psittaci) | Sera | CF | |

**Table 24-3.** Bacterial Diseases—Sexually Transmitted*

| AGENT OR DISEASE | SPECIMEN(S) TO COLLECT | METHOD OF CONFIRMATION OR IDENTIFICATION | COMMENTS |
|---|---|---|---|
| Chancroid | Swab from lesion | PCR | Investigational test |
| Lymphogranuloma venereum (LGV) (*C. trachomatis*) | Lesion, endourethral, endocervical, rectal swabs | Culture, NAAT | Rectal swabs from women and MSM<br>Culture: maintain at 4 °C or −70 °C if transport time >24 hr<br>NAAT: investigational, PCR can differentiate between LGV and other *C. trachomatis* biovars |
| | Lymph node biopsy | Pathology | |
| | Sera | MIF | Negative MIF test rules out LGV |
| Genital (non-LGV) *C. trachomatis* | Endourethral, endocervical swab | Culture, NAAT | Culture: maintain at −70 °C in sucrose-phosphate transport medium |
| | Urine | NAAT | Investigational test |
| | Vaginal, rectal swabs | NAAT | |
| Gonorrhea | Endourethral, endocervical, vaginal, rectal, pharyngeal swab | Culture | Vaginal swab from prepubescent girls<br>Rectal swab from women and MSM<br>Direct inoculation of specimen onto selective medium; transport at room temperature in $CO_2$-enhanced atmosphere; incubate within 8h |
| | Urine | NAAT | Vaginal, pharyngeal, rectal: investigational test |
| | Urethral, cervical, vaginal, pharyngeal, rectal swabs | | NAATs cannot be used for medicolegal purposes |

| | | Nontreponemal/treponemal tests, DNA and Reiter absorption, WB | Treponemal tests available on postmortem bloods |
|---|---|---|---|
| Syphilis | Sera | | |
| | Autopsy, biopsy, lesional material | Darkfield microscopy<br>DFA-TP<br>PCR | Darkfield microscopy at point-of-care site only<br>DFA-TP: paraffin blocks, slides, or fixed material acceptable; must state fixative<br>PCR: investigational use only |
| Congenital | Sera | FTA-ABS,<br>IgM EIA | Mother's and baby's serum and history requested<br>IgM EIA investigational only |
| | Autopsy, biopsy, lesional material | Darkfield microscopy<br>DFA-TP | Darkfield microscopy at point-of-care site only<br>DFA-TP: paraffin blocks, slides, or fixed material acceptable; must state fixative<br>PCR: investigational use only |
| Neurosyphilis | CSF | FTA-ABS CSF,<br>VDRL (CSF),<br>WB | |

*See Appendix 24–3 for definitions of acronyms.

**Table 24-4.** Bacterial Diseases—Food-Borne[a, b]

| AGENT OR DISEASE | SPECIMEN(S) TO COLLECT | METHOD OF CONFIRMATION OR IDENTIFICATION | COMMENTS |
|---|---|---|---|
| *Bacillus cereus* | Stool | Culture | Isolation of organism from stool of two or more ill persons and not from stool of control patients |
| | Food | Culture, assay for toxin | Isolation of $10^5$ organisms/g from epidemiologically implicated food, provided specimen is properly handled; commercial immunoassay may also be used to detect diarrheal toxin in food |
| *Campylobacter jejuni* | Stool | Culture | Isolation of organism from clinical specimens from two or more ill persons or isolation of organism from epidemiologically implicated food. Isolates may be sent to the state PulseNet laboratory for PFGE subtyping |
| | Food | | |
| Botulism (*Clostridium botulinum*) | Stool | Culture, mouse assay for toxin | Call CDC if you suspect botulism |
| | NG aspirate | | |
| | Food | | |
| | Serum | Mouse assay for toxin | |
| *Clostridium perfringens* | Stool | Culture | Isolation of $10^6$ organisms/g from stool of two or more ill persons, provided specimen is properly handled followed by PCR detection of toxin genes |
| | Food | Culture, assay for toxin | Isolation of $10^5$ organisms/g from epidemiologically implicated food, provided specimen is properly handled. |

| Organism | Specimen | Test | Criteria / Comments |
|---|---|---|---|
| *Escherichia coli* O157:H7 and other Shiga toxin-producing *E. coli* | Stool, Food | Culture | Isolation of *E. coli* O157:H7 or other Shiga toxin-producing *E. coli* from clinical specimen from two or more ill persons or from food..Isolates should be sent to the state PulseNet laboratory for PFGE subtyping. Serotyping of non O157:H7 strains performed at CDC. |
| | Serum | Assay for lipopolysaccharide (LPS) antibody | Serodiagnosis at CDC only for outbreak or HUS cases |
| Enterotoxigenic *E. coli* and other Diarrheagenic *E. coli* | Stool, Food | Culture | Isolation of organism of same serotype, demonstrated by PCR to have enterotoxin genes (heat-labile and/or heat-stable) or other virulence marker, from stool of two or more ill persons or from food |
| *Enterobacter sakazakii* | CSF, Blood, rectal swab, stool, Powdered infant formula, powdered breast milk supplement | Culture, PCR | Molecular subtyping (e.g., PFGE) is done to confirm epidemiologic link to formula fed to the infant. |
| *Salmonella* sp. | Stool, Food | Culture, serotyping | Isolation of organism of same serotype from clinical specimens from two or more ill persons or from food. Isolates should be sent to the state PulseNet laboratory for PFGE subtyping. |
| *Shigella* sp. | Stool, Food | Culture, serogrouping | Isolation of organism of same serotype from clinical specimens from two or more ill persons or from food.. Isolates should be sent to the state PulseNet laboratory for PFGE subtyping |

*Continued*

**Table 24-4.** Bacterial Diseases—Food-Borne[a, b]—Continued

| AGENT OR DISEASE | SPECIMEN(S) TO COLLECT | METHOD OF CONFIRMATION OR IDENTIFICATION | COMMENTS |
|---|---|---|---|
| *Staphylococcus aureus* | Stool<br>Food<br>Vomitus<br>Nasal swabs | Culture, assay for toxin | Need $10^5$ organisms per gram of incriminated food. PCR detection of enterotoxin genes. Molecular typing (e.g., PFGE) to determine lineage |
| *Vibrio cholerae* O1 and O139 | Stool<br>Food | Culture | Isolation of toxigenic organism from stool or vomitus of two or more ill persons or from food. Send isolates to CDC for toxin testing and serogrouping. Call the CDC if you suspect cholera. |
| | Sera | Vibriocidal and antitoxic antibodies | Serodiagnosis is performed at CDC in special circumstances |
| *Vibrio cholerae* non-01 | Stool<br>Food | Culture | Isolation of toxigenic organism from stool or vomitus of two or more ill persons or from food. Send isolates to CDC for toxin testing and serogrouping. |
| *Vibrio parahemolyticus* | Stool<br>Food | Culture | Isolation of organisms of the same serotype from clinical specimens from two or more ill persons or from food. Isolates should be sent to CDC for serotyping. |
| *Yersinia enterocolitica* | Stool<br>Food | Culture | Isolation of organisms of the same serotype from clinical specimens from two or more ill persons or from food. Isolates may be sent to CDC for serotyping |

[a] For more information, refer to CDC website, "Guide to Confirming a Diagnosis in Foodborne Disease": http://www.cdc.gov/foodborneoutbreaks/guide_fd.htm.
[b] For more information on collection of stool specimens, refer to the CDC website, "Guidelines for Specimen Collection": http://www.cdc.gov/foodborneoutbreaks/guide_sc.htm.

**Table 24-5.** Viral Diseases—General*

| AGENT OR DISEASE | SPECIMEN(S) TO COLLECT | METHOD OF CONFIRMATION OR IDENTIFICATION | COMMENTS |
|---|---|---|---|
| Adenovirus | Respiratory, stool, eye swab | Culture, EIA, IFA, PCR | Respiratory specimens: nasal pharyngeal swabs, aspirates or washes are preferred over throat swabs; for suspected lower respiratory tract infections, bronchoalveolar lavage and transtracheal aspirates are preferred over sputum. Biopsy or autopsy specimens may be useful in some circumstances. |
| | Sera | HI, CF, NT, EIA, IIF | |
| Human immunodeficiency virus types 1 and 2 (HIV-1/2) | Plasma, sera, saliva, or urine | EIA, WB | |
| | Whole blood, plasma, sera, or saliva | Rapid tests | |
| | Plasma | NAAT | |
| Cytomegalovirus (CMV) | Urine, throat swab | Culture, PCR | Serologic tests of limited diagnostic value |
| | Sera | EIA, NT, IgM capture EIA | |
| Coronaviruses | Respiratory | Culture, RT-PCR | Respiratory specimens: nasal pharyngeal swabs, aspirates or washes are preferred over throat swabs; for suspected lower respiratory tract infections, bronchoalveolar lavage and transtracheal aspirates are preferred over sputum. Biopsy or autopsy specimens may be useful in some circumstances. Culture suitable for only some coronaviruses. |
| | Sera | NT, EIA | |

*Continued*

**Table 24-5.** Viral Diseases—General*—Continued

| AGENT OR DISEASE | SPECIMEN(S) TO COLLECT | METHOD OF CONFIRMATION OR IDENTIFICATION | COMMENTS |
|---|---|---|---|
| Coxsackieviruses | CSF, stool, rectal swab, throat swab | Culture, RT-PCR | Serologic tests of limited diagnostic value |
| Epstein-Barr virus | Blood, throat swab<br>Sera | Culture, PCR<br>EIA | |
| Echoviruses | CSF, stool, rectal swab, throat swab | Culture, RT-PCR | Serologic tests of limited diagnostic value |
| Hantaviruses | Serum | ELISA, Immunoblot | |
| | Blood | ELISA, Immunoblot, RT-PCR | |
| Hepatitis A | Plasma<br>Serum | EIA^ | IgG and IgM assays available |
| Hepatitis B | Plasma<br>Serum | EIA^ | • Markers available: anti-HBs, total anti-HBc, IgM anti-HBc, and HbsAg<br>• HBsAg confirmatory assay is a neutralization assay |
| Hepatitis (Delta) | Plasma<br>Serum | EIA^ | |
| Hepatitis C | Plasma<br>Serum | EIA^ and Immunoblot (RIBA) | Confirmatory assay results are important to due false positive EIA results in populations with low prevalence of disease |

| | | | |
|---|---|---|---|
| Hepatitis E | Plasma<br>Serum | EIA^ | |
| *Herpes simplex* | Vesicular fluid, brain biopsy<br>Sera | Culture, PCR, DFA<br>IgG-EIA | Serologic tests of limited diagnostic value |
| Human metapneumovirus | Respiratory<br>Sera | Culture, PCR<br>EIA, NT | Respiratory specimens: nasal pharyngeal swabs, aspirates or washes are preferred over throat swabs; for suspected lower respiratory tract infections, bronchoalveolar lavage and transtracheal aspirates are preferred over sputum. Biopsy or autopsy specimens may be useful in some circumstances. Commercial antigen detection assays still not widely available. |
| Human parainfluenza viruses | Respiratory<br>Sera | Culture, EIA/IFA, PCR<br>EIA, NT | Respiratory specimens: nasal pharyngeal swabs, aspirates or washes are preferred over throat swabs; for suspected lower respiratory tract infections, bronchoalveolar lavage and transtracheal aspirates are preferred over sputum. Biopsy or autopsy specimens may be useful in some circumstances. |
| Influenza virus | Throat swab<br>Sera | Culture, EIA<br>CF, HI, EIA | |
| Lymphocytic choriomeningitis | Brain<br>Sera<br>CSF | Culture, RT-PCR<br>ELISA, NT<br>Culture, RT-PCR, ELISA | |

*Continued*

**Table 24-5.** Viral Diseases—General*—Continued

| AGENT OR DISEASE | SPECIMEN(S) TO COLLECT | METHOD OF CONFIRMATION OR IDENTIFICATION | COMMENTS |
|---|---|---|---|
| Measles | NP swab, Throat swab, urine | Culture, EIA, RT-PCR | Serology preferred for diagnosis |
| | Sera | EIA, HI, CF, NT | |
| Mumps | Throat swab; Stensons duct swab, urine | Culture, EIA, RT-PCR | |
| | Sera | HI, CF, NT, EIA | |
| Norovirus | Stool | Real-time RT-PCR, immune electron microscopy | |
| | Sera | EIA | |
| Parainfluenza | Throat swab | Culture, EIA | |
| | Sera | CF, HI, EIA, IIF | |
| Parvovirus B19 | Blood, sera | PCR | |
| | Sera | EIA, IFA | |
| Picornaviruses (parechoviruses, cardioviruses) | Stool, rectal swab, throat swab | Culture, RT-PCR | Serologic tests of limited diagnostic value |
| Polioviruses | Stool, rectal swab, throat swab, CNS tissue | Culture, RT-PCR | |
| | Sera | NT | |

| Agent | Specimen | Methods | Comments |
|---|---|---|---|
| Rabies | Brain, skin biopsy | Culture, DFA | |
| | Sera | RFFIT, IFA | |
| Respiratory syncytial virus | Respiratory | Culture, EIA, IFA, RT-PCR | |
| | Sera | EIA, NT | |
| Rhinoviruses | Respiratory | Culture, PCR | Respiratory specimens: nasal pharyngeal swabs, aspirates or washes are preferred over throat swabs; for suspected lower respiratory tract infections, bronchoalveolar lavage and transtracheal aspirates are preferred over sputum. Biopsy or autopsy specimens may be useful in some circumstances. Serologic tests of limited diagnostic value. |
| | Sera | EIA, NT | |
| Rotavirus | Stool | EIA, culture, electron microscopy, gel electrophoresis | |
| | Sera | EIA, NT, RT-PCR | |
| Rubella | Throat swab | Culture, EIA, RT-PCR | Serology preferred for diagnosis |
| | Sera | EIA, HI, Latex Agglutination, IIF | |
| Vaccinia | Vesicular fluid, scabs, brain | Culture, Electron microscopy | |
| | Sera | EIA, HI, NT | |
| Varicella-zoster | Vesicular fluid | PCR, DFA, electron microscopy Culture | PCR preferred method, EM only identifies as herpes family virus: not VZV specific; serology not useful for identification—need direct detection method |
| | Sera | EIA | |

*See Appendix 24–3 for definitions of acronyms.
^Other Enzyme immunoassay formats available—Chemiluminescent (CIA) and Microparticle (MEIA)

**Table 24-6.** Diagnostic Testing Algorithm for Medically Important Arthropod-Borne Viral Diseases in North America *

| AGENT OR DISEASE | SPECIMEN(S) TO COLLECT | METHOD OF CONFIRMATION OR IDENTIFICATION** | COMMENTS |
|---|---|---|---|
| California encephalitis/ La Crosse encephalitis | Sera | IgM ELISA, NT | Except where noted, freeze specimens for virus isolation at −70°C (dry ice) |
| | Brain | Real-time RT-PCR, Virus isolation | |
| | CSF | IgM ELISA, NT, Real-time RT-PCR,† Virus isolation† | |
| | Mosquitoes | Real-time RT-PCR, Virus isolation | |
| Colorado tick fever | Whole blood/clot | Real-time RT-PCR, Virus isolation | Do not freeze samples for CTF virus isolation. |
| | Sera | Real-time RT-PCR, Virus isolation, paired NT | |
| | Ticks | Real-time RT-PCR, Virus isolation | |
| Dengue Serotypes 1–4 | Sera | IgM ELISA, NT, Real-time RT-PCR,‡ Virus isolation‡ | |
| | Liver, lung, lymph nodes | Real-time RT-PCR, Virus isolation | |
| Eastern equine encephalitis/ | Sera | IgM ELISA, NT, Real-time RT-PCR,† virus isolation† | Isolation requires biosafety level 3 containment with additional PPE recommended for all non-immune personnel; Venezuelan equine encephalitis virus requires HEPA filtered exhaust air flow |
| | Brain | Real-time RT-PCR, Virus isolation | |
| Venezuelan equine encephalitis/ | CSF | IgM ELISA, NT, Real-time RT-PCR,† Virus isolation† | |
| | Mosquitoes | Real-time RT-PCR, Virus isolation | |
| Western equine encephalitis | Horse sera | IgM ELISA, NT, Real-time RT-PCR, Virus isolation | |

| Disease | Specimen | Test | Comments |
|---|---|---|---|
| St. Louis encephalitis | Sera | MIA/IgM ELISA, NT, Real-time RT-PCR† | Isolation requires biosafety level 3 containment |
| | Brain | Real-time RT-PCR, virus isolation | |
| | CSF | IgM ELISA, NT, Real-time RT-PCR,† virus isolation† | |
| West Nile virus | Sera | MIA/IgM ELISA, NT, Real-time RT-PCR† | Isolation requires biosafety level 3 containment |
| | Brain, brain stem, spinal cord | Real-time RT-PCR, Virus isolation | |
| | CSF | IgM ELISA, NT, Real-time RT-PCR,† Virus isolation† | |
| | Mosquitoes | Real-time RT-PCR, Virus isolation, Dipstick, RAMP | |
| Yellow fever§ | Sera | IgM ELISA, NT, Real-time RT-PCR,† Virus isolation† | Isolation requires biosafety level 3 containment with HEPA filtered exhaust air flow; Yellow fever immunization required |
| | Liver | Real-time RT-PCR, Virus isolation, histopathology | |
| | Mosquitoes | Real-time RT-PCR, Virus isolation | |

*See Appendix 24–3 for definitions of acronyms.
**Listed in order of priority.
†If specimen is acute and volume allows for both serology and molecular testing.
‡In acute specimens up to 7 days post-onset of fever.
§Imported cases only; international travel history to yellow fever endemic areas.

**Table 24–7.** Rickettsial Diseases*

| AGENT OR DISEASE | SPECIMEN(S) TO COLLECT | METHOD OF CONFIRMATION OR IDENTIFICATION | COMMENTS |
|---|---|---|---|
| Q fever | Sera | CF, IIF | Isolation of organisms in lab requires biosafety level 3 containment |
| | Lung, blood | Culture | |
| Rocky Mountain spotted fever | Sera | IIF | Isolation of organisms in lab requires biosafety level 3 containment |
| | Brain, spleen, blood | Culture, FA | |
| Murine typhus | Sera | IIF | |
| | Blood | Culture | |
| Ehrlichiosis | Blood, spleen | Culture | |
| | Sera | IIF | |

*See Appendix 24–3 for definitions of acronyms.

**Table 24–8.** Mycotic Infections*

| AGENT OR DISEASE | SPECIMEN(S) TO COLLECT | METHOD OF CONFIRMATION OR IDENTIFICATION | COMMENTS |
|---|---|---|---|
| Aspergillus and Zygomycetes | Tissue | Immunohistochemistry | |
| Candidiasis | Sera | ID, LA, EIA | |
| | Tissue | Histology, culture | |
| Coccidioidomycosis | Tissue, site of infection | Gene Probe Test | |
| Cryptococcosis | Sera | TA, LA | |
| | Tissue, site of infection, CSF | Histology, FA, direct exam, culture | |
| Histoplasmosis | Sera | ID, CF | |
| | Tissue, site of infection | Direct exam, culture, ID, histology, GenProbe Test | |

**Table 24–8.**  Mycotic Infections*—Continued

| AGENT OR DISEASE | SPECIMEN(S) TO COLLECT | METHOD OF CONFIRMATION OR IDENTIFICATION | COMMENTS |
|---|---|---|---|
| Nocardiasis | Sera | ID | |
| | Tissue, site of infection | Direct exam, culture | |
| Sporotrichosis | Sera | LA | |
| | Tissue, site of infection | Culture | |

*See Appendix 24–3 for definitions of acronyms.

**Table 24–9.**  Parasitic Infections*

| AGENT OR DISEASE | SPECIMEN(S) TO COLLECT | METHOD OF CONFIRMATION OR IDENTIFICATION | COMMENTS |
|---|---|---|---|
| Amoebiasis, intestinal | Sera | EIA | |
| | Tissue | Direct examination | |
| | Formalin- and PVA-preserved stool | Trichrome stain | |
| | Unpreserved stool | PCR | |
| | Water from suspect source | | |
| Free-living amoebic infections | CSF | PCR | |
| | Tissue | Culture; IFA (for confirmation of species) | |

*Continued*

**Table 24–9.**   Parasitic Infections*—Continued

| AGENT OR DISEASE | SPECIMEN(S) TO COLLECT | METHOD OF CONFIRMATION OR IDENTIFICATION | COMMENTS |
|---|---|---|---|
| Cryptosporidiosis | Formalin-preserved stool | Direct examination of concentrated stool stain by modified Kinyoun (acid-fast) stain or DFA | |
| | Unpreserved or potassium dichromate preserved stool | PCR or direct exam | |
| | Tissue | Histopathology | |
| | Sera | | |
| | Water from suspect source | PCR, IFA, or direct exam | |
| Cyclospora | Formalin-preserved stool | Direct exam of concentrated stool by Kinyoun modified acid-fast stain, hot safranin stain, or UV | |
| | Potassium dichromate-preserved stool | PCR or direct exam | |
| | Suspect food sample | PCR | |
| Giardiasis | Formalin-preserved stool | Direct examination of concentrated stool or DFA | |
| | PVA-preserved stool | Trichrome stain | |
| | Unpreserved or potassium dichromate preserved stools | PCR | |
| Leishmaniasis | Sera | IFA | |
| | Tissue Tissue impression smears | Direct exam of H&E or Giemsa stained tissue or impression smears | |
| | Whole blood | Culture | |

**Table 24–9.**  Parasitic Infections*

| AGENT OR DISEASE | SPECIMEN(S) TO COLLECT | METHOD OF CONFIRMATION OR IDENTIFICATION | COMMENTS |
|---|---|---|---|
| Malaria | Blood smear | Direct exam of Giemsa stained smear | |
| | Sera | IFA | |
| | Blood | PCR | EDTA, do not freeze |
| Schistosomiasis | Formalin-preserved stool | Exam of concentrated stool for eggs | Tissue diagnosis occasionally necessary for diagnosis; rectal biopsy more common |
| | Fresh urine (examine within 45 minutes or preserve with formalin) | Examination of centrifuged urine sediment | Serologic tests helpful in acute or ectopic schistosomiasis |
| | Sera | EIA | |
| Trichinellosis | Sera | EIA | In addition to pork, other meats such as bear, cougar, moose, walrus, and horse meat have been implicated as the source of infection |
| | Tissue sample of suspect meat | Direct exam of biopsied tissue | |

For more detailed instructions on how to collect specimens for specific parasites, please go to http://www.dpd.cdc.gov/dpdx/.

## Whole blood

When whole blood is sent for isolation of certain viral and parasitic agents, the blood should be kept cold, but not frozen, prior to shipping, and shipped in wet ice, not dry ice. Blood for bacteria culture should never be refrigerated prior to incubation. If the blood is to be cultured at a local or distant facility, the blood should be collected directly in the blood bottle used by the facility in which the blood culture will be performed. This will also dictate how best to transport the specimens by courier. If whole blood is submitted for PCR only, follow the directions in LRN protocols. The investigative group should contact DEOC at CDC (see instructions above), or the state lab they are in and find out where the nearest LRN lab is, since it may be in a hospital. Water ice should not be used for packing when taken directly from the ice maker or ice trays. Rather, the, wet ice should be held in a container until some liquid water collects, indicating the ice is starting to thaw. The liquid may be poured off and the specimen containers packed with the remaining solid ice with less fear of ruining the specimen by freezing en route. Provision should be made to prevent leakage of the water as the wet ice melts and to keep this water from contaminating the specimen containers (a good sealed container such as using gallon-sized resealable plastic bags will suffice). Be sure that the specimen containers are packaged so that they will not be broken by the solid ice in which they are packed. Whole blood submitted for rickettsial isolation must be packed in dry ice and shipped frozen. Because some microbial specimens require different handling procedures, be sure to check with the diagnostic laboratory prior to shipping.

## Slides

Slides with tissue sections, blood films, and smears of clinical material should be dry, free of immersion oil, properly labeled, and carefully packed in a slide mailing container. If a smear is unstained, it should be fixed prior to shipping to minimize the chance of sending live organisms. If a cardboard slide mailer is the only mailer available, it should be placed in another shipping container to ensure that the slides are not broken in transit.

## Other specimens

Digital images of suspected parasitic organisms may now be submitted electronically for evaluation to DPDx via the link http://www.dpd.cdc.gov/DPDx/htm.

Cultures of etiologic agents should be incubated and shipped in a medium that will protect and ensure the viability of the microorganism during transit. This medium is used to minimize growth of both the organism and unwanted contaminants during transport.

Optimum containers for different groups of etiologic agents vary depending upon the agent and the distance involved in shipment. In all instances, the primary container should be of a durable material that, when properly packaged, is leakproof and can withstand the temperature and pressure variations likely to occur in the air and on the ground during shipment.

When in doubt about what to collect, when to collect, and how to handle specimens, consult your support laboratory or the CCID laboratory contact. If time is of the essence and that person(s) cannot be reached, refer to a standard microbiology text for this information, such as *A Guide to Specimen Management in Clinical Microbiology*, 2nd edition, J. Michael Miller, ASM Press, Washington, D.C., 1999.

## LABORATORY RESPONSE NETWORK

The Laboratory Response Network (LRN) is a partnership between the CDC, the Association of Public Health Laboratories (APHL), and the Federal Bureau of Investigation (FBI) to provide a network of laboratories throughout the United States that have the capability to identify microbial and chemical agents most likely to be used in biological or chemical terrorism. The LRN was established in 1999, and by 2006, nearly 150 laboratories worldwide (>140 in the U.S.) were members. The LRN laboratories will provide to users a standard operational plan, algorithms, protocols for standardized testing, proprietary reagents (for detection of biological agents), reporting requirements, and a secure network for sharing information. These laboratories use molecular tests to rapidly confirm the presence of biological and chemical agents in human specimens. Additionally, most LRNs can identify biological agents in environmental specimens. For detection of chemical agents most likely to be used in a terrorist event, currently 41 laboratories have instrumentation and trained personnel to detect cyanide and toxic metals; five of those laboratories are also capable of detecting mustard gas and nerve agents as well as ricin. Most of the laboratories are public health laboratories (all chemical LRN laboratories are state public health laboratories), though some are federal laboratories.

For biological agents, the hospital and clinical laboratories are considered sentinel laboratories, having the capability to rule out many of the agents likely to be used for terrorism. They are to submit suspicious isolates and specimens to the nearest LRN laboratory for confirmation. The CDC will provide a secondary confirmation and will characterize the agent to determine whether the outbreak or incident has a common source.

For possible chemical terrorism incidents, chemical LRN Level 3 labs (similar to the sentinel laboratories for biological agents) are instructed to package and ship specimens. The CDC DLS laboratory will conduct a rapid toxic screen for the first 40 specimens to identify possible chemical or radionuclide agent(s), and the chemical LRN laboratories will analyze overflow specimens according to their capabilities, using the validated DLS assays.

## SPECIMEN SHIPPING PROTOCOL

This protocol applies for specimens to be tested for potential chemical or microbial exposures. Shipping regulations have changed over the years, so it is prudent to call the nearest LRN laboratory or to refer to current regulations prior to shipping specimens. For assistance in determining how to ship specimens, contact your support laboratory or consult either of the following CDC websites: http://www.cdc.gov/od/ohs/biosfty/biosfty.htm; http://www.cdc.gov/ncidod/srp/specimens/reference-testing.html.

Consultations for packaging, marking and labeling specimens for shipment to CDC may also be obtained from:

Packing, Marking, Labeling Consultation
CDC Shipping Activity
Yvonne Stifel: 404–639–3355

### Temperature Requirements

It is critical that specimens be shipped at temperatures appropriate for the analyte to be tested; guidance as to the method of shipment of specimens should be obtained from the laboratory in which the specimens will be processed. Usually, the following types of specimens must be shipped frozen in containers with dry ice:

- Serum/plasma (when directed by protocol)
- Urine
- Frozen food
- Tissue
- Red blood cell hemolysates (if prepared by special protocol)
- CSF

The following types of specimens must be sent refrigerated, in containers with reusable cold-packs:

- Whole blood (e.g., the tubes collected for heavy metals such as Pb or for VOCs)
- Red blood cells (if separated for a special protocol)

- Food
- Serum/plasma (when directed by protocol)
- Urine (when directed by protocol)

The following types of specimens may be sent refrigerated or frozen:

- Water
- Soil[aa*]
- Fecal specimens (depending on protocol)

The following specimens must be shipped without cooling or freezing:

- Blood bottles containing whole blood for bacterial culture
- Blood for hematology determinations

## List of Materials Needed

Available locally (e.g., at local hospitals, cryogenic companies, or with several days notice, from CDC's STAT Laboratory): 10–12 pounds of dry ice per shipping container (for frozen specimens) or enough dry ice to ensure that the specimens remain frozen until received in the diagnostic laboratory. Shipping materials supplied by DLS for analysis of chemical toxins (for infectious specimens, refer to CCID laboratory for necessary materials):

- Styrofoam™-insulated shipping container
- Cardboard storage boxes with dividers or foam inserts for anticoagulated blood collection tubes or processed specimens
- "Bubble" wrap packing material (additional paper material such as paper towels or newspaper will be needed.)
- Clear or reinforced packaging tape
- Reusable cold-packs for refrigerated specimens: These must be placed in a –20 °C freezer for a minimum of two hours before use.
- Air express courier shipping labels (with CDC's account number)

Animal specimens or specimens believed to contain pathogens of importance to livestock and poultry being shipped from outside the United States

---

[aa*] If soil is being sent from an international field site for chemical testing, DLS has a USDA-approved soil importation certificate. Contact the laboratory (770–488–4305) for a copy and the required stickers for the soil container.

(e.g., for investigation of potential zoonotic disease) or between states require a USDA import permit for the laboratory receiving such specimens. The receiving laboratory must provide a copy of a current, appropriate USDA Veterinary Services permit to the sending laboratory.

## APPENDIX 24–2. SHIPPING INSTRUCTIONS FOR SPECIMENS COLLECTED FROM PEOPLE POTENTIALLY EXPOSED TO CHEMICAL & RADIOLOGICAL TERRORISM AGENTS

### COLLECTING SPECIMENS

### Required Specimens

*Unless you are otherwise directed, collect the following specimens from each person who may have been exposed:*

- *Urine*: Collect at least 30 mL, if possible. Use a screw-capped plastic container. Please do not overfill. **Freeze as soon as possible** (–70 °C or dry ice preferred). If possible, ship the specimen on dry ice. If dry ice is not available, you may ship frozen specimens with freezer ice packs. For pediatric patients, collect urine only, unless otherwise directed by CDC.
- *Whole blood*: Use three 4-mL or larger purple-top (EDTA) tubes, vacuum-fill only (unopened). **If collecting in 3-mL purple top tubes, please collect a *fourth* tube**.
- *Whole blood*: Use one 3-, 5-, or 7-mL gray-top (Na oxalate/NaF anticoagulant) or one 3-, 5-, or 7-mL green-top tube (heparin anticoagulant), vacuum-fill tube only (unopened). **If possible, *glass*, rather than plastic, collection tubes are preferred to minimize background contamination. Please also submit several empty tubes of type used for the laboratory to use as "blanks" to assess background contamination levels.**

### Order of Collection

Please mark the first purple-top tube of whole blood collected with a "1" ("one") using indelible ink. The first purple-top tube of whole blood collected will be used to analyze for blood metals.

## Blanks

For **each lot number** of tubes and urine cups used for collection, please provide two empty unopened purple-top tubes, two empty unopened green- or gray-top tubes, and two empty unopened urine cups to serve as blanks for measuring background contamination. **Note: Although blanks do not have to be labeled, please secure their container tops in the same fashion as described below for collected blood tubes and urine cups**.

## Labeling

Label specimens with labels generated by your facility. These labels may include the following information: medical records number, specimen identification number, collector's initials, and date and time of collection. Follow your facility's procedures for proper specimen labeling. The collector's initials and date and time of collection will allow law enforcement officials to trace the specimen back to the collector should the case go to court and the collector be needed to testify that they collected the specimen.

Information provided on labels may prove helpful in correlating the results obtained from the Rapid Toxic Screen and subsequent analysis with the people from whom the specimens were collected.

Place a single, unbroken strip of waterproof, tamper-evident forensic evidence tape over each specimen top, being careful not to cover the specimen ID labels. This tape must make contact with the specimen container at two points. **The individuals placing the evidence tape must identify themselves by writing their initials on the container and on the evidence tape**.

Maintain a list of names with corresponding specimen identification numbers at the collection site to enable results to be reported to the patients.

## SPECIMEN SHIPPING PROTOCOL

This protocol applies for specimens to be tested for chemical or microbial exposures. For shipping purposes, specimens may be categorized into *infectious substances* and *patient specimens.*

*Infectious substances* are substances known to contain, or reasonably expected to contain, pathogens. *Pathogens* are microorganisms (including bacteria, viruses, rickettsia, parasites, and fungi) or recombinant microorganisms (hybrid or mutant) that are known or reasonably expected to cause infectious disease in humans or animals. For transport purposes, agents are classified into two classes,

Category A or Category B, based on their ability to cause permanent disability or life-threatening or fatal disease in healthy humans or animals (This category includes CDC-defined Select Agents and USDA animal pathogens.). Category A agents pose a higher degree of danger than Category B agents. These guidelines were recently updated in the 49 Code of Federal Regulations (CFR), parts 171, 172, 173, and 175, Hazardous Materials: Infectious Substances: Harmonization with the United Nations Recommendations; Final Rule (http://edocket.access. gpo.org). Lists of Category A agents affecting humans and animals are available in this document.

## CATEGORY A INFECTIOUS SUBSTANCES—49 CFR 173.199

A *Category A Infectious Substance* is defined as "an infectious substance in a form capable of causing permanent disability or life-threatening or fatal disease to otherwise healthy humans or animals when exposure to it occurs." Exposure occurs when an infectious substance is released outside of its protective packaging, resulting in physical contact with humans or animals. The infectious substance determination must be based on the known medical history or symptoms of the source patient or animal, endemic local conditions, or professional judgment concerning the individual circumstances of the source human or animal.

A Category A Infectious Substance must be assigned one of the following proper shipping names:

- *"Infectious substances, affecting humans, 6.2, UN2814"*
(for substances causing disease in humans or in both humans and animals)
- *"Infectious substances, affecting animals only, 6.2, UN2900"*
(for substances causing disease in animals only).

For unknown samples of infectious substances strongly believed to contain a Category A infectious substance, the words "suspected Category A infectious substance" must be entered in parentheses in place of the technical name as part of the proper shipping description. For known Category A pathogens, the technical name of the pathogen must be indicated.

## CATEGORY B INFECTIOUS SUBSTANCES—49 CFR 173.199

A *Category B Infectious Substance* is defined as "an infectious substance that is not in a form generally capable of causing permanent disability or life-threatening or fatal disease in otherwise healthy humans or animals when exposure to it occurs."

Most infectious substances currently shipped as Risk Group 2 or 3 will be shipped as Category B infectious substances under this final rule. Category B infectious substances do NOT include "Regulated Medical Waste." The proper shipping name for Category B infectious substances is:

## "BIOLOGICAL SUBSTANCE, CATEGORY B, 6.2, UN3373"

The packaging for a Category B infectious substance must be a triple packaging consisting of the primary receptacle, a secondary packaging and a rigid outer packaging (49 CFR 173.199). The packaging is NOT required to be a UN-specification packaging; however, it must be capable of passing the drop tests in 49 CFR 178.609.

Shipping regulations may change over the years, so it is prudent to call the nearest LRN laboratory, contact CCEHIP or CCID, or to refer to current regulations prior to shipping specimens.

## Packaging

Packaging specimens for shipment consists of three components:

- a primary specimen container (blood tubes, urine cups, culture tube or plate);
- secondary packaging, including materials for protecting the primary receptacles from breakage, absorbent material that protects the primary containers and absorbs all material that may leak from the primary container, and waterproof packaging that prevents materials leaking into the outer packaging), and
- an outer packaging container (Styrofoam™-insulated corrugated, fiberboard box). Examples of packaging for Category A and Category B materials are described and illustrated in U.S. Department of Transportation publication *Transporting Infectious Substances Safely* (http://hazmat.dot. gov/training/Transporting_Infectious_Substances_Safely.pdf).

For Category A materials (infectious substances), either the primary receptacle or secondary packaging must be capable of withstanding, without leakage, temperatures in the range of $-40\,°C$ to $+55\,°C$ ($-40\,°F$ to $+131\,°F$), (49 CFR 173.196 (6). According to 49 CFR 173.199(b), if specimens are to be transported by air, either the primary receptacle or the secondary packaging used must be capable of withstanding without leakage an internal pressure producing a pressure differential of not less than 95 kPa (0.95 bar, 14 psi). Verify in advance that the manufacturer of either the primary specimen container or the secondary packaging used in your facility is in compliance with the pressure differential requirement.

## Primary packaging

Everything in the primary container, including transport media, is considered the infectious substance or patient specimen. To facilitate processing, package specimens such as blood tubes so that similar tubes are packaged together, e.g., all purple-tops together in one primary package and all grey-top tubes in another primary package; do not mix purple-top and green/gray-top tubes in the same primary package.

The primary container must be watertight; seal screw-top containers with Parafilm™, adhesive tape, or a similar material. Separate each container from other containers to prevent contact between tubes and minimize the chance for breakage. Containers may be separated in a variety of ways, such as wrapping each container to prevent contact between them. Place each in a gridded box wrapped with absorbent material and sealed inside a plastic bag–sealable Styrofoam™ container, shipment sleeve and transport tube, or individually wrapped tubes sealed inside a plastic bag.

Assemble shipping container, packing materials, and dry ice. Work quickly so the frozen specimens will not be exposed to ambient temperatures for more than 5 to 10 minutes, if possible. It is imperative that the specimens be kept in a hard-frozen state. Package specimens according to the temperature at which they must be transported. **Do not ship frozen specimens and specimens to be shipped at 4 ˚C in the same package**. Several primary packages to be shipped under the same temperature conditions may be contained in the same secondary package if space permits. Similarly, specimens to be shipped under the same temperature conditions to different laboratories at the same final destination should be packaged in separate secondary packages and clearly labeled with the name of the laboratory to facilitate timely delivery to the appropriate laboratory. Such packages should be shipped under the labeling for the most hazardous specimen category contained in the outer container.

## Secondary packaging

Place the absorbent material between the primary receptacle(s) and the secondary packaging. Use enough absorbent material to absorb the entire contents of all primary containers in case of leakage from or damage to the primary specimen containers. Secondary packaging must be watertight (liquids) or sift-proof (solids). Follow the instructions included with the secondary packaging material by the packaging manufacturer or other authorized party's packing.

## Outer Packaging

Use Styrofoam™-insulated corrugated fiberboard boxes (may be available from your transfusion service or send-outs department). The outer packaging must be large enough for all markings, labels, and shipping documents (e.g., airway bill and shipper's declaration for dangerous goods) and must be at least 100 mm (4 inches) in the smallest overall external dimension.

Note also that there are restrictions on the volume of material that may be contained in the outer containers. Containers with Category A substances may not exceed 50 mL or 50 g when shipped by passenger aircraft or rail, and 4 L or 4 kg when shipped by cargo aircraft; containers with Category B substances cannot contain more than 4 L or 4 kg when shipped either by passenger or cargo aircraft or rail.

Both dry ice and wet ice must be placed outside the secondary packaging. Specimens packaged in dry ice must permit the release of carbon dioxide gas and not allow a build-up of pressure that could rupture the packaging. Cold packs must be leak-proof.

For refrigerated shipments (4 °C), place absorbent material in the bottom of the outer packaging. Add a layer of frozen cold packs on the absorbent material. Place the secondary packages containing the specimen containers (e.g., blood tubes) on top of the cold packs. Place additional cold packs or absorbent material between the secondary packages to reduce their movement within the outer packaging. Place a layer of frozen cold packs on top of the secondary packages. Place additional absorbent material around and on top of the frozen cold packs to fill any remaining space and prevent movement of the contents in the outer package. Secure the outer packaging tops and bottoms with filamented shipping/strapping tape.

For frozen (dry ice) shipments, place absorbent material in the bottom of the outer packaging. Add a layer of dry ice. Do not use large chunks of dry ice because these may shatter the primary specimen containers during transport. (To break dry ice into small pieces, wrap the large chunks of dry ice in a towel to contain the pieces, and use a hammer or other heavy object to break the dry ice into smaller chunks one to two inches in diameter). Place the secondary packages containing the specimen containers (e.g., urine containers) on top of the cold packs. Place additional dry ice or absorbent material between the secondary containers to reduce their movement within the outer packaging. Place a layer of dry ice on top of the secondary packages. Place additional absorbent material around and on top of the frozen cold packs to fill any remaining space and prevent movement of the contents in the outer package. Secure the outer packaging tops and bottoms with filamentous shipping/strapping tape. Label the top of each box with identifying information (e.g., study number), and "Box 1 of 3" (etc.) if multiple packages are being shipped as part of a single investigation.

## Preparing Documentation

Since packages of primary specimens (e.g., blood tubes and urine cups) are shipped separately, prepare a separate shipping manifest for each shipment or

**separate secondary package in each shipment.** Place each shipping manifest (with specimen identification numbers) in a plastic zippered bag on top of the specimens before closing the Styrofoam™ lid of the corrugated fiberboard box. If multiple secondary packages—either of different types of tubes or of specimens for different laboratories—are shipped in the same outer container, prepare a shipping manifest (with specimen identification numbers) for each secondary package in a separate plastic zippered bag clearly labeled with either the tube type or laboratory name and place on top of the absorbent material before closing the outer package container.

## Chain of Custody

**Chain of custody forms may be required for some shipments. Chain of custody forms *do not* need to be transported with specimens**. Each entity/organization handling the specimens is responsible for the specimens only during the time that they have control of the specimens. Each entity/organization receiving the specimens must sign off on the chain of custody form of the entity/organization relinquishing the specimens to close that chain. When receiving specimens, each new entity/organization must begin their own chain of custody and have the entity/organization relinquishing the specimens sign their chain of custody to start the chain and indicate that they have transferred the specimens. **When specimens are transferred between entities/organizations, each entity/organization retains its own chain of custody forms**.

    **Note:** When the individual relinquishing the specimens (relinquisher) and the individual receiving the specimens (receiver) are not together at the time of specimen transfer, the relinquisher will document on their chain of custody that the receiver is [FedEx Tracking Number] or have the individual transporting the specimens sign the chain of custody to indicate that they have taken control of the specimens. Likewise, when the receiver receives the specimens, they will document on their chain of custody that the relinquisher is [FedEx Tracking Number] or the have the individual transporting the specimens sign the chain of custody.

## Labeling and Documentation for Shipment

Instructions for labeling and documentation of infectious substances shipments meeting Category A specifications may be found at: http://www.asm.org/Policy/index.asp?bid=6342 (Download Revised Packing and Shipping Guideline [Packing&Shipping11–18–05.pdf]). Instructions for the placement of labels for the shipment of Category A specimens are illustrated in

Packing&Shipping11–18–05.pdf, Figure 12. Packages containing Category A specimens must conform to the following requirements:

- The address label should include the complete name of person, complete name of facility, shipping address (street address), and telephone number (no toll-free numbers) of both shipper and consignee.
- The name and telephone number of the person responsible for the shipment must be on the package. The person responsible for shipment must know the contents of the shipment and the emergency response procedures. A 24-hour emergency contact telephone number must be included.
- All hazardous markings and labels must be on the same side of the box, adjacent to the address label so that they can be seen at the same time.
- Labels must include an Infectious Substances label, the proper shipping name (Infectious Substance, affecting humans, UN2814; Infectious Substance, affecting animals, UN2900), and the UN specification package certification mark, e.g., UN 4G/CLASS 6.2/99/GB/2450
- If the package contains dry ice, a UN1845 label and a label indicating how much dry ice (weight) is in the package must be placed on the package.
- "Orientation arrows" indicating which side is up must be placed on opposite sides of the package.
- Include two (three for Federal Express) copies of the completed Shipper's Declaration for Dangerous Goods. You must use the original form with red and white striped border; copies are not acceptable. An example of the Shipper's Declaration for Dangerous Goods form and instructions for completing the form may be found at: http://www.asm.org/Policy/index. asp?bid=6342 (Download Revised Packing and Shipping Guideline [Packing&Shipping11–18–05.pdf])
- Transport Details box: if your package contains less than 50 mL or 50 g, mark through the box containing the words "cargo aircraft only." If your package contains more than 50 mL or 50 g, mark through the box containing the words "passenger and cargo aircraft."
- Nature and Quantity of Dangerous Goods box: The comma after the word *substance*, as in "Infectious Substance, affecting humans, UN2814," is required; note the spelling of *fibreboard*; the genus/species or technical name must be in parentheses. For unidentified infectious substances, use 'suspected Category A infectious substance" for the technical name. Also, use this for the technical name on the itemized list of contents.
- The shipper's Declaration for Dangerous Goods is a legal document—*You must sign the form.*

- Telephone DLS (call 770–488–4305 or 770–488–7950; fax 770–488–4609) or the appropriate CCID laboratory to alert them how specimens are being sent and when and where they will arrive. This is especially important if it is unavoidable that the specimens will be delivered on weekends or holidays.

Guidelines for labeling of shipments of Category B substances may be found at: http://www.asm.org/Policy/index.asp?bid=6342 (Download Revised Packing and Shipping Guideline [Packing&Shipping11–18–05.pdf; Figure 11]). Packages containing Category B specimens must conform to the following requirements:

- Place labels with the addresses of the shipper and the consignee in the upper left-hand corner of the package.
- Place a UN3373 diamond marking on the outer package.
- Place the proper shipping name, "Biological substances, Category B" on the outer packaging below the UN3373 marking.
- For packages containing dry ice, place a Class 9 Hazard label on the same side of the outer packaging as the UN3373 marking. If the proper shipping name, either "dry ice" or "carbon dioxide solid," and "UN1845" is not preprinted on the hazard label, add it adjacent to the label. Note the weight of dry ice in the packaging on the preprinted area of the hazard label or place that information adjacent to the Class 9 Hazard label and proper shipping name.
- Orientation arrows are not required on an outer packaging containing Category B infectious substances. If orientation arrows are present, be sure to orient the inner packaging with their closures in the proper orientation with the arrows.
- The name, address, and telephone number of a person knowledgeable about the shipment must be provided on a written document accompanying the shipment, or on the package itself.
- If the package will be transported by a commercial air carrier, complete an airway bill. On the airway bill, note the proper shipping name and UN number for each hazardous material, and identify a person responsible for the package per IATA packing instruction 650.

## Shipping Specimens

*Follow the guidance provided in your state's chemical terrorism comprehensive response plan. If you are directed to ship the specimens to CCEHIP at CDC, please ship the specimens to the following address:*

CDC Division of Laboratory Sciences
Attn: Specimen Coordinator

4770 Buford Hwy.
Building 110 Loading Dock
Atlanta, GA 30341–3724
(770) 488–4305
*Specimens to be shipped to CCID laboratories for the investigation of infectious disease agents should be shipped to:*

CENTERS FOR DISEASE CONTROL AND PREVENTION

STAT
Attn: (Unit #/disease agent)
1600 Clifton Road, N.E.
Atlanta, GA 30333
(404) 639–3931

## Questions

If you have any questions or problems with specimen packaging or shipment, please e-mail or call one of the following contacts at the CDC's Division of Laboratory Sciences (DLS), National Center for Environmental Health, CCEHIP:

- Dr. John Osterloh, DLS Chief Medical Officer, 770–488–7367
- Dr. Jerry Thomas, ERAT Medical Officer, 770–488–7279
- DLS administrative office, 770–488–7950

Consultations for packaging, marking, and labeling specimens for shipment to CCID laboratories CDC may also be obtained from:

Packing, Marking, Labeling Consultation
CDC Shipping Activity
Yvonne Stifel: 404–639–3355

## APPENDIX 24–3: ABBREVIATIONS

| | |
|---|---|
| APHL | Association of Public Health Laboratories |
| CCID | Coordinating Center for Infectious Diseases |
| CDC | Centers for Disease Control and Prevention |
| CF | Complement fixation |
| CFR | Code of Federal Regulations |
| CMV | Cytomegalovirus |
| CSF | Cerebrospinal fluid |
| CTF | Colorado tick fever |

| | |
|---|---|
| DEOC | [CDC] Director's Emergency Operations Center |
| DFA | Direct fluorescent antibody test |
| DFA-TP | Direct fluorescent antibody test for *T. pallidum* |
| DHL | DHL International GmbH |
| DLS | Division of Laboratory Sciences |
| DNA | Deoxyribonucleic acid |
| DPDx | Website: Laboratory identification of parasites of public health concern |
| EDTA | Ethylenediaminetetraacetic acid |
| EIA | Enzyme immunoassay |
| ELISA | Enzyme-linked immunosorbent assay |
| ERAT | Emergency Response and Air Toxicants Branch |
| FA | Fluorescent antibody test (direct or indirect) |
| FTA-ABS | Fluorescent treponemal antibody-absorption |
| H&E | Hematoxylin and eosin stain |
| HI | Hemagglutination inhibition |
| HUS | Hemolytic uremic syndrome |
| ICT | Immunochromatographic test |
| ID | Immunodiffusion |
| IEP | Immune electrophoresis |
| IFA | Indirect fluorescent antibody test |
| IgG | Immunoglobulin G |
| IgM | Immunoglobulin M |
| IIF | Indirect immune fluorescence |
| LA | Latex agglutination |
| LGV | *Lymphogranuloma venereum* |
| LIMS | Laboratory information management system |
| LPS | Lipopolysaccharide |
| LRN | Laboratory Response Network |
| MAT | Microscopic agglutination |
| MIA | Microsphere immunoassay |
| MIF | Microimmunofluorescence test |
| MSM | Men who have sex with men |
| NAAT | Nucleic acid amplification test |
| CCEHIP | National Center for Environmental Health |
| NT | Neutralization test |
| PAH | Polyaromatic hydrocarbons |
| PCB | Polychlorinated bisphenol compounds |
| PCR | Polymerase chain reaction |
| PFGE | Pulsed field gel electrophoresis |
| PVA | Polyvinyl alcohol |

| RAMP | Rapid analyte measurement platform |
| Resp. | Respiratory |
| RFFIT | Rapid fluorescent focus inhibition test |
| RRAT | Rapid Response and Advanced Technology |
| RT-PCR | Reverse transcriptase-polymerase chain reaction |
| SBA | Sheep blood agar |
| TA | Tube agglutination |
| UN | United Nations |
| UPS | United Parcel Service |
| VDRL | Venereal disease research laboratory |
| VOC | Volatile organic compounds |
| WB | Western blot |

# APPENDIX A WALK-THROUGH EXERCISE: A FOOD-BORNE EPIDEMIC IN OSWEGO COUNTY, NEW YORK

Michael B. Gregg

Chapter 5 describes in some detail how to investigate an epidemic. Although not "chipped in stone," the steps described in that chapter lead you logically through a broad series of actions and thought processes that virtually every field epidemiologist will take during an investigation. However, the beginner, the neophyte epidemiologist, may need a more detailed explanation of what to do, when to do it, and how to think. In other words, a "walk-through" kind of exercise might be of use to some of the readers of this book—particularly those who are local food inspectors responsible for investigating sicknesses associated with social functions and food establishments. This Appendix attempts to do just that.

The following story is true, and, although old in time, it represents a typical outbreak and subsequent investigation still performed by many local and state health departments to this day. Designed as the first exercise for introductory courses in epidemiology, the "Oswego problem," as it is known, has probably taught more budding epidemiologists than any other exercise of its kind in existence. It has been translated into many languages, is still used at CDC, and has weathered well the test of time as a true "classic."

Before we begin unraveling the story in Oswego County, New York, let us review the critical steps in a field investigation referred to in Chapter 5.

- Establish the existence of the epidemic
- Verify the diagnosis
- Define a case and count cases
- Describe the epidemic in terms of time, place, and person
- Determine who is at risk
- Develop a hypothesis
- Test the hypothesis
- Compare the hypothesis with the established facts
- Plan a more systematic study
- Prepare a written report
- Execute control and prevention measures

For our purposes here, we concentrate on all the steps that you will actually perform while you are in the field; therefore, we omit the steps of planning a study and writing a report.

Recall several important things:

- The order you do these steps will vary from epidemic to epidemic depending on many factors. You actually may do several steps at the same time. However different the circumstances may be, you will ultimately do them all to a greater or lesser degree.
- In this particular "walk-through" exercise, Dr. Rubin, the investigator in Oswego, was given, right at the beginning, some preliminary time, place, and person information that he necessarily had to take at face value. He did not collect the data, but, then, he would not have responded to the outbreak unless he thought that there was some reasonable chance a problem existed. This is true for all field investigations. You usually will have received "tip-of-the-iceberg" data, preliminary assessments, even rumors that will soon need verification and amplification.
- Some investigators might find it useful to think along two lines of activity: operational and epidemiologic. *Operationally*, as you investigate the epidemic, think of where you are "on that list," where you have been, and where you will be going next. Take the time to orient yourself to the tasks accomplished and those ahead of you. There is nothing more useful than a framework or a defined context to help you plan and execute your work. So take a deep breath now and then! *Epidemiologically*, think of the need for and the value of the hard facts of time, place, and person and how you will build the strongest possible case for your analyses, interpretations, and conclusions. Be sure of your data, for you may be challenged. So consider where you want to "do battle": on the quality of the data or on their analysis and interpretation.

In this walk-through, we describe the events much as they are written in the Oswego exercise and taken from Dr. Rubin's report, which is found in the records of the New York State Department of Health (CDC, unpublished data). Some minor changes have been made to enhance the flow and logic of the exercise. Periodically, we take stock of where we are in the investigative process by asking questions, looking at what we *know* and what we can *infer* or what we think the information is suggesting. It is quite important to keep these two processes very separate in your mind.

## THE OUTBREAK

On April 19. 1940, the local health officer in Lycoming, Oswego County, New York, reported the occurrence of an outbreak of acute gastrointestinal (GI) illness to the District Health Officer in Syracuse. Dr. A. M. Rubin, epidemiologist-in-training, was assigned to conduct an investigation.

When Dr. Rubin arrived in the field that day he immediately went to the local health officer and was told that all per\sons known to be ill had attended a church supper on the previous evening and that most of them became ill the early morning of April 19. Eighty persons were known to have attended the supper and over 40 were ill. Family members who did not attend the supper did not become ill.

## Would You Call This an Epidemic? Would You Call It an Outbreak?

Both terms, *epidemic* and *outbreak*, are usually defined as the occurrence of more cases of illness in a place (or population) and time than is normally expected. Here, 40 or more cases of GI illness spanning a 24 hour period, seemingly among a social group, are clearly more than one would expect.

The words "epidemic" and "outbreak" are used interchangeably by many epidemiologists, although some consider the term "outbreak" to refer to a more localized situation, and "epidemic" to a more widespread—and perhaps prolonged—occurrence. Try not to use the word "epidemic" when you are in the field; it can be very frightening to some and real fodder for the press.

## What Do You Know Now?

- This is *an outbreak*, or epidemic, if you wish, because 40 plus cases of GI illness in such a short period of time is clearly unusual.
- *A probable time frame*: most identified illnesses occurred during one night.
- Most of the known ill had some kind of *GI illness*.
- The ill people *shared a common experience* the night before.

- GI illnesses, particularly those that start fairly soon after eating, often come from eating contaminated food.
- As of April 19, the day Dr. Rubin arrived, no family members who did not attend the supper had become ill.

## What Can You Realistically Infer from This Information So Far?

- The 40 or more cases were probably the majority of church supper–related cases, yet there certainly could have been other cases not yet reported or found.
- Since there were no known cases among family members, this suggests a noncommunicable illness. However, remember, Dr. Rubin arrived less than 24 hours after the outbreak—for many communicable diseases, too short a time for secondary cases to appear.
- So, with an acute GI disease affecting some people who shared a common meal, in the absence of known disease elsewhere in the community, the logical inference is that these people were exposed to something at the supper—probably something they ate.

## What Should You Do Now?

There are several possibilities, but, since your preliminary data suggest a possible food-borne epidemic, *one of the first things to do is to collect food, stool, and vomitus specimens*, if available, for laboratory testing. You do not know if these specimens will be needed, but time is critical in this kind of an outbreak, and it is better to have specimens you do not need than none at all, when you wish you had them.

Now, back to Oswego and the steps in the outline above: so far the facts and inferences strongly point to a food-borne outbreak among church members, but *you know very little about the disease* these people had, only that they had an acute GI problem. In no way have you made, much less confirmed, the diagnosis. And in order to develop a reasonable idea of what specific agent might have caused the epidemic, where it came from, and how it was transmitted—in short, its epidemiologic characteristics—you should try to get some idea of the clinical disease and what it resembles. If you are not clinically trained, you may very likely need a physician or health professional to help you in the differential diagnosis. But below is what Dr. Rubin reported:

According to Dr. Rubin the onset of illness in all cases was acute, characterized chiefly by nausea, vomiting, diarrhea, and abdominal pain. None of the ill persons reported having an elevated temperature; all recovered within 24 to 30 hours. Approximately 20% of the ill persons visited physicians. No fecal specimens were obtained for bacteriologic examination. (Whether Dr. Rubin actually saw some cases, we do not know. If you had been he, before investigating any further, it would have been a good idea to visit several cases or, at least, to talk to the physicians who saw some cases.)

## What Do You Know Now?

- Among those you know about, the illness was not severe or life threatening but very short-lived.
- The agent affected both the upper and lower GI tract without fever.
- The laboratory probably will not be of help; therefore you will have to rely heavily on the clinical picture and the epidemiologic findings for a presumptive diagnosis.

## What Can You Infer?

- That all the cases have been reported to Dr. Rubin. (If you had serious doubts, you would throw the net wide and find as many cases as possible.) (See Chapters 3 and 5.)
- That all cases are related in some way and that their illnesses are probably due to the same agent.
- That no one died or was hospitalized. This may or may not be true, because you do not know how the local health officer conducted case finding. However, for our purposes, you can assume these are all the cases.
- The agent caused illness within a few hours after exposure. In other words, the agent probably has a relatively short *incubation period*—the time from exposure to the time of onset of illness.

## What Should You Do Now?

This is where you will need someone clinically trained to help in the differential diagnosis. But before you look at the table below, there are a few things you should know that can be very useful. The major categories of agents that cause acute onset of GI diseases are:

- Infectious—caused by bacteria, viruses, or parasites
- Toxic/environmental—such as heavy metals, herbicides, household cleaning agents, or certain fish toxins
- Sociogenic—such as mass hysteria

When you try to "diagnose" an acute food poisoning outbreak, recall that nausea, vomiting, and diarrhea are normal body defense mechanisms designed to rid the body of harmful substances. So think of how and where in the GI tract the agent might affect the body. Ingestion of toxins predominantly affects the upper GI tract—the stomach, where their effect is usually within hours, causing nausea, vomiting, and, not infrequently, diarrhea. At the other extreme, bacteria, like salmonella and shigella, take more time—24 to 48 hours—to invade intestinal tissue (usually small and/or large bowel), to reproduce, and often to cause fever, cramps, diarrhea, and other symptoms. Fever is usually a sign that an agent or toxin has actually entered or invaded the body tissues—not just irritated the lining of the intestine. Many other agents exhibit considerable variations in their pathogenesis and presentation. Several of the more frequently encountered ones are listed in Table A–1.

## What Are Some Important Things You Have Learned from This Table?

- Many agents have fairly similar presentations.
- Toxins predominately affect the upper GI tract.
- Staphylococcus produces a toxin that can have a very short incubation period.
- Finally, more clinical details on those who ate at the supper would help in the diagnosis.

## What Should You Do Next?

With some general ideas about the time, place, and person of the epidemic; a good idea of who might be at risk; and a fairly reasonable hypothesis that the church supper could be responsible; you should get a list of the church supper participants, draw up a questionnaire, and ask the participants a series of questions primarily to focus on what unique exposures they may have had that made them ill. This is exactly what Dr. Rubin did.

## What Information Do You Want To Know?

Minimally, for this investigation you would like to know (see Chapters 11 and 12):

- Identifying information: name, address, phone number, and respondent (self, parent, spouse)
- Demographic information: birth date or age, gender

**Table A-I.** Some common and food-borne and water-borne agents that cause Acute Gastroenteritis

| AGENT | INCUBATION PERIOD | SYMPTOMS | PATHOPHYSIOLOGY | TYPICAL FOODS |
|---|---|---|---|---|
| Staphylococcus aureus | 2–4 hours | Sudden vomiting, cramps, diarrhea, no fever | Preformed enterotoxin | Ham, meats, custards, cream fillings |
| Clostridium perfringens | 6–24 hours, usually 10–12 hours | Abdominal pain, diarrhea. nausea, vomiting, fever usually absent | Enterotoxin formed in vivo | Meat, poultry |
| Salmonella (nontyphoid) | 6–48 hours | Diarrhea, fever, cramps | Intestinal invasion of bacteria | Poultry, eggs, meat |
| Shigella species | 2–4 days | Diarrhea, often bloody, cramps, little or no fever | Intestinal invasion of bacteria | Foods contaminated by food handler, usually not food-borne |
| E. Coli *Escherichia coli* (OI57:H7 and others) | 3–4 days | Diarrhea, abdominal cramps, little or no fever | Cytotoxin | Beef, raw milk, water |
| Norwalk-like viruses | 24–48 hours | Vomiting, cramps, headache, fever | Unknown | Raw or undercooked shellfish, sandwiches, salads, water |
| Heavy metals (antimony, cadmium, copper, lead, tin, zinc) | Usually less than 1 hour | Vomiting | Chemical irritation | Foods and beverages prepared/stored/ cooked in containers contaminated with offending metal. |

- Clinical information: signs/symptoms, severity, time of onset, and duration of illness
- Epidemiologic information:
  - Did you attend the supper?
  - Did you eat food at the supper?
  - When did you eat?
  - What did you eat and drink?

From Dr. Rubin's investigation we learn:

The supper was held in the basement of the village church. Foods were contributed by numerous members of the congregation. The supper began at 6:00 p.m. and continued until 11:00 p.m. Food was spread out on a table and consumed over a period of several hours. Data were collected regarding onset of illness and food eaten or water drunk by each of the 75 persons interviewed.

Dr. Rubin put his data into what is called a *line-listing*—a presentation or a spread sheet of results of the questionnaires displayed in considerable detail. A line-listing is a grid containing information about persons who are under study. Each row shows data on a single case. Each column represents a variable such as identifying information, clinical data, and epidemiologic information, such as risk and exposure factors. Such a list can be very useful, particularly at the beginning of an investigation, to help you view the entire database as time progresses, to fill in gaps of information, to share the results with others on your team, and simply to "eyeball" for obvious errors, outliers, and trends. Table A–2 is Dr. Rubin's line-listing.

## What Can You Glean from This Line-List?

Not a great deal; it is really a working document. Most of the ill attendees were adults, and many could not remember when they ate the meal; however, all remembered when they became ill, and all but two knew what they ate. This latter observation is truly remarkable. In many food-borne outbreaks there will almost always be persons who forget most or some of what they ate, particularly those who were not ill. Several things, however, may have come into play here: (*1*) the number of food items was small, making it easy to remember; (*2*) the questionnaire may not have had a space for the respondent to answer: "Don't know," thus forcing the respondent to give an answer, "yes" or "no"; (*3*) the outbreak was quite a vivid experience for everyone, thus sharpening their memory; and (*4*) since all the food was prepared by church members, they would have a better recollection of who prepared what foods and what they ate.

**Table A–2.** Line-listing from investigation of an outbreak of gastroenteritis, Oswego, New York, 1940

| ID | AGE | SEX | TIME OF MEAL | ILL | DATE OF ONSET | TIME OF ONSET | BAKED HAM | SPINACH | MASHED POTATOES | CABBAGE SALAD | JELLO | ROLLS | BROWN BREAD | MILK | COFFEE | WATER | CAKES | VAN. ICE CREAM | CHOC. ICE CREAM | FRUIT SALAD |
|----|-----|-----|--------------|-----|---------------|---------------|-----------|---------|------------------|----------------|-------|-------|-------------|------|--------|-------|-------|----------------|------------------|-------------|
| 1 | 11 | M | UNK | N | | | N | N | N | N | N | N | N | N | N | N | N | N | Y | N |
| 2 | 52 | F | 8:00 PM | Y | 4/19 | 12:30 AM | Y | Y | Y | N | N | Y | N | N | Y | N | N | Y | N | N |
| 3 | 65 | M | 6:30 PM | Y | 4/19 | 12:30 AM | Y | Y | Y | Y | N | N | N | N | Y | N | N | Y | Y | N |
| 4 | 59 | F | 6:30 PM | Y | 4/19 | 12:30 AM | Y | Y | N | N | Y | Y | N | N | Y | N | Y | Y | Y | N |
| 5 | 13 | F | UNK | N | | | N | N | N | N | N | N | N | N | N | N | N | N | Y | N |
| 6 | 63 | F | 7:30 PM | Y | 4/18 | 10:30 PM | Y | Y | N | Y | N | Y | N | N | N | Y | N | Y | N | N |
| 7 | 70 | M | 7:30 PM | Y | 4/18 | 10:30 PM | Y | Y | Y | Y | Y | N | Y | N | Y | Y | N | Y | N | N |
| 8 | 40 | F | 7:30 PM | Y | 4/19 | 2:00 AM | N | N | N | N | N | N | N | N | N | N | N | Y | Y | N |
| 9 | 15 | F | 10:00 PM | Y | 4/19 | 1:00 AM | N | N | Y | N | N | N | N | N | N | N | Y | N | Y | N |
| 10 | 33 | F | 7:00 PM | Y | 4/18 | 11:00 PM | Y | Y | Y | Y | Y | Y | N | N | N | N | N | Y | Y | Y |
| 11 | 65 | M | UNK | N | | | Y | Y | Y | Y | Y | N | N | N | N | Y | N | N | N | N |
| 12 | 38 | F | UNK | N | | | Y | Y | N | N | N | N | N | N | N | Y | N | N | N | N |
| 13 | 62 | F | UNK | N | | | Y | Y | N | N | N | N | Y | N | N | Y | N | N | N | N |
| 14 | 10 | M | 7:30 PM | Y | 4/19 | 2:00 AM | N | N | N | Y | N | N | N | N | N | N | N | Y | Y | N |
| 15 | 25 | M | UNK | N | | | Y | Y | Y | Y | Y | Y | Y | N | Y | Y | Y | Y | N | N |

| No. | Age | Sex | | | Date | Time | | | | | | | | | | | | | | |
|---|---|---|---|---|---|---|---|---|---|---|---|---|---|---|---|---|---|---|---|---|
| 16 | 32 | F | UNK | Y | 4/19 | 10:30 AM | Y | Y | N | Y | N | N | N | Y | N | N | Y | Y | Y | N |
| 17 | 62 | F | UNK | Y | 4/19 | 12:30 AM | N | N | N | N | N | N | N | N | N | N | N | N | Y | N |
| 18 | 36 | M | UNK | Y | 4/18 | 10:15 PM | Y | Y | N | Y | Y | N | N | N | N | Y | N | Y | N | N |
| 19 | 11 | M | UNK | N | | | Y | Y | ? | Y | Y | Y | N | Y | Y | Y | Y | N | N | N |
| 20 | 33 | F | UNK | Y | 4/18 | 10:00 PM | Y | Y | Y | Y | N | Y | N | Y | Y | N | Y | Y | Y | N |
| 21 | 13 | F | 10:00 PM | Y | 4/19 | 1:00 AM | N | N | N | N | N | N | N | N | N | N | N | N | N | N |
| 22 | 7 | M | UNK | Y | 4/18 | 11:00 PM | Y | Y | Y | Y | N | Y | N | Y | Y | Y | Y | Y | Y | N |
| 23 | 64 | M | UNK | N | | | N | N | N | N | N | N | N | N | N | N | N | N | N | N |
| 24 | 3 | M | UNK | Y | 4/18 | 9:45 PM | N | Y | Y | Y | N | Y | N | N: | N | N | Y | N | Y | N |
| 25 | 65 | F | UNK | N | | | Y | N | Y | N | Y | N | Y | Y | Y | Y | Y | Y | Y | N |
| 26 | 59 | F | UNK | Y | 4/18 | 9:45 PM | N | Y | Y | Y | N | Y | N | N | Y | N | Y | Y | Y | N |
| 27 | 15 | F | 10:00 PM | Y | 4/19 | 1:00 AM | N | N | N | N | N | N | N | N | N | N | N | N | N | N |
| 28 | 62 | M | UNK | N | | | Y | N | N | N | Y | N | Y | Y | Y | Y | Y | Y | Y | N |
| 29 | 37 | F | UNK | Y | 4/18 | 11:00 PM | Y | Y | Y | Y | N | Y | N | Y | Y | N | Y | Y | Y | N |
| 30 | 17 | M | 10:00 PM | N | | | N | N | N | N | N | N | N | N | N | N | N | N | N | N |
| 31 | 35 | M | UNK | Y | 4/18 | 9:00 PM | Y | Y | Y | Y | N | Y | Y | Y | Y | Y | Y | Y | Y | N |
| 32 | 15 | M | 10:00 PM | Y | 4/19 | 1:00 AM | N | N | N | N | N | N | N | N | N | N | N | N | N | N |
| 33 | 50 | F | 10:00 PM | Y | 4/19 | 1:00 AM | Y | N | N | N | N | N | N | Y | N | N | Y | N | N | N |
| 34 | 40 | M | UNK | N | | | Y | Y | N | Y | N | Y | Y | Y | Y | Y | Y | Y | Y | Y |
| 35 | 35 | F | UNK | N | | | Y | Y | Y | Y | Y | Y | Y | Y | N | Y | Y | N | N | N |

Continued

**Table A-2.** Line-listing from investigation of an outbreak of gastroenteritis, Oswego, New York, 1940—Continued

| ID | AGE | SEX | TIME OF MEAL | ILL | DATE OF ONSET | TIME OF ONSET | BAKED HAM | SPINACH | MASHED POTATOES | CABBAGE SALAD | JELLO | ROLLS | BROWN BREAD | MILK | COFFEE | WATER | CAKES | VAN. ICE CREAM | CHOC. ICE CREAM | FRUIT SALAD |
|----|-----|-----|------|-----|------|------|---|---|---|---|---|---|---|---|---|---|---|---|---|---|
| 36 | 35 | F | UNK | Y | 4/18 | 9:15 PM | Y | Y | Y | Y | N | Y | Y | N | Y | N | N | Y | N | N |
| 37 | 36 | M | UNK | N |  |  | Y | N | Y | Y | N | Y | Y | N | Y | N | N | N | Y | N |
| 38 | 57 | F | UNK | Y | 4/18 | 11:30 PM | Y | Y | N | Y | Y | Y | Y | N | Y | N | Y | Y | Y | N |
| 39 | 16 | F | 10:00 PM | Y | 4/19 | 1:00 AM | N | N | N | N | N | N | N | N | N | N | Y | N | Y | N |
| 40 | 68 | M | UNK | Y | 4/18 | 9:30 PM | Y | N | Y | Y | N | Y | Y | N | Y | N | Y | Y | Y | N |
| 41 | 54 | F | UNK | N |  |  | Y | Y | Y | Y | N | Y | N | N | N | N | N | N | N | Y |
| 42 | 77 | M | UNK | Y | 4/19 | 2:30 AM | N | N | N | N | Y | N | N | N | Y | N | Y | Y | Y | Y |
| 44 | 58 | M | UNK | Y | 4/18 | 9:30 PM | Y | Y | Y | N | N | Y | Y | N | Y | N | N | Y | N | N |
| 45 | 20 | M | 10:00 PM | N |  |  | N | N | N | N | N | N | N | N | N | Y | Y | Y | ? | N |
| 46 | 17 | M | UNK | N |  |  | Y | Y | Y | N | N | Y | N | N | N | Y | N | Y | Y | N |
| 47 | 62 | F | UNK | Y | 4/19 | 12:30 AM | Y | N | N | N | N | N | N | N | N | N | N | Y | Y | N |
| 48 | 20 | F | 7:00 PM | Y | 4/19 | 1:00 AM | N | N | N | N | N | N | N | N | Y | N | N | Y | N | N |
| 49 | 52 | F | UNK | Y | 4/18 | 10:30 PM | Y | Y | Y | Y | N | Y | N | N | N | Y | Y | N | N | N |
| 50 | 9 | F | UNK | N |  |  | N | N | N | Y | N | Y | N | Y | N | Y | Y | N | Y | N |
| 51 | 50 | M | UNK | N |  |  | Y | Y | Y | Y | N | Y | Y | Y | Y | Y | Y | N | Y | N |

| ID | Age | Sex | Onset Time | Y/N | Date | Time | | | | | | | | | | | | | | | | | | |
|---|---|---|---|---|---|---|---|---|---|---|---|---|---|---|---|---|---|---|---|---|---|---|---|---|
| 52 | 8 | M | 11:00 PM | Y | 4/18 | 3:00 PM | N | N | N | N | N | N | N | N | N | N | N | N | N | Y | Y | N |
| 53 | 35 | F | UNK | N | | | N | N | N | N | N | N | N | N | N | N | N | N | N | Y | Y | N |
| 54 | 48 | F | UNK | Y | 4/18 | 12:00 MN | Y | Y | Y | Y | Y | Y | Y | Y | Y | Y | Y | Y | Y | Y | Y | N |
| 55 | 25 | M | UNK | Y | 4/18 | 11:00 PM | Y | N | Y | Y | Y | Y | Y | Y | Y | Y | Y | Y | Y | Y | Y | N |
| 56 | 11 | F | UNK | N | | | N | N | N | N | N | N | N | N | N | N | N | N | N | N | N | N |
| 57 | 74 | M | UNK | Y | 4/18 | 10:30 PM | Y | Y | Y | Y | Y | Y | Y | Y | Y | Y | Y | Y | Y | Y | Y | N |
| 58 | 12 | F | 10:00 PM | Y | 4/19 | 1:00 AM | N | N | N | N | N | N | N | N | N | N | N | N | N | Y | Y | N |
| 59 | 44 | F | 7:30 PM | Y | 4/19 | 2:30 AM | Y | Y | Y | Y | Y | Y | Y | Y | Y | Y | Y | Y | Y | Y | Y | N |
| 60 | 53 | F | 7:30 PM | Y | 4/18 | 11:30 PM | Y | Y | Y | Y | Y | Y | Y | Y | Y | Y | Y | Y | Y | Y | Y | N |
| 61 | 37 | M | UNK | N | | | N | N | N | N | N | N | N | N | N | N | N | N | N | N | N | N |
| 62 | 24 | F | UNK | N | | | Y | Y | Y | Y | Y | Y | Y | Y | Y | Y | Y | Y | Y | Y | Y | N |
| 63 | 69 | F | UNK | N | | | N | N | N | N | N | N | N | N | N | N | N | N | N | N | N | N |
| 64 | 7 | M | UNK | N | | | Y | Y | Y | Y | Y | Y | Y | Y | Y | Y | Y | Y | Y | Y | Y | N |
| 65 | 17 | F | 10:00 PM | Y | 4/19 | 1:00 AM | N | N | Y | Y | Y | Y | Y | Y | Y | Y | Y | Y | Y | Y | Y | N |
| 66 | 8 | F | UNK | Y | 4/19 | 12:30 AM | Y | Y | Y | Y | Y | Y | Y | Y | Y | Y | Y | Y | Y | Y | Y | N |
| 67 | 11 | F | 7:30 PM | N | | | Y | Y | Y | Y | Y | Y | Y | Y | Y | Y | Y | Y | Y | Y | Y | N |
| 68 | 17 | M | 7:30 PM | N | | | N | N | Y | Y | Y | Y | Y | Y | Y | Y | Y | Y | Y | Y | Y | N |
| 69 | 36 | F | UNK | N | | | N | N | N | N | N | N | N | N | N | N | N | N | N | Y | Y | N |
| 70 | 21 | F | UNK | Y | 4/19 | 12:30 AM | N | N | Y | Y | Y | Y | Y | Y | Y | Y | Y | Y | Y | Y | N | N |
| 71 | 60 | M | 7:30 PM | Y | 4/19 | 1:00 AM | N | N | Y | Y | Y | Y | Y | Y | Y | Y | Y | Y | Y | N | N | N |

Continued

**Table A-2.**  Line-listing from investigation of an outbreak of gastroenteritis, Oswego, New York, 1940—Continued

| ID | AGE | SEX | TIME OF MEAL | ILL | DATE OF ONSET | TIME OF ONSET | BAKED HAM | SPINACH | MASHED POTATOES | CABBAGE SALAD | JELLO | ROLLS | BROWN BREAD | MILK | COFFEE | WATER | CAKES | VAN. ICE CREAM | CHOC. ICE CREAM | FRUIT SALAD |
|----|-----|-----|--------------|-----|---------------|---------------|-----------|---------|------------------|----------------|-------|-------|-------------|------|--------|-------|-------|----------------|-----------------|-------------|
| 72 | 18 | F | 7:30 PM | Y | 4/18 | 12:00 MN | Y | Y | Y | Y | Y | N | N | N | N | Y | Y | Y | Y | N |
| 73 | 14 | F | 10:00 PM | N | | | N | N | N | N | N | N | N | N | N | N | Y | Y | N | N |
| 74 | 52 | M | UNK | Y | 4/19 | 2:15 AM | Y | N | Y | Y | Y | Y | Y | N | Y | Y | Y | Y | Y | N |
| 75 | 45 | F | UNK | Y | 4/18 | 11:00 PM | Y | Y | Y | Y | Y | Y | Y | N | Y | N | Y | Y | N | Y |

## What Should You Do Next?

Now you have the necessary information to describe the epidemic in terms of time, place, and person—the essentials for developing hypotheses of why the epidemic occurred, who was at risk, and what was the definitive exposure. As was described in Chapters 5 and 6, one of the most useful ways to depict the *time aspect* of an epidemic is to draw an *epidemic curve*. By plotting cases of illness on the vertical (*y*) axis and a suitable time frame on the horizontal (*x*) axis you create a graph that gives you an idea of the size of the epidemic, its relation to endemic cases, its time course, its pattern of spread, and where you are in the course of the epidemic—the upslope or the downslope of the curve. Figure A–1 shows the epidemic curve for the Oswego outbreak.

## What Can You Learn from This Graph?

- Most cases form a tight cluster within a 6-hour interval, suggesting a single common exposure.
- There are two "outliers"—one very early and one late in the epidemic. Either one or both could represent background or endemic cases not related to the epidemic at all; or the early case could be the "source" of the epidemic; the late case could be a secondary case.
- You will want to investigate these cases later, but there are still much more important things to do.

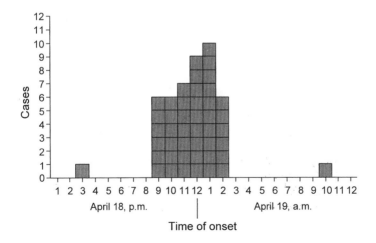

**Figure A–1.** Cases of gastrointestinal illness by time of onset of symptoms, Oswego County, New York, April 18–19, 1940. (CDC, Unpublished data).

Another aspect of *time* focuses on when the ill persons became sick in relation to when they ate or were exposed: the incubation period. Virtually all infectious diseases and many toxins have known or estimated incubation periods—a characteristic that can help you identify what agent caused the disease.

Dr. Rubin's questionnaire provides the data needed to determine the incubation periods of those ill persons (only 22 of the 46 ill persons) who remembered when they ate and when they became ill. See Figure A–2.

## What Can You Learn from Figure A-2?

- It is hard to generalize with such small numbers, but it looks as though there are two clusters of occurrence in time, one at 3 hours and one at about 6 to 6½ hours. Overall the median incubation period is 4 hours.

- Interestingly, the incubation period was shorter for those who ate later in the evening than those who ate earlier in the evening. This difference could be explained by a continuing production of enterotoxin by staphylococci in a food. It could also be explained by the fact that younger people ate later and perhaps ate more than the older folks who ate earlier. (This is an excellent example of a simple, creative analysis of basic demographic and epidemiologic data that can uncover fascinating and sometimes important aspects of a very common type of outbreak.)

- But most important, an incubation period of 4 hours fits well with incubation periods of agents such as staphylococcus, some fish toxins, and *Bacillus cereus*. Fish toxins can be ruled out, because fish was not served; *B. cereus* seems unlikely, because the foods usually associated with it (rice, custards, cereals) were not served either. So staphylococcal toxin seems

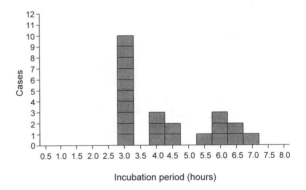

**Figure A–2.** Cases of gastrointestinal illness by incubation period in hours, Oswego County, New York, April 18–19, 1940. (CDC, Unpublished data).

the most likely agent, although it would be helpful to have more detailed clinical information.

Next, you will want to orient the data in terms of *place*. According to Dr. Rubin's report, all 75 respondents to the questionnaire ate at the supper, which strongly suggests the risk and exposure occurred there. However, you should view the two outliers, patient No. 16 and patient No. 52, with some skepticism simply because their onsets are so different from the rest.

In terms of *person* characteristics, the age and gender profiles appear normal, though age- and gender-specific attack rates might be revealing. But at this time in the investigation your attention should be focused on food exposures among the attendees.

So, with all the evidence at hand, what is your hypothesis as to what happened? Initially, always think in terms of single factors causing outbreaks: in this instance, one agent, one contaminated food, and one specific population at risk. Avoid muddying the waters with multifactorial hypotheses. In the great majority of instances you will be dealing with one agent, one specific exposure, and one well-defined group of people.

To put it in more epidemiologic terms: what do you think was the critical exposure that caused illness? Your hypothesis would be: "I think a single food or drink was contaminated with some agent, probably staphylococcal enterotoxin, that caused the illness in those who attended and ate at the church supper." In this context the word *exposure* means a food or drink eaten at the supper.

## What Next?

You now should extract from the questionnaire data that will identify which possible exposures (foods, drinks) the persons might have had at the supper that made them ill. In other words, you will need to study and analyze these data in such a way as to be able to test and verify your hypothesis.

## How Will the Information on the Questionnaire Help Test Your Hypothesis?

Your initial reflex might be to choose one of two approaches in hopes of finding out what item caused the outbreak. To do these analyses more easily, however, you might first want to separate the supper participants into two groups: the ill and the well. Table A–3 shows a new line-listing with such a breakdown.

- *Approach 1*: Look at the food and drink list and see which one(s) were associated with the most number of ill persons. If one item was associated

**Table A–3.** Line-listing from an investigation of an outbreak of gastroenteritis, Oswego, New York, 1940

| ID | AGE | SEX | TIME OF MEAL | ILL | DATE OF ONSET | TIME OF ONSET | BAKED HAM | SPINACH | MASHED POTATOES | CABBAGE SALAD | JELLO | ROLLS | BROWN BREAD | MILK | COFFEE | WATER | CAKES | VAN. ICE CREAM | CHOC. ICE CREAM | FRUIT SALAD |
|----|-----|-----|--------------|-----|---------------|---------------|-----------|---------|-----------------|---------------|-------|-------|-------------|------|--------|-------|-------|----------------|-----------------|-------------|
| 52 | 8  | M | 11:00 PM | Y | 4/18 | 3:00 PM  | N | N | N | N | N | N | N | N | N | N | N | Y | Y | N |
| 31 | 35 | M | UNK     | Y | 4/18 | 9:00 PM  | Y | Y | Y | N | Y | Y | Y | N | Y | N | Y | Y | N | Y |
| 36 | 35 | F | UNK     | Y | 4/18 | 9:15 PM  | Y | Y | Y | Y | N | Y | Y | N | Y | N | N | Y | N | N |
| 40 | 68 | M | UNK     | Y | 4/18 | 9:30 PM  | Y | N | Y | Y | N | N | Y | N | Y | N | N | Y | N | N |
| 44 | 58 | M | UNK     | Y | 4/18 | 9:30 PM  | Y | Y | Y | N | N | Y | Y | N | Y | N | N | Y | ? | Y |
| 24 | 3  | M | UNK     | Y | 4/18 | 9:45 PM  | N | Y | Y | N | N | Y | N | N | N | Y | Y | Y | N | N |
| 26 | 59 | F | UNK     | Y | 4/18 | 9:45 PM  | N | Y | Y | Y | Y | Y | Y | N | N | Y | Y | Y | N | N |
| 20 | 33 | F | UNK     | Y | 4/18 | 10:00 PM | Y | Y | N | Y | N | N | N | N | N | N | Y | Y | Y | N |
| 18 | 36 | M | UNK     | Y | 4/18 | 10:15 PM | Y | Y | N | Y | Y | Y | Y | N | N | Y | N | Y | N | N |
| 6  | 63 | F | 7:30 PM | Y | 4/18 | 10:30 PM | Y | Y | Y | N | Y | N | N | N | Y | Y | N | Y | N | N |
| 7  | 70 | M | 7:30 PM | Y | 4/18 | 10:30 PM | Y | Y | Y | Y | Y | Y | Y | N | Y | N | N | Y | N | N |
| 49 | 52 | F | UNK     | Y | 4/18 | 10:30 PM | Y | Y | Y | Y | N | Y | N | N | Y | N | N | Y | Y | N |

| | | | | | | | | | | | | | | | | | | | | | |
|---|---|---|---|---|---|---|---|---|---|---|---|---|---|---|---|---|---|---|---|---|---|
| 57 | 74 | M | UNK | Y | 4/18 | 10:30 PM | N | N | Y | Y | N | Y | N | Y | Y | Y | Y | Y | N | N |
| 10 | 33 | F | 7:00 PM | Y | 4/18 | 11:00 PM | N | Y | Y | N | Y | N | N | Y | Y | N | Y | Y | Y | N |
| 22 | 7 | M | UNK | Y | 4/18 | 11:00 PM | N | Y | Y | Y | Y | N | N | Y | Y | Y | Y | Y | Y | N |
| 29 | 37 | F | UNK | Y | 4/18 | 11:00 PM | N | N | Y | Y | N | Y | N | Y | Y | N | Y | Y | N | N |
| 55 | 25 | M | UNK | Y | 4/18 | 11:00 PM | N | Y | Y | Y | Y | N | N | Y | Y | N | N | Y | Y | N |
| 75 | 45 | F | UNK | Y | 4/18 | 11:00 PM | Y | N | Y | Y | N | Y | N | Y | Y | Y | Y | Y | N | Y |
| 38 | 57 | F | UNK | Y | 4/18 | 11:30 PM | N | Y | Y | Y | Y | Y | N | N | Y | Y | Y | Y | Y | N |
| 60 | 53 | F | 7:30 PM | Y | 4/18 | 11:30 PM | N | Y | Y | Y | Y | Y | Y | Y | N | Y | Y | Y | Y | N |
| 72 | 18 | F | 7:30 PM | Y | 4/18 | 12:00 MN | N | Y | Y | Y | N | N | N | Y | Y | N | Y | Y | Y | N |
| 54 | 48 | F | UNK | Y | 4/18 | 12:00 MN | N | Y | Y | N | Y | Y | N | N | Y | Y | Y | Y | Y | N |
| 2 | 52 | F | 8:00 PM | Y | 4/19 | 12:30 AM | N | N | Y | N | N | N | N | N | N | Y | Y | Y | N | N |
| 3 | 65 | M | 6:30 PM | Y | 4/19 | 12:30 AM | N | Y | Y | Y | Y | Y | N | N | Y | Y | Y | Y | Y | N |
| 4 | 59 | F | 6:30 PM | Y | 4/19 | 12:30 AM | N | Y | Y | N | N | N | N | N | N | N | Y | Y | Y | N |
| 17 | 62 | F | UNK | Y | 4/19 | 12:30 AM | N | N | Y | N | N | N | N | N | N | Y | N | Y | N | N |
| 47 | 62 | F | UNK | Y | 4/19 | 12:30 AM | N | Y | Y | Y | N | N | N | N | N | N | Y | Y | Y | N |
| 66 | 8 | F | UNK | Y | 4/19 | 12:30 AM | N | Y | Y | N | N | N | N | N | N | N | N | Y | N | N |
| 70 | 21 | F | UNK | Y | 4/19 | 12:30 AM | N | N | Y | Y | Y | Y | N | Y | Y | Y | N | Y | Y | N |
| 71 | 60 | M | 7:30 PM | Y | 4/19 | 1:00 AM | N | Y | Y | Y | N | N | N | N | N | N | N | Y | N | N |
| 21 | 13 | F | 10:00 PM | Y | 4/19 | 1:00 AM | N | N | Y | N | N | N | N | N | N | N | N | Y | N | N |
| 27 | 15 | F | 10:00 PM | Y | 4/19 | 1:00 AM | N | Y | Y | Y | N | N | N | N | N | N | N | Y | Y | Y |

*Continued*

**Table A-3.**  Line-listing from an investigation of an outbreak of gastroenteritis, Oswego, New York, 1940—Continued

| ID | AGE | SEX | TIME OF MEAL | ILL | DATE OF ONSET | TIME OF ONSET | BAKED HAM | SPINACH | MASHED POTATOES | CABBAGE SALAD | JELLO | ROLLS | BROWN BREAD | MILK | COFFE | WATER | CAKES | VAN. ICE CREAM | CHOC. ICE CREAM | FRUIT SALAD |
|----|-----|-----|--------------|-----|---------------|---------------|-----------|---------|-----------------|---------------|-------|-------|-------------|------|-------|-------|-------|----------------|-----------------|-------------|
| 32 | 15 | M | 10:00 PM | Y | 4/19 | 1:00 AM | N | N | N | N | N | N | N | N | N | N | Y | Y | N | N |
| 33 | 50 | F | 10:00 PM | Y | 4/19 | 1:00 AM | N | N | N | N | N | N | N | N | N | N | N | Y | N | N |
| 39 | 16 | F | 10:00 PM | Y | 4/19 | 1:00 AM | N | N | N | N | N | N | N | N | N | N | Y | N | Y | N |
| 9 | 15 | F | 10:00 PM | Y | 4/19 | 1:00 AM | N | N | N | N | N | N | N | N | N | N | Y | N | Y | N |
| 48 | 20 | F | 7:00 PM | Y | 4/19 | 1:00 AM | N | N | N | N | N | N | N | N | N | N | N | Y | N | N |
| 58 | 12 | F | 10:00 PM | Y | 4/19 | 1:00 AM | N | N | N | N | N | N | N | N | N | N | Y | Y | Y | N |
| 65 | 17 | F | 10:00 PM | Y | 4/19 | 1:00 AM | N | N | N | N | N | N | N | N | N | N | Y | Y | Y | N |
| 8 | 40 | F | 7:30 PM | Y | 4/19 | 2:00 AM | N | N | N | N | N | N | N | N | N | N | N | Y | Y | N |
| 14 | 10 | M | 7:30 PM | Y | 4/19 | 2:00 AM | N | N | N | N | N | N | N | N | N | N | N | Y | Y | N |
| 43 | 72 | F | UNK | Y | 4/19V | 2:00 AM | Y | Y | Y | Y | Y | Y | Y | N | Y | Y | Y | Y | Y | N |
| 74 | 52 | M | UNK | Y | 4/19 | 2:15 AM | Y | N | Y | N | Y | Y | Y | N | Y | Y | Y | N | Y | N |
| 59 | 44 | F | 7:30 PM | Y | 4/19 | 2:30 AM | Y | Y | N | N | N | Y | N | N | N | N | Y | Y | Y | N |
| 16 | 32 | F | UNK | Y | 4/19 | 10:30 AM | Y | Y | N | N | N | N | N | N | Y | N | Y | N | Y | N |
| 1 | 11 | M | UNK | N |  |  |  | N | N | N | N | N | N | N | N | N | N | N | Y | N |

| | | | | | | | | | | | | | | | | | | |
|---|---|---|---|---|---|---|---|---|---|---|---|---|---|---|---|---|---|---|
| 5 | 13 | F | UNX | N | | N | N | N | N | N | N | N | N | N | N | N | N | N |
| 11 | 65 | M | UNK | N | | Y | Y | Y | Y | Y | Y | N | Y | N | Y | Y | Y | Y |
| 12 | 38 | F | UNK | N | | Y | Y | Y | Y | Y | Y | Y | Y | Y | Y | Y | N | N |
| 13 | 62 | F | UNK | N | | Y | Y | N | Y | Y | Y | Y | Y | Y | Y | Y | Y | Y |
| 15 | 25 | M | UNK | N | | Y | Y | N | Y | Y | Y | Y | Y | Y | Y | Y | N | Y |
| 19 | 11 | M | UNK | N | | Y | Y | Y | Y | Y | Y | ? | Y | Y | Y | Y | Y | N |
| 23 | 64 | M | UNK | N | | N | N | N | N | N | N | N | N | N | N | Y | N | N |
| 25 | 65 | F | UNK | N | | Y | Y | Y | Y | Y | Y | Y | Y | Y | Y | Y | N | Y |
| 28 | 62 | M | UNK | N | | Y | Y | Y | Y | Y | Y | Y | Y | Y | Y | Y | N | Y |
| 30 | 17 | M | 10:00 PM | N | | N | N | N | N | N | N | N | N | N | N | Y | N | N |
| 34 | 40 | M | UNK | N | | Y | Y | Y | Y | Y | Y | Y | Y | Y | Y | Y | N | Y |
| 35 | 35 | F | UNK | N | | Y | N | Y | Y | Y | Y | Y | Y | Y | Y | Y | N | Y |
| 37 | 36 | M | UNK | N | | Y | Y | Y | Y | Y | Y | Y | Y | Y | Y | Y | N | N |
| 41 | 54 | F | UNK | N | | Y | N | Y | Y | Y | Y | Y | Y | Y | Y | Y | Y | Y |
| 45 | 20 | M | 10:00 PM | N | | N | N | N | N | N | N | N | N | N | N | Y | N | N |
| 46 | 17 | M | UNK | N | | Y | Y | Y | Y | Y | Y | Y | Y | Y | Y | Y | N | N |
| 50 | 9 | F | UNK | N | | N | N | N | N | N | N | N | N | N | N | Y | N | N |
| 51 | 50 | M | UNK | N | | Y | Y | Y | Y | Y | Y | Y | Y | Y | Y | Y | N | Y |

Continued

**Table A-3.** Line-listing from an investigation of an outbreak of gastroenteritis, Oswego, New York, 1940—Continued

| ID | AGE | SEX | TIME OF MEAL | ILL | DATE OF ONSET | TIME OF ONSET | BAKED HAM | SPINACH | MASHED POTATOES | CABBAGE SALAD | JELLO | ROLLS | BROWN BREAD | MILK | COFFE | WATER | CAKES | VAN. ICE CREAM | CHOC. ICE CREAM | FRUIT SALAD |
|---|---|---|---|---|---|---|---|---|---|---|---|---|---|---|---|---|---|---|---|---|
| 53 | 35 | F | UNK | N | | | N | N | N | N | N | N | N | N | N | N | N | Y | Y | N |
| 56 | 11 | F | UNK | N | | | N | N | N | N | N | N | N | N | N | N | N | N | Y | N |
| 61 | 37 | M | UNK | N | | | N | N | N | N | N | N | N | N | N | N | N | N | Y | N |
| 62 | 24 | F | UWK | N | | | Y | Y | Y | N | N | Y | N | N | Y | N | N | N | N | N |
| 63 | 69 | F | UNK | N | | | N | Y | Y | Y | Y | N | Y | N | N | Y | Y | N | Y | N |
| 64 | 7 | M | UNK | N | | | Y | Y | Y | Y | Y | Y | N | N | N | Y | Y | N | Y | N |
| 67 | 11 | F | 7:30 PM | N | | | Y | Y | Y | Y | N | Y | N | N | Y | Y | N | N | Y | N |
| 68 | 17 | M | 7:30 PM | N | | | Y | Y | Y | Y | N | Y | N | N | Y | N | Y | Y | N | N |
| 69 | 36 | F | UNK | N | | | N | N | N | N | N | N | N | N | N | N | N | N | Y | N |
| 73 | 14 | F | 10:00 PM | N | | | N | N | N | N | N | N | N | N | N | N | Y | Y | N | N |

with more sick people than another item, then that might incriminate that item.

- *Approach 2*: Look at all the ill persons and see what they ate. Again, using similar logic as above, if more ill people ate a particular item more than other items, that might identify the contaminated food or drink.

## Problems with Approaches 1 and 2

### Approach 1

Simply because one food is associated with more illness than another food does not establish that one food is more likely to cause illness than another. Among the 46 who ate ham, 29 were ill; among the 54 who ate vanilla ice cream, 43 became ill; and 16 of 23 who ate Jell-o developed GI illness. What do these numbers really mean? How can you reconcile the fact that some persons became ill when they ate one food, but they also ate other foods too, and they became ill after eating them? Persuasive or not as the case may be, these numbers alone cannot validly explain or identify a contaminated food.

### Approach 2

If you now look only at the ill persons, you will see that 29 ate the ham, 26 had spinach, and 45 had vanilla ice cream. These were quite popular foods. But do these numbers alone help you find out what item might have caused the outbreak? It is pretty clear that they do not. All the numbers tell you is what were the most popular or most frequently consumed items eaten by the ill persons. In no way can you validly implicate ham more than spinach just because more ill people ate ham than spinach. Moreover, what about those ill people who ate rolls or mashed potato? How do you explain them? In sum, there really is no logical or scientific way to incriminate a specific food or drink by this analysis either.

## THE SOLUTION TO APPROACHES 1 AND 2—THE CRITICAL ANALYSIS

You have now arrived at the most critical juncture in your investigation of the outbreak. Your hypothesis seems very defensible and reasonable, but your analysis thus far has not established much of anything—perhaps only what foods were popular at the supper. Specifically, neither of the above approaches helped you incriminate a food item.

So here is the logic behind the correct way to solve the problem. If you are thinking (hypothesizing) that a single food, among several, caused illness, then you might expect that that food would cause illness more frequently among those who ate that food than among those who did not eat it. If that makes sense, then, next, you should determine the rates of illness or attack rates among those who ate the food and those who did not. This is what Dr. Rubin did. See Table A–4.

Here you can see attack rates for each food item among those who ate the food in one column and among those who did not eat the food in the opposite column. *If you compare the attack rates between the two, you are performing the quintessential operation of all epidemiologic analysis: the comparison of rates.* In this instance you are comparing attack rates between those exposed (who ate a food) and those not exposed (who did not eat a food).

Now if you "eyeball" these attack rates for each food in both columns on Table A–4, you will see that for all foods, except one, the attack rates were fairly similar. For example, the attack rate for those who ate ham was 63%, for those not eating ham it was 59%; for those who ate spinach it was 66%, for those not eating spinach it was 62%; and for mashed potatoes the percentages were 62% and 62%, respectively. These rates certainly do not implicate any of these foods.

However, for vanilla ice cream the comparison of attack rates showed a great difference: 80% for those who ate it compared to 14% who did not. This comparison is striking, so much so that you should ask yourself, "How often would we expect to see such a difference in attack rates if vanilla ice cream had nothing to do with the outbreak?" Or to put it another way," Assuming no relationship between eating vanilla ice cream and getting sick, how often would we see such a difference in attack rates simply by chance alone?" With some experience in this kind of "eyeballing" and a little statistical background you would likely say, "Not very often." And, indeed, you would be right. For if you perform some simple statistical tests, you could say that this difference in attack rates for vanilla ice cream would occur in less than 1 in 100,000 instances such as this, assuming that the ice cream had nothing to do with the illness.

## What Should You Do Next?

- Unless you are quite familiar with the appropriate statistical function to perform, you should have your "eyeball" assessment verified by a trusted statistician.
- The statistician will confirm your conclusion that such a difference in attack rates would occur less than 1 out of 100,000 or more times (assuming no association between the ice cream and illness)—a statistic good enough, along with all the other data—for field epidemiologists worth their salt to look immediately for any remaining vanilla ice cream, culture it, and throw it out. Of course, if it was a commercially prepared ice cream, you should immediately notify your local health department of your findings.

**Table A–4.** Illness rates among church supper attendees according to foods/drinks consumed, Oswego County, New York, April 1940

| FOOD ITEMS SERVED | NUMBER OF PERSONS WHO ATE SPECIFIED FOOD | | | | NUMBER OF PERSONS WHO DID NOT EAT SPECIFIED FOOD | | | |
|---|---|---|---|---|---|---|---|---|
| | ILL | NOT ILL | TOTAL | PERCENT ILL (ATTACK RATE) | ILL | NOT ILL | TOTAL | PERCENT ILL (ATTACK RATE) |
| Baked ham | 29 | 17 | 46 | 63% | 17 | 12 | 29 | 59% |
| Spinach | 26 | 17 | 43 | 60% | 20 | 12 | 32 | 62% |
| Mashed potato* | 23 | 14 | 37 | 62% | 23 | 14 | 37 | 62% |
| Cabbage salad | 18 | 10 | 28 | 64% | 28 | 19 | 47 | 60% |
| Jello | 16 | 7 | 23 | 70% | 30 | 22 | 52 | 58% |
| Rolls | 21 | 16 | 37 | 57% | 25 | 13 | 38 | 66% |
| Brown bread | 18 | 9 | 27 | 67% | 28 | 20 | 48 | 58% |
| Milk | 2 | 2 | 4 | 50% | 44 | 27 | 71 | 62% |
| Coffee | 19 | 12 | 31 | 61% | 27 | 17 | 44 | 61% |
| Water | 13 | 11 | 24 | 54% | 33 | 18 | 51 | 65% |
| Cakes | 27 | 13 | 40 | 67% | 19 | 16 | 35 | 54% |
| Ice cream, vanilla | 43 | 11 | 54 | 80% | 3 | 18 | 21 | 14% |
| Ice cream, chocolate* | 25 | 22 | 47 | 53% | 20 | 7 | 27 | 74% |
| Fruit salad | 4 | 2 | 6 | 67% | 42 | 27 | 69 | 61% |

* Excludes one person with indefinite history of consumption of that food.

They, in turn, should call the local or regional Food and Drug Administration Office.

- You should now try to find out how the vanilla ice cream became contaminated with staphylococcus. This means locating those responsible for preparing the vanilla ice cream, asking them exactly how they prepared the ice cream, examining them for any possible infections, and culturing them for staphylococci. Here, again, are Dr. Rubin's findings:

The ice cream was prepared by the Petrie sisters as follows:

On the afternoon of April 17 raw milk from the Petrie farm at Lycoming was brought to boil over a water bath, sugar and eggs were then added and a little flour to add body to the mix. The chocolate and vanilla ice cream were prepared separately. Hershey's chocolate was necessarily added to the chocolate mix. At 6 p.m. the two mixes were taken in covered containers to the church basement and allowed to stand overnight. They were presumably not touched by anyone during this period. On the morning of April 18, Mr. Coe added five ounces of vanilla and two cans of condensed milk to the vanilla mix, and three ounces of vanilla and one can of condensed milk to the chocolate mix. Then the vanilla mix was transferred to a freezing can and placed in an electrical freezer for 20 minutes, after which the vanilla ice cream was removed from the freezer can and packed into another can which had been previously washed with boiling water. Then the chocolate mix was put into the freezer can, which had been rinsed out with tap water and allowed to freeze for 20 minutes. At the conclusion of this both cans were covered and placed in large wooden receptacles which were packed with ice. As noted, the chocolate ice cream remained in the one freezer can.

All handlers of the ice cream were examined. No external lesions or upper respiratory infections were noted. Nose and throat cultures were taken from two individuals who prepared the ice cream. Bacterial examinations ... were made on both ice creams .... Large numbers of *Staphylococcus aureus* and *albus* were found in the specimens of vanilla ice cream. Only a few staphylococci were demonstrated in the chocolate ice cream .... *Staphylococcus aureus* ... [was] isolated from [the] nose culture and *Staphylococcus albus* from [the] throat culture of Grace Petrie. *Staphylococcus albus* was isolated from the nose culture of Marian Petrie....

*Discussion as to Source*: The source of bacterial contamination of the vanilla ice cream is not clear. Whatever the method of the introduction of the staphylococci, it appears reasonable to assume it must have occurred between the evening of April 17 and the morning of April 18. No reason for contamination peculiar to the vanilla ice cream is known.

In dispensing the ice creams, the same scooper was used. It is therefore not unlikely to assume that some contamination to the chocolate ice cream occurred in this way. This would appear to be the most plausible explanation for the illness in the three individuals who did not eat the vanilla ice cream.

*Control Measures*: Later, all remaining ice cream was condemned. All other food at the church supper had been consumed.

*Conclusions*: An attack of gastroenteritis occurred following a church supper at Lycoming. The cause of the outbreak was contaminated vanilla ice cream. The method of contamination of ice cream is not clearly understood. Whether the positive

Staphylococcus nose and throat cultures had anything to do with the contamination is a matter of conjecture.

## What About the Two Outliers?

Patient No. 52 was a child who, while watching the freezing procedure, was given a dish of vanilla ice cream at 11:00 a.m. on April 18.

Patient No. 16 was a 32-year-old woman, whose time of eating is not known. Did she take the ice cream home to eat later, was this an unrelated illness, was this human error by the interviewer or transcriber, was this a secondary case (highly unlikely), or did she just have a long incubation period (also highly unlikely)?

## What Are Some of the Important "Take-home" Messages of this Walk-through?

- This is a very typical outbreak and investigation.
- You were given a fair amount of information—simple time, place, and person data—that very often you will not have at the beginning of your fieldwork. You may know that there is an outbreak, but you will not know that the ill shared a meal, that they all became sick shortly thereafter, and that no one else became ill. These were all "givens," right up front. So be prepared.
- Recognize the limitations of a retrospective investigation:
- Poor recall of study subjects
- Study subjects may not understand the interview form or questions
- Food handlers or those responsible for the meal may hide facts because of guilt, real or imagined
- Well people tend to remember less well and less completely; also they may be questioned differently by the interviewer
- Avoid using the word "proof." Epidemiologic investigations like this one show only an association between vanilla ice cream and illness. True, it is a very strong association, but, nevertheless, it does not prove a causal relationship.

## EPILOGUE

Some 32 years later a CDC epidemiologist visited Lycoming. The church was there, annual suppers were still being given, homemade ice cream was still the chief attraction, and the same two sisters were still helping out. "Although the installation of refrigeration in the early 1950s put an end to overnight incubation of the ice cream mix, they readily admit that their lapse in proper foodhandling continued until then. But a second epidemic did not occur."[1]

## REFERENCE

1. Gross, M. (1976). Oswego revisited. *Public Health Rep* 91, 168–70.

# INDEX

Note: Page numbers followed by *f* and *t* indicate figures and tables, respectively.